EVIDENCE-BASED CARDIOLOGY

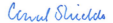
EVIDENCE-BASED CARDIOLOGY

Peter J. Sharis, M.D.
Boston University Medical Center
Boston, Massachusetts

Christopher P. Cannon, M.D.
Assistant Professor of Medicine
Harvard Medical School
Brigham and Women's Hospital
Boston, Massachusetts

LIPPINCOTT WILLIAMS & WILKINS
A **Wolters Kluwer** Company

Philadelphia · Baltimore · New York · London
Buenos Aires · Hong Kong · Sydney · Tokyo

Acquisitions Editor: Ruth W. Weinberg
Developmental Editor: Selina M. Bush
Production Editor: Frank Aversa
Manufacturing Manager: Kevin Watt
Cover Designer: Joan Greenfield
Compositor: Circle Graphics
Printer: RR Donnelley–Crawfordsville

© 2000 by **LIPPINCOTT WILLIAMS & WILKINS**
227 East Washington Square
Philadelphia, PA 19106-3780 USA
LWW.com

Printed in the USA

Library of Congress Cataloging-in-Publication Data

Sharis, Peter J.
    Evidence-based cardiology / Peter J. Sharis, Christopher P. Cannon.
      p. cm.
    Includes bibliographical references and index.
    ISBN 0-7817-1613-6
    1. Heart—Diseases Handbooks, manuals, etc. 2. Heart—Diseases
Bibliography.   I. Cannon, Christopher P. II. Title.
    [DNLM: 1. Heart Diseases—therapy. 2. Evidence-Based
Medicine—methods.   3. Heart Diseases—diagnosis.
WG 210 S5307e 1999]
RC692.S46   1999
616.1'2—dc21
DNLM/DLC
for Library of Congress   99-38949
                                             CIP

10   9   8   7   6   5   4   3   2   1

Contents

Preface

In the field of cardiology, pharmacologic agents and procedures increasingly undergo extensive evaluation in large clinical trials. The first goal of this handbook, *Evidence-Based Cardiology,* is to summarize the data from many of these studies. The results of major randomized trials in six major topic areas are presented in a systematic fashion, including the design, study population, exclusion criteria, treatment regimen, and results. Meta-analyses, review articles, and nonrandomized and less important trials have more abbreviated summaries. The second goal of this handbook is to place all of these annotated references into context, so that the book is not just a compendium of trials. Each chapter begins with an overview that includes a discussion of the importance and relevance of most of these studies.

Chapter 1 emphasizes lipid management, as numerous large, randomized trials have been conducted in this area. Other sections review established cardiac risk factors and emerging, potential risk factors. Chapter 2 focuses on the three best studied revascularization procedures: balloon angioplasty, stenting, and bypass surgery. Chapters 3 and 4 cover the wealth of trial information on unstable angina and myocardial infarction. Chapter 5 focuses on the pharmacologic management of heart failure, including the numerous recent trials supporting the use of beta-blockers. The subject of the final chapter is ventricular arrhythmias and atrial fibrillation. Space constraints did not permit us to fully discuss other arrhythmias and antiarrhythmic devices, such as defibrillators or pacemakers; however, we have included a brief overview of several major trials in the treatment of ventricular arrhythmias. We plan to expand this section in the next edition of *Evidence-Based Cardiology.*

The earliest version of this handbook was an extensive bibliography compiled by Peter Sharis during his internal medicine residency. The bibliography gradually progressed to a compendium of annotated references. When several residents, fellows, and cardiologists recommended the work be published, a nearly two-year-long effort ensued to produce a compact, up-to-date handbook that is targeted to general cardiologists, medical students, residents, internists, and others with an interest in cardiology and a desire to keep current with the vast amount of evidence-based literature.

We acknowledge several cardiologists who provided extremely helpful comments and suggestions on specific chapters: Jorge Plutzky (Chapter 1), Campbell Rogers (Chapter 2), James DeLemos (Chapters 3 and 4), Elliott Antman (Chapter 4), and James Fang (Chapter 5). We also thank Eugene Braunwald, whose expert leadership of the Thrombolysis in Myocardial Infarction (TIMI) Study Group has provided us with a greater appreciation and understanding of the importance of well-designed clinical trials, and the careful, considerate analysis and interpretation needed to appropriately incorporate their results into current practice.

Peter J. Sharis, M.D.
Christopher P. Cannon, M.D.

1

Risk Factors for Coronary Artery Disease and Primary and Secondary Prevention Trials

LIPIDS, CHOLESTEROL, AND DIET

Epidemiology (see pages 21–24, 44)

A 10% decrease in total cholesterol (TC) is associated with an approximately 10% to 15% lower coronary heart disease (CHD) mortality rate and an approximately 20% decrease in the risk of myocardial infarction (MI) (3,11,16). When TC levels are lowered by life-style modification (e.g., diet, exercise) and/or pharmacologic intervention, it appears that more benefit is derived in younger individuals and that the full benefits of a sustained decrease are not achieved for at least 5 years (13–15). Very low TC levels have been associated with higher mortality rates than than found with normal TC levels (17), which is likely due to the higher prevalence of cancer in such individuals. The Framingham Heart Study showed that low-density lipoprotein (LDL) is an even stronger predictor of CHD than TC. High levels of high-density lipoproteins (HDLs) are associated with a decreased risk of CHD mortality (83), and the National Cholesterol Education Program (NCEP) guidelines consider an HDL level of 60 mg/dL to be a negative cardiac risk factor (Table 1-1). A meta-analysis of 35 randomized cholesterol-lowering trials (3) showed that a 10% reduction in TC was associated with a 13% lower CHD mortality rate and a 10% lower all-cause mortality rate ($p < 0.002$). A more recent meta-analysis of 59 randomized, controlled trials found that several classes of lipid agents lower cholesterol—but only 3-hydroxy-3-methylglutaryl–coenzyme A (HMG-CoA) reductase inhibitors (statins)—significantly reduced CHD-related and all-cause mortality [34% and 25% relative risk reductions (RRRs), respectively] (10). In another meta-analysis of only statin trials (9), statin-treated patients had a 22% lower overall mortality rate, a 28% lower cardiovascular mortality rate, and 29% fewer strokes. Niacin and bile acid sequestrants also appear to reduce CHD events, whereas the available data on fibrates are inconclusive.

Cardiac risk tables have been created to estimate the risk of CHD death at various cholesterol levels and in combination with other major cardiac risk factors. For example, the Sheffield risk and treatment table provides risk factor combinations that are associated with 1.5% per year risk of CHD death in patients 52 to 70 years of age (18) (Table 1-2).

NCEP Guidelines (see pages 21,23)

NCEP II guidelines recommend that all adults undergo a lipid panel analysis at least once every 5 years (4,8).

Table 1-1. NCEP recommendations for drug treatment based on LDL cholesterol level

Risk Factors	LDL Threshold Level	Goal LDL
No CHD, <2 risk factors	≥190 mg/dL	<160 mg/dL
No CHD, ≥2 risk factors	≥160 mg/dL	<130 mg/dL
Known CHD	≥130 mg/dL	<100 mg/dL

Positive risk factors include current smoking; hypertension; diabetes; family history of premature CHD (men ≤55 years, women ≤65 years of age), HDL <35 mg/dL; and age (men ≤45 years, women ≥55 years or premature menopause without estrogen replacement therapy).
Negative risk factors include HDL ≥60 mg/dL.

NCEP LDL Goals (*see* Table 1-1) are listed as follows:

1. No CHD and fewer than two other cardiac risk factors: LDL less than 160 mg/dL; start drug therapy if 190 mg/dL after 6 months of diet.
2. No CHD but two other risk factors: LDL less than 130 mg/dL; initiate drug therapy if >160 mg/dL after 6 months of diet.
3. Definite CHD or other atherosclerotic disease: LDL less than or equal to 100 mg/dL; if 130 mg/dL, start drug therapy immediately if no contraindications exist.

American College of Physicians Guidelines (see page 22)

These controversial evidence-based guidelines recommend no routine testing in men under 35 years of age and women under 45 years of age or in individuals of either sex over 65 years of age (7).

Evaluation of Lipid Disorders

1. Obtain family history (e.g., of familial heterozygous hypercholesterolemia and other disorders).
2. Rule out hypothyroidism (increased TC, triglycerides), diabetes (increased triglycerides), thiazides or β-blockers (increased triglycerides), and renal or liver disease (increased triglycerides, TC).

Diet

Unless LDL is greater than 220 mg/dL, the NCEP step I dictates that the patient should be restricted to less than 30% fat calories, 8% to 10% saturated fat calories (use olive oil), less than 300 mg/ day cholesterol; step II calls for less than 30%, less than 7%, and less than 200 mg/day, respectively. Of note, fiber has minimal impact on cholesterol, and approximately 25% of compliant patients have no response. The average response is a reduction in TC of only 10% to 15%.

Vitamin E (see pages 39–41)

Several epidemiologic studies, including the Nurses Health Study, have shown increased vitamin E intake to be associated with less cardiovascular disease (65). In the Cambridge Heart Antioxidant Study (CHAOS) (62), a randomized study of 2,002 patients with known coronary artery disease (CAD), the vitamin E supplement group (400–800 IU/day) had a significantly lower incidence of cardiovascular death and MI. In the Alpha-Tocopherol Beta-Carotene Cancer Prevention (ATBC) trial (66), the α-tocopherol group (only 50 mg/day) had fewer nonfatal MIs but no reduction in primary end point of cardiovascular death and MI. Gruppo Italiano per lo Studio della Sopravivenza nell' Infarto miocardico (GISSI) Prevention Study (67) showed that vitamin E supplementation (300 mg/day) was associated with a nonsignificant reduction in overall mortality (odds ratio 0.86, $p = 0.081$). Preliminary results of the Heart Outcome Prevention Evaluation (HOPE) study found no benefit associated with vitamin E use (68).

Vitamin C (see page 38)

The National Health and Nutrition Examination Survey (NHANES) Epidemiologic Follow-up Study found that individuals with the highest intake had lower all-cause mortality and cardiovascular mortality rates at 10 years (60). Of note, the reduction in the all-cause mortality rate was not significant in women, and the preliminary results from a study of over 34,000 women showed no significant association between vitamin C intake and major events.

Beta Carotene (see pages 39,40)

No benefit of beta carotene supplementation was observed in the Physicians Health Study (63), whereas the Beta-Carotene and Retinol Efficacy Trial (CARET) was stopped early due to an excess of lung cancer, lung cancer deaths, and all-cause mortality (64), and the ATBC trial found a significant excess of cardiac deaths (66).

n-3 Polyunsaturated Fatty Acids (see page 41)

The GISSI Prevention Study (70) found n-3 polyunsaturated fatty acids (PUFA) supplementation (1 g/day) to be associated with a significant reduction (15%) in death, MI, and stroke ($p = 0.024$), as well as lower risks of all-cause mortality (21%) and cardiovascular death (30%).

Special Diets (see pages 41,42)

1. Mediterranean (includes more bread, fruit, and margarine, and less meat, butter, and cream): in a prospective study of 605 patients, a 73% reduction in death and MI, at a 2.3 year follow-up was observed (69).
2. High fish consumption: In a study of 852 Dutch men, the mortality rate was more than 50% lower among those consuming over 30 g of fish per day (equivalent of one to two dishes per week) (see *N Engl J Med* 1985;312:1305); however, in the much larger Health Professionals Follow-up Study, with 6-year follow-up data on approximately 45,000 individuals, there was no significant association between fish intake and risk of coronary disease (70).
3. High fiber: Analysis of 21,930 ABTC patients showed the risk of CHD death to be inversely related to fiber intake [highest quintile (34.8 g/day) vs. lowest quintile (16.1 g/day); relative risk (RR) of CHD death 0.69] (72). A recent Nurses' Health Study analysis also found a significant association between

Table 1-2. Sheffield risk and treatment table for primary prevention of coronary heart disease

Men

	Cholesterol concentration (mmol/L)											
Hypertension	Yes	Yes	Yes	Yes	Yes	Yes	No	No	Yes	Yes	No	No
Smoking	Yes	Yes	Yes	No	Yes	No	Yes	Yes	No	No	No	No
Diabetes	Yes	No	Yes	Yes	No	No	Yes	No	Yes	No	Yes	No
LVH	Yes	Yes	No	Yes	No	Yes	No	No	No	No	No	No
Age (years)												
70	5.5	5.5	5.7	5.9	6.5	6.8	7.2	8.3	8.4			
69	5.5	5.5	5.9	6.1	6.8	7.0	7.5	8.6	8.8			
68	5.5	5.5	6.3	6.4	7.1	7.3	7.8	9.0	9.1			
67	5.5	5.5	6.4	6.7	7.3	7.6	8.1	9.3				
66	5.5	5.5	6.7	6.9	7.7	8.0	8.5					
65	5.5	5.6	7.0	7.2	8.0	8.3	8.8					
64	5.5	5.8	7.3	7.5	8.3	8.6	9.2					
63	5.5	6.1	7.6	7.9	8.7	9.0						
62	5.5	6.3	7.9	8.2	9.1							
61	5.8	6.6	8.3	8.6								
60	6.0	6.9	8.7	9.0								
59	6.3	7.3	9.1									
58	6.6	7.6										

(continued)

Men

Hypertension	Yes	Yes	Yes	Yes	Yes	Yes	No	No	Yes	Yes	No	No
Smoking	Yes	Yes	Yes	No	Yes	No	Yes	Yes	No	No	No	No
Diabetes	Yes	No	Yes	Yes	No	No	Yes	No	Yes	No	Yes	No
LVH	Yes	Yes	No	Yes	No	Yes	No	No	No	No	No	No
Age (years)												
57	7.0	8.0	7.4	9.0								
56	7.3	8.4	7.7	9.4								
55	7.7	8.8	8.0	9.8								
54	8.1	9.3	8.3									
53	8.5											
52	9.0											
<52												

Women

Hypertension	Yes	Yes	Yes	No	Yes	Yes	No	Yes	Yes	No	Yes	No
Smoking	Yes	Yes	No	Yes	No	Yes	No	Yes	No	Yes	No	No
Diabetes	Yes	Yes	Yes	Yes	Yes	No	Yes	No	No	No	No	No
LVH	Yes	No	Yes	No	No	Yes	No	No	Yes	No	No	No
Age (years)												
70	5.5	7.1	7.4	9.0								
69	5.5	7.4	7.7	9.4								
68	5.5	7.7	8.0	9.8								
67	5.6	8.0	8.3									

(continued)

Table 1-2. *Continued*

Women

	Cholesterol concentration (mmol/L)										
Hypertension	Yes	Yes	No	Yes	Yes	No	Yes	Yes	No	Yes	No
Smoking	Yes	No	Yes	Yes	No	No	Yes	No	Yes	No	No
Diabetes	Yes	Yes	Yes	No	Yes	Yes	No	No	No	No	No
LVH	No	Yes	No	Yes	No	No	No	Yes	No	No	No
Age (years)											
66	8.4	8.7									
65	8.7	9.1									
64	9.1	9.4									
63	9.5	9.9									
62	9.9										
61	5.8										
60	6.1										
59	6.4										
58	6.6										
57	6.9										
56	7.2										
55	7.6										
54	7.9										
<54	8.3										
	8.7										
	9.2										
	9.6										
	10.1										

A patient whose value falls in the unshaded area has an estimated risk of coronary death of less than 1.5%.

fiber intake and CHD events. A 10 g/day increase in daily fiber intake was associated with a multivariate relative risk of 0.81 (95% CI 0.66–0.99) [see *JAMA* 1999;281:1998]. Further studies are needed to determine if this association is attributable to the low fiber diet or a healthy life-style effect.

DRUGS

Bile Resins (e.g., Cholestyramine, Colestipol)
(see pages 25–30)

These agents lower lipid levels by binding and blocking the reabsorption of bile acids. These agents typically decrease LDL cholesterol by 15% to 30%, increase HDL by 3% to 5%, and possibly increase triglyceride levels. Compliance is often problematic because of their poor taste and gastrointestinal side effects, such as bloating. There are also numerous drug interactions, and use is associated with an increased risk of gallstones. In the Lipid Research Clinic Coronary Primary Prevention Trial (20), cholestyramine use in 3,806 men with a mean TC of 291 mg/dL and LDL of 215 mg/dL resulted in 17% fewer MIs and a 19% reduction in CHD death and MI over the 7.4-year follow-up period. However, the all-cause mortality rate was not significantly different. The Cholesterol Lowering Atherosclerosis Study (CLAS) (32) was a smaller angiographic study that evaluated the combination of colestipol and niacin in 162 men with prior coronary artery bypass graft (CABG) surgery. Drug treatment resulted in lower TC (26%) and LDL levels (43%), higher HDL levels (37%), a higher atherosclerosis regression rate (16.2% vs. 2.4%), and fewer new lesions in bypass grafts. The Familial Atherosclerosis Treatment Study (FATS) (33) and a National Heart, Lung, and Blood Institute study (31) were angiographic studies that both showed beneficial lipid-lowering effects and better angiographic outcomes in colestipol-treated patients.

Niacin (see page 27)

Niacin is a B vitamin that typically decreases LDL by 10% to 25%, increases HDL by 15% to 35%, decreases triglycerides by 20% to 50%, and decreases lipoprotein (a) [Lp(a)]. A common side effect is flushing, which is often controllable by daily aspirin use. Also, a long-acting formulation of niacin is now available that appears to reduce flushing. Other side effects of niacin include hyperglycemia, increased uric acid levels, increased liver function tests, exacerbation of peptic ulcer disease, and rhabdomyolysis (rare). In the Coronary Drug Project (24), a randomized trial enrolling over 8,000 men with prior MI, the use of niacin 3 g/day was associated with a 27% lower nonfatal MI rate at 5-year follow-up and a significant 11% reduction in overall mortality at 15 years. Other trials evaluating the use of niacin in combination with other agents (e.g. CLAS, FATS) also have shown significant favorable changes in lipid levels and reduced rates of CHD mortality.

Fibric Acid Derivatives (see pages 25–30)

These agents typically increase HDL levels by 10% to 15%, decrease triglycerides by 20% to 50%, and have a variable effect on LDL levels. They are usually well tolerated. The Helsinki Heart Study (21) evaluated the effect of gemfibrozil in 4,081 asymptomatic hypercholesterolemic men. At 5-year follow-up, gemfibrozil use was associated with 34% fewer cardiac events and a 26% lower CHD mortality rate. However, the overall mortality rate was not significantly different because of more deaths due to accidents, violence, and intracranial hemorrhage in the gemfibrozil group. The Veterans Administration HDL Intervention Trial (VA-HIT), which was a secondary prevention trial of 2,531 patients, found that gemfibrozil was associated with a nonsignificant 10% mortality reduction and 20% reduction in the incidence of CAD-related death and MI (30).

The World Health Organization Cooperative Study (19) evaluated clofibrate in 10,627 hypercholesterolemic men. At an average follow-up of 5.3 years, the clofibrate group had 25% fewer nonfatal MIs, but there was a 47% increase in overall mortality ($p < 0.05$). The Coronary Drug Project showed that clofibrate use had no significant effect on all-cause mortality.

HMG-CoA Reductase Inhibitors (*statins*) (see pages 23–35)

These agents inhibit the rate-limiting step of cholesterol synthesis in the liver and typically decrease LDL by 20% to 60%, increase HDL by 5% to 15%, and decrease triglycerides by 10% to 20%. Potency (weakest to strongest on mg-per-mg basis) may be characterized as follows: fluvastatin, lovastatin, pravastatin and simvastatin, atorvastatin, and cerivastatin. Side effects are uncommon (approximately 1%–2%) and include mild gastrointestinal intolerance, increased liver function tests, myositis (rare and usually with concurrent niacin, cyclosporine, gemfibrozil, or erythromycin). It is important to titrate or increase the dose of a specific agent until the NCEP LDL goal is reached because an analysis of approximately 5,000 CAD patients found that only 25% had met the NCEP LDL goal of less than 100 mg/dL.

There are several proposed mechanisms of action by which these agents achieve significant reductions in CHD and overall mortality:

1. Increased luminal diameter—unlikely because most angiographic trials [NHLBI, CLAS-I, FATS, MARS, CCAIT, SCRIP, HARP, MAAS, PLAC-I, REGRESS, and LCAS (31–39,41,42)] demonstrate minimal or no changes.
2. Restoration of endothelial-dependent vasodilatation: a recent small study (*Circulation* 1999;99:3227–3233) found initiation early after acute coronary syndromes (10.4 ± 0.7 days) rapidly improved endothelial function after 6 weeks of therapy (*see* also *Circulation* 1994;89:2519 and *N Engl J Med* 1995; 332: 481,488).
3. Decreased cholesterol content in lesions, leading to more stable fibrous cap and other plaque-stabilization effects.
4. Inhibition of thrombus formation (*see JAMA* 1998;279:1643 and *J Am Coll Cardiol* 1999;93:1294).
5. Decreased oxidative stress (limited evidence available).

A meta-analysis of 16 trials with approximately 29,000 patients with an average follow-up of 3.3 years showed the use of statins to be associated with 22% lower all-cause mortality rates, 28% lower cardiovascular mortality rates, and 29% fewer strokes (9)

(Table 1–3). Another analysis of randomized found that the full effect of these agents is not achieved until at least 5 years after initiation of therapy (approximately 25% lower mortality vs. 7% in the first 2 years) (14).

Primary Prevention Trials (see page 26)

The West of Scotland Coronary Prevention Study (WOSCOPS) (22) was a randomized, placebo-controlled trial of 6,595 patients with an average TC of 272 mg/dL. At 5 years, the pravastatin group had 29% fewer nonfatal MIs ($p < 0.001$), a 32% lower cardiovascular mortality rate ($p = 0.033$), and a 22% lower overall mortality rate ($p = 0.051$). The Air Force/Texas Coronary Atherosclerosis Prevention Study (AFCAPS/TexCAPS) (23) randomized 9,605 men and postmenopausal women with average TC and LDL levels and below average HDL levels to lovastatin or placebo. At average follow-up of 5.2 years, the lovastatin group experienced a 37% reduction ($p < 0.001$) in the risk for acute major coronary events. Of note, only 17% of AFCAPS/TexCAPS patients met NCEP guidelines for drug therapy.

Secondary Prevention Trials (see pages 28–33)

The Scandinavian Simvastatin Survival Study (4S) (26) was a randomized, placebo-controlled trial enrolling 4,444 patients with an elevated TC (≥ 213 mg/dL) and a history of CAD. At 5.4-year follow-up, the use of simvastatin 40 mg/day was associated with 25% lower TC, 35% lower LDL, a 42% lower CHD mortality rate, and a highly significant 30% relative reduction in lower overall mortality rate ($p = 0.0003$). Also, simvastatin patients underwent 34% less coronary revascularization procedures and had fewer fatal and nonfatal cerebrovascular events.

The Cholesterol and Recurrent Events (CARE) trial (27) examined the use of pravastatin (40 mg/day) in patients with normal or mildly elevated TC (<240 mg/dL). At 5 years, pravastatin was associated with 24% fewer cardiac deaths and nonfatal MIs ($p = 0.003$) and 20% lower overall mortality ($p = 0.10$). No significant beneficial effect was seen if the baseline LDL level was less than 125 mg/dL.

The Long-term Intervention with Pravastatin in Ischemic Disease (LIPID) trial (28) enrolled over 9,000 patients with known CAD and average TC levels (155–271 mg/dL). Pravastatin (40 mg/day) was associated with a 24% RRR in CHD mortality ($p < 0.001$), 22% RRR in overall mortality rate ($p < 0.001$), 19% RRR in strokes ($p = 0.048$), and 20% RRR in revascularization procedures ($p < 0.001$). Thus, both the LIPID and CARE trials provide compelling data to support aggressive lipid lowering with statins in CAD patients with normal TC levels.

The Post-CABG trial (40) was an angiographic trial of 1,351 patients with one patent saphenous venous coronary bypass graft that showed that aggressive LDL-lowering therapy with lovastatin 40 to 80 mg/day (and cholestyramine added if necessary) to achieve a target LDL of less than 85 mg/dL was associated with less graft atherosclerotic progression and 29% fewer revascularization procedures ($p = 0.03$). These data suggest that achieving very low LDL levels in post-CABG patients is important.

The Atorvastatin versus Revascularization Treatments (AVERT) trial (29) randomized patients with stable one- or two-vessel CAD referred for percutaneous coronary intervention (PCI) to aggres-

Table 1-3. All deaths, CVD deaths, and non-CVD deaths in 16 randomized trials using statin drugs

| | Allocated Active Treatment (n) | | | | Allocated Control Treatment (n) | | | | Calculations for Treatment Groups | | | | | |
| | | | | | | | | | All Deaths | | CVD Deaths | | Non-CVD Deaths | |
Study Name	All Deaths	CVD Deaths	Non-CVD Deaths	Random-ized	All Deaths	CVD Deaths	Non-CVD Deaths	Random-ized	O–E	Var (O–E)	O–E	Var (O–E)	O–E	Var (O–E)
Major trials														
4S	182	136	46	2,221	256	207	49	2,223	−36.9	98.7	−35.4	79.1	−1.5	23.2
WOSCOP	106	50	56	3,302	135	73	62	3,293	−14.7	58.1	−11.8	30.2	−3.1	29.0
CARE	180	112	68	2,081	196	130	64	2,078	−8.1	85.5	−9.1	57.0	2.0	32.0
Subtotal	468	298	170	7,604	587	410	175	7,594	−59.7	242.3	−56.1	166.3	−2.6	84.2
Other trials														
Sahni	3	1	2	79	4	3	1	78	−0.5	1.7	−1.0	1.0	0.5	0.7
EXCEL	33‡	32‡	1‡	6,582	3‡	3‡	0‡	1,663	4.3	5.8	4.1	5.6	0.2	0.2
MARS	2‡	1‡	1‡	134	1‡	1‡	0‡	136	0.5	0.7	0.0	0.5	0.5	0.2
Jones	1	1	0	83§	0	0	0	42§	0.3	0.2	0.3	0.2	—	—
Pravastatin Multi-national	0	0	0	530	3	3	0	532	−1.5	0.7	−1.5	0.7	—	—

CCAIT	2‡	2‡	0‡	165	2‡	1‡	1‡	166	0.0	1.0	0.5	0.7	-0.5	0.2
PLAC-I	4	3	1	206	6	3	3	202	-1.0	2.4	0.0	1.5	-1.0	1.0
PLAC-II	3‡	2‡	1‡	75	5‡	3‡	2‡	76	-1.0	1.9	-0.5	1.2	-0.5	0.7
MAAS	4	4	0	193	11	6	5	188	-3.6	3.6	-1.1	2.4	-2.5	1.2
ACAPS	1	0	1	460	8	6	2	459	-3.5	2.2	-3.0	1.5	-0.5	0.7
Lovastatin Restenosis	3	NR	NR	203	1	NR	NR	201	1.0	1.0	—	—	—	—
REGRESS	5	3	2	450	8	5	3	435	-1.6	3.2	-1.1	2.0	-0.5	1.2
KAPS	3	2	1	224	4	3	1	223	-0.5	1.7	-0.5	1.2	0.0	0.5
Subtotal	64	51	10	9,384	56	37	18	4,401	-7.1	26.1	-3.8	18.5	-4.3	6.6
Total	532	349	180	16,988	643	447	193	11,995	-66.8	268.4	-59.9	184.8	-6.9	90.8
Odds ratio	—	—	—	—	—	—	—	—	0.78	—	0.72	—	0.93	—
95% CI	—	—	—	—	—	—	—	—	0.69–0.88	—	0.63–0.84	—	0.75–1.14	—

‡ Numbers provided by investigators.

§ Numbers randomized to treatment groups provided only for those who remained on assigned treatment.

For explanation of trial names, see text.

CVD, cardiovascular disease; O–E, observed–expected events; Var (O–E), variance of observed–expected events; NR, not reported; CI, confidence interval.

Adapted from Herbert PR, et al., with permission.

sive LDL lowering with atorvastatin 80 mg/day or PCI. At 18-month follow-up, the atorvastatin group had a nonsignificant 36% reduction in cardiovascular events. The results of this study are controversial, with critics pointing out its small size and that enrolled patients were not ideal PCI candidates. To help determine if aggressive lipid-lowering therapy and PCI are the best care pathway, the Clinical Outcomes Utilizing Revascularization and Aggressive Drug Evaluation (COURAGE) trial will randomize 3,200 patients to PCI, medical therapy, and aggressive life-style modification versus medical therapy alone.

Triglycerides (see pages 35–38)

NCEP Guidelines classify triglyceride levels of less than 200 mg/dL as desirable, 200 to 400 mg/dL as borderline, 400 to 1,000 mg/dL as high, more than 1,000 mg/dL as very high. Obesity, physical inactivity, glucose intolerance, hypothyroidism, and the use of β-blockers, estrogen, and diuretics are associated with an increased risk of hypertriglyceridemia. Agents that are effective in lowering triglyceride levels are fibric acid derivatives and niacin. There is mounting evidence that high triglyceride levels are an independent predictor of increased CHD mortality (51,57). A recent analysis of studies with nearly 60,000 participants found that even after adjustment for multiple cardiac risk factors, high triglyceride levels are associated with significant 14% and 37% reductions in cardiovascular risk in men and women, respectively (44).

A Helsinki Heart Study analysis determined that a subgroup of patients with triglyceride levels of more than 200 mg/dL and an LDL:HDL ratio of more than 5:1 had a 3.8-fold higher risk of cardiac events; furthermore, such patients had their risk reduced by 71% with gemfibrozil treatment (*see Circulation* 1992;85:37). The importance of this ratio has been confirmed in other studies, including a case-control study that found patients with the higher triglyceride:HDL ratios were 16 times more likely to suffer an MI (56).

Lipoprotein(a) (see pages 36,37)

Lipoprotein(a) is structurally similar to LDL except for the addition of a single apolipoprotein(a) [apo(a)] molecule; levels are difficult to measure, and various measurement and storage techniques have been used in different studies. There is conflicting evidence on whether Lp(a) is an independent risk factor for CAD, and the majority of studies have involved only men. In one large case-control study [Lipid Research Clinics Coronary Primary Prevention Trial (LRC-CPPT) (49)], Lp(a) levels were 21% higher in CHD cases, whereas an analysis of 2,191 Framingham Study participants showed an Lp(a) level of more than 30 mg/dL to be associated with an RR of CHD of 1.9 (52). Other studies also have suggested increased risk with higher Lp(a) levels (53–55; *see* also *BMJ* 1990;301:1948 and *Am J Cardiol* 1992;69:1251). However, three nested case-control studies, including one of the Physician Health Study participants, showed no significant increased MI risk with higher Lp(a) levels (47; *see* also *Atherosclerosis* 1991; 89:57 and *Atherosclerosis* 1993;98:139). One major study in women involved 3,103 Framingham Heart Study participants and found Lp(a) to be an independent predictor of MI and cardiovascular disease (50). Of note, Lp(a) was indirectly measured using an electrophoresis technique. Most importantly, it is difficult to significantly reduce Lp(a) levels with lipid-lowering agents (niacin and estrogen appear best), and the clinical significance of lowering Lp(a) levels is unknown.

SMOKING (see pages 42–44)

Current smoking is associated with an approximately threefold increased risk of MI (74–82) and an approximately twofold increased risk of CHD-related death (75). Smoking in combination with another major cardiac risk factor (e.g., hypertension, diabetes, hypercholesterolemia) results in an approximately 20-fold increase in death and MI (77). Among those who quit smoking, the risk gradually returns to baseline after several years (79). Passive or second-hand smoke exposure results in an average 20% to 25% increase in CHD mortality (80, 82), whereas frequent or heavy exposure can result in a nearly twofold increased risk (81).

DIABETES (see pages 44,45)

Approximately 15 million individuals in the United States have diabetes mellitus, of whom more than 95% have the non–insulin-dependent variety of diabetes mellitus (NIDDM). The significant decline in CHD mortality seen in the general population in recent decades has not occurred in diabetes (87). NIDDM is associated with approximately two- and threefold increased risks of CHD death in men and women, respectively (84). The risks of death from MI and CHD are as high in diabetics without prior MI as in nondiabetics with prior MI (86). As a result, guidelines recommend that all diabetics over 30 years of age take aspirin (≥81 mg daily). Diabetics also have an approximately twofold increased risk of stroke.

Diabetics frequently have other modifiable risk factors, most often hypertension and obesity. Addressing these risk factors (e.g., by exercise, dietary modification or pharmacologic agent(s)) is essential to reducing an individual's cardiac risk (85). Intensive glycemic control of individuals with IDDM in the Diabetes Control and Complications Trial (DCCT) resulted in a 34% reduction in LDL levels and a 41% reduction in major cardiovascular and peripheral vascular events (*see N Engl J Med* 1993;329:977). Current American Diabetes Association guidelines (*see Diabetes Care* 1998;21:179) recommend target goals of LDL cholesterol of less than 100 mg/dL, HDL more than 45 mg/dL, and triglycerides less than 200 mg/dL.

HYPERTENSION

Epidemiology (see pages 46,47)

From age 30 to 65 years, systemic blood pressure (SBP) and diastolic blood pressure (DBP) increase by approximately 20 and 10 mm Hg, respectively (92). Hypertension occurs in the absence of other cardiac risk factors in 20%. A Framingham Heart Study analysis showed the age-adjusted prevalence of Stage II or III hypertension (SBP ≥ 160 mm Hg or DBP ≥ 100 mm Hg) declined significantly from 1950 to 1989 (men: 18.5% to 9.2%; women: 28.0% to 7.7%) (95). However, data from the Framingham Heart Study and Physicians Health Study show that even borderline isolated systolic hypertension (SBP 140–159 mm Hg) is associated with a 50% to 60% higher incidence of cardiovascular death (90,94).

Etiology (see pages 46–47)

Approximately 90% to 95% of cases have no known cause (essential hypertension). Secondary causes include renal parenchymal disease (2%–5%), renovascular hypertension (approximately 1%), primary aldosteronism (adrenal adenoma, 60%; bilateral hyperplasia, 40%), Cushing's syndrome, pheochromocytoma [10% malignancy, 10% bilateral, 10% familial (MEN II)], coarctation of aorta, numerous drugs [e.g. glucocorticoids, anabolic steroids, nonsteroidal antiinflammatory drugs (NSAIDs) (96), alcohol (91), oral contraceptives, cocaine, cyclosporine, sympathomimetics, tricyclic antidepressants, and amphetamines], hyperparathyroidism, and acromegaly.

Diagnosis (see pages 49–51)

Unless blood pressure is markedly elevated, it be should measured on three separate occasions before initiating therapy. The current Joint National Committee (JNC VI) classification is as follows:

Stage I hypertension: SBP 140 to 159 mm Hg, DBP 90 to 99 mm Hg
Stage II: SBP 160 to 179 mm Hg, DBP 100 to 109 mm Hg
Stage III: SBP greater than or equal to 180 mm Hg, DBP greater than or equal to 110 mm Hg

Isolated systolic hypertension, which is more common in elderly patients, also warrants treatment (102,107).

Treatment

Nonpharmacologic (see pages 48,53)

Weight loss has been shown to reduce the need for anti-hypertensive medication(s) (115). Sodium restriction also appears to have a modest beneficial effect. One meta-analysis of 56 trials showing a 100 mg/day reduction in urinary sodium excretion was associated with a reduction of 3.7 mm Hg in SBP ($p<0.001$) (98,115).

Pharmacologic (see pages 45–50)

The recent JNC VI guidelines continue to advocate the use of β-blockers and diuretics as first-line agents (89) (Table 1–4). A meta-analysis of 18 randomized trials enrolling a total of over 48,000 patients showed that the use of β-blockers and low-dose diuretics was associated with fewer strokes (RRs 0.71, 0.49, and 0.66) and less congestive heart failure (RRs 0.58, 0.17, and 0.58). Low-dose diuretics were also associated with less CAD and lower all-cause mortality rates [RR 0.90; 95% confidence interval (CI) 0.81–0.99] (99).

These latest JNC guidelines allow for the consideration of different agents in specific types of patients or conditions. For instance, elderly patients with isolated systolic hypertension may be treated with calcium-channel antagonists (long-acting dihydropyridines) (106). The use of ACE inhibitors should be considered in individuals with diabetes, congestive heart failure with left ventricular (LV) dysfunction, or MI complicated by LV dys-

Table 1-4. JNC VI risk stratification and treatment guidelines

Blood Pressure Stages (mm Hg)	Risk Group A (No Risk Factors and No TOD/CCD)	Risk Group B (≥1 Risk Factor, Not Including DM and No TOD/CCD)	Risk Group C (TOD/CCD and/or DM, With or Without Other Risk Factors)
High normal (130–139/85–89)	Life-style modification	Life-style modification	Drug therapy*
Stage 1 (140–159/90–99)	Life-style modification (up to 1 yr)	Life-style modification† (up to 6 mo)	Drug therapy
Stages 2 and 3 (≥160/≥100)	Drug therapy	Drug therapy	Drug therapy

Risk factors include smoking, dyslipidemia, diabetes, age >60 years, sex (mean and postmenopausal women), family history of cardiovascular disease (women <65 years, men <55 years of age).
* For patients with heart failure, renal insufficiency, or diabetes
† For patients with multiple risk factors, consider drugs as initial therapy in addition to life-style modifications
DM, diabetes mellitus, TOD/CCD, target organ damage/clinical cardiovascular disease (left ventricular hypertrophy, angina or prior MI, prior coronary revascularization, heart failure, stroke or transient ischemic attack, nephropathy, peripheral arterial disease, or retinopathy).
Adapted from *Arch Intern Med* 1997;157:2413(89).

function. In pregnancy, safe agents include labetolol, hydralazine, and methyldopa.

Target Blood Pressure (see page 51)

The Hypertension Optimal Treatment (HOT) study (108) randomized 18,790 patients to target DBP levels of less than or equal to 90, less than or equal to 85, or less than or equal to 80 mm Hg. The incidence of major events did not differ between the three groups. However, the power to detect such a difference was less than planned for two reasons: (a) actual mean blood pressures were approximately 2 mm Hg apart instead of 5 mm Hg apart and (b) only 724 major cardiovascular events occurred over 3.8 years versus the projected 1,100 over 2.5 years. Thus, the trial was not adequately powered to determine if a target DBP of approximately 80 mm Hg results in the fewest major events. Nevertheless, there were significantly fewer cardiovascular events and deaths among diabetic patients assigned to a target DBP of less than or equal to 80 mm Hg compared with less than or equal to 90 mm Hg ($p = 0.005, p = 0.016$).

Treatment of Hypertensive Crisis

1. Labetalol (best all-around choice): 20 mg intravenously, then 40 to 80 mg intravenously every 10 minutes as needed (maximum 300 mg) or continuous infusion at 2 to 5 mg/h.
2. Nitroprusside: 0.5 to 10 µg/kg/min; avoid in MI (use nitroglycerin); side effects include thiocyanate poisoning, which usually occurs at levels above 12 mg/dl (see somnolence, weakness, aphasia, twitching, diaphoresis, and tinnitus); minimize risk by avoiding in renal failure and limiting use to 24 to 48 hours.
3. Esmolol: 500 µg/kg loading dose, then 50 to 300 µg/kg/min; side effects include wheezing.
4. Phentolamine (specific uses include monoamine oxidase inhibitor/tyramine crisis, pheochromocytoma and cocaine toxicity): 5 to 10 mg intravenously, repeated as needed up to 20 mg.
5. Enalaprilat (use in scleroderma crisis): 1.25 to 5.0 mg every 6 hours; when converting to oral agent, high-doses are often beneficial (e.g., captopril 100–150 four times daily).
6. Propranolol (useful in thyroid storm): 2 to 10 mg intravenously every 3 to 4 hours, 0.5 to 1.0 mg/min continuous intravenous infusion, or 40 to 80 mg orally every 6 hours.
7. Other: clonidine 0.1 to 0.2 mg orally then 0.05 to 0.1 mg every hour until DBP is below 110 mm Hg, nimopidine 60 mg every 4 hours (useful in subarachnoid hemorrhage).

OBESITY (see page 54)

Data from the Nurses Health Study showed that even modest gains over 18 years resulted in significantly higher risks of CHD death and nonfatal MI; RRs ranged from 1.25 for a 5- to 7.9-kg gain to 2.65 for a 20-kg gain (117). It appears that the excess mortality associated with obesity diminishes with increasing age (120). Other studies have shown that a higher waist:hip ratio and greater waist circumference are independent predictors of CHD death and MI (119). In the Framingham Study, variability in weight was associated with increased all-cause and CHD mortality rates (116).

SEDENTARY LIFESTYLE AND EXERCISE (see pages 55,56)

Observational studies have shown individuals with low fitness levels have a 25% to 100% increased mortality risk. One meta-analysis showed a nearly twofold risk of CHD death among individuals in sedentary (vs. active) occupations (121), whereas an analysis of Multiple Risk Factor Intervention Trial (MRFIT) subjects showed a 27% lower CAD mortality rate among subjects with moderate versus less active physical activity (122). Two recent studies of middle-aged women and elderly men have found substantial benefits associated with walking (127,128). A Nurses' Health Study analysis of over 72,000 women found brisk walking (more than 3 hours a week) was associated with a 35% reduction in coronary events, a benefit comparable to that seen with vigorous exercise (128).

Formal exercise testing can provide a more accurate risk assessment. In the Lipid Research Clinics Mortality Follow-up Study, the least fit quartile on a standard treadmill test had a greater than eightfold risk of CAD mortality compared with the fittest quartile. Other studies have shown that exertion is a trigger of acute MI, with a markedly increased RR of MI (>100 times) in the 1 hour after heavy exertion in those who exercise infrequently (no more than once per week) (123,124). Thus, although exercise is protective, the initiation of any exercise program should generally be preceded by evaluation or consultation with a physician and initiated gradually.

NONMODIFIABLE RISK FACTORS

Family History (see page 56)

A positive family history is most important in those otherwise at low risk (128). One analysis of 45,317 physicians showed that if a parent had an MI before 70 years of age, the RRs of cardiac death, percutaneous transluminal coronary angioplasty (PTCA), and revascularization procedures were approximately twofold higher (129), whereas a study of 21,004 Swedish twins showed the risk of CHD death was as high as eightfold greater if the other monozygous twin died of CHD before 55 years of age (131).

Age (see page 56)

Advancing age is associated with a gradual deterioration in cardiovascular function (e.g., diastolic function, blood pressure regulation) and increasing risks of CHD death (130).

Gender

Coronary artery disease–related events are more common in men. This gender disparity is largely due to a later onset of symptomatic CAD in women (approximately 10 years), which is likely related to the protective effects of estrogen.

ALCOHOL (see page 57)

Several observational studies have shown that moderate alcohol consumption (e.g., one to two drinks per day) is associated with a significant reduction in CHD and overall mortality (136,137). A Physicians Health Study analysis reported adjusted relative mortality risks of 0.79 and 0.84 in those consuming one and 2 drinks per day, respectively (137). However, because of the significant health risks associated with more substantial alcohol consumption, many physicians are hesitant to recommend alcohol consumption as a means to reduce cardiovascular risk. American Heart Association (AHA) Nutrition Committee recommendations include consulting a physician to assess the risks and benefits of alcohol consumption, with contraindications including family history of alcoholism, hypertriglyceridemia, liver disease, uncontrolled hypertension, and pregnancy (135).

HORMONAL STATUS AND HORMONAL THERAPY (see pages 58,59)

Estrogen replacement therapy in postmenopausal women results in an approximately 15% to 20% reduction in LDL and 15% to 20% elevation in HDL levels. Significant epidemiologic data suggest that estrogen replacement is associated with an approximately 40% to 50% decrease in CHD mortality (138,139,141). However, breast cancer rates are 10% to 30% higher and endometrial cancer occurs up to six times more often (143). Despite these substantial epidemiologic data, the first large prospective, randomized trial [Heart and Estrogen/Progestin Replacement Study (HERS)] showed that a combination of estrogen and progestin in 2,763 women with a CHD event in the preceding 6 months did *not* result in a significant reduction in cardiovascular death and MI (relative hazard 0.99) (142). A detailed analysis of the HERS data showed that the hormone group had more events in year 1 but fewer events in years 4 and 5; as a result, the accompanying editorial advocated that current users should not stop and that the other benefits of hormone replacement (e.g., bone and menopausal symptoms) should be taken into consideration. Two ongoing studies will provide additional information about hormone replacement: the Women's Health Initiative (results expected in 2005) and WELL-HART (angiographic endpoint).

OTHER POTENTIAL RISK FACTORS

Homocysteine (see pages 60–62)

Hyperhomocysteinemia appears to be an independent risk factor for CAD, cerebrovascular disease, and peripheral vascular disease. Most studies have confirmed that high homocysteine levels are associated with an increased CAD mortality rate (147,149,150, 153); however, other studies have shown no association (154; *see* also *Stroke* 1994;25:1924). A meta-analysis of 27 nonrandomized studies showed each 5 μM increment in homocysteine levels was associated with 1.6- and 1.8-fold increased CAD risks in men and women, respectively (146). Two recent studies have reported that folic acid fortification and multivitamin use are associated with lower homocysteine levels (151,152). Randomized trials are needed to determine if lowering homocysteine levels through folate supplementation will result in a reduction in CHD-related events.

C-Reactive Protein (see pages 63,64)

Recent studies have shown that elevated CRP levels are strongly associated with an increased risk of cardiovascular events. In a nested case-control study of Women's Health Study participants, the highest C-reactive protein (CRP) levels were associated with a sevenfold increased risk of MI and stroke (160), whereas an analysis of 936 men in the Monitoring Trends and Determinants in

Cardiovascular Disease (MONICA) study found that a 1 standard deviation increase in CRP level was associated with an age- and smoking-adjusted risk of CHD events of 1.50 (164). A nested case-control study of CARE patients suggested that treatment with an HMG-CoA reductase inhibitor attenuates the risk associated with high CRP levels; pravastatin-treated patients had an RR of CHD events of only 1.29 versus 2.11 for placebo patients (162) (see also *Circulation* 1999;100:230). A Physicians Health Study analysis found the use of aspirin was most beneficial among men in the highest quartile of CRP values (56% reduction in MI vs 14% [lowest quartile]) (159).

Fibrinogen (see pages 62,63)

Several prospective epidemiologic studies have shown fibrinogen to be an independent CAD risk factor (157,158; *see* also *N Engl J Med* 1984;311:511, *JAMA* 1987;258:1183, and *Circulation* 1991; 83:836). One meta-analysis of six large studies showed a greater than twofold risk of subsequent MI or stroke in patients with high fibrinogen levels (156). While a more recent analysis of 18 prospective studies showed a 1 to 8-fold higher CHD risk among those in the top third of fibrinogen levels (161). No long-term pharmacologic intervention has been shown to significantly reduce fibrinogen levels.

Plasminogen Activator Inhibitor 1 (see page 64)

Many observational studies have shown plasminogen activator inhibitor 1 (PAI-1) levels to be elevated in CAD patients (163; *see* also *N Engl J Med* 1985, *Lancet* 1987, *Circulation* 1998).

Infection (see pages 64,65)

Some studies have demonstrated an increased risk of CAD in individuals who are seropositive for certain infectious agents. The most compelling evidence to date is for *Chlamydia pneumoniae* (166,167–169). However, a nested case-control study of Physician Health Study subjects found no increased risk of future MI in those with rising immunoglobulin G titers to *C. pneumoniae* (170). Also, the results of the ACADEMIC (Azithromycin in Coronary Artery Disease: Elimination of Myocardial Infection with Chlamydia) trial, which treated patients with CAD and elevated *C. pneumoniae* titers with azithromycin, showed no difference between the treated and placebo groups in a 3-month composite of four inflammatory markers and clinical outcomes at 6 months (171).

Personality Characteristics (see page 66)

Some observational studies have reported an association between type A personality characteristics and increased CHD risk (*see JAMA* 1975;233:872), whereas others have shown no increased risk (MRFIT, Framingham Heart Study). Other studies have reported an association between mental stress, depression, and submissiveness and increased cardiac events (172,173–176).

Genetic Markers (see page 67)

The Pl A1/A2 polymorphism of platelet glycoprotein IIIa and the ACE gene have been most extensively studied. Observational studies of the Pl A1/A2 polymorphism reported an increased risk of cardiac events among those with the P1 A2 allele, whereas larger studies have shown no significant relationship (179,180). A meta-analysis of 15 studies found an approximately 25% increased risk of MI among those homozygous for the deletion allele of the ACE gene (178).

ANTIPLATELET DRUGS FOR PRIMARY AND SECONDARY PREVENTION

Aspirin

Primary Prevention Trials (see pages 68,69)

The Physicians Health Study found that aspirin-treated patients (325 mg every other day) had 44% fewer nonfatal MIs and a non-significant 4% reduction in cardiovascular deaths (186). Of note, this study was stopped prematurely due to concerns about the high stroke rate (RR 2.1). A study of 5,139 British physicians found that aspirin use (500 mg/day) resulted resulted in a non-significant 10% mortality reduction and no effect on the incidence of nonfatal MI (185). In the Swedish Angina Pectoris Aspirin Trial (SAPAT) (188), which randomized 2,035 patients to aspirin 75 mg/day or placebo, aspirin was associated with a 34% reduction in MI and sudden death, but there was a nonsignificant increase in major bleeds (1.0% vs 0.7%). It should be noted that the recent American Diabetes Association guidelines recommend that all individuals with diabetes over 30 years of age should take aspirin (minimum 81 mg/day; *see Diabetes Care* 1997;20:1772).

Secondary Prevention Trials (see pages 69,70)

In the second Persantine-Aspirin Reinfarction Study (PARIS II) (189), the aspirin plus persantine group had a 30% lower 1-year mortality rate. An early meta-analysis that includes the PARIS II results found a similar reduction in mortality with aspirin use. In a recent observational study of elderly patients, with no con-traindications to aspirin, aspirin use was associated with a 23% lower mortality rate (190); however, only 76% were given this ben-eficial therapy hospital discharge.

Clopidogrel (see page 70)

The Clopidogrel versus Aspirin in Patients at Risk of Ischaemic Events (CAPRIE) trial randomized over 19,000 patients with a recent MI, ischemic stroke, or peripheral arterial disease to clopi-dogrel 75 mg once daily or aspirin 325 once daily (191). Overall, clopidogrel was associated with a significantly lower incidence in the primary composite end point, consisting of ischemic stroke, MI, or vascular death (5.32% vs. 5.83%/yr; $p = 0.043$). Among the subgroup of patients with a recent MI, clopidogrel was associated with a statistically insignificant 3.7% increase in the composite end point. However, in a post hoc secondary analysis of all 8,446 patients with any history of MI, clopidogrel was associated with a statistically insignificant 7.4% decrease in the combined end point. Interestingly, another analysis of all enrolled patients has shown a statistically significant 19.2% reduction in the MI event rate (*see Circulation* 1997;96(suppl I):I-467). Based on these data, the use of clopidogrel in all patients with recent MI or stroke or documented peripheral arterial disease appears to result in a reduced risk of subsequent MI. Future studies of only MI patients who are enrolled in the acute setting will help better define the role of clopidogrel in the management of patients with MI. Also, the role of clopidogrel in combination with aspirin needs to be evaluated to determine if the two agents have additive benefits.

REFERENCES

General Articles

1. **Forrester JS**, et al. 27th Bethesda Conference. Task Force 4. Efficacy of risk factor management. *J Am Coll Cardiol* 1998; 27:991–1006.

   Numerous topics are covered, including diet and lipid levels, hypertension, smoking, diabetes, physical inactivity, hormone replacement therapy, psychosocial factors, and family history. A detailed review is provided of all the major cholesterol-lowering trials.

2. **Daviglus ML**, et al. Benefit of a favorable cardiovascular risk-factor profile in middle age with respect to Medicare costs. *N Engl J Med* 1998;339:1122–1129.

   This is a cohort study of 7,039 men and 6,757 women who were 40 to 64 years of age when they were surveyed between 1967 and 1973 and who survived to have 2 years of Medicare coverage from 1984 through 1994. Low-risk patients were defined as those with TC less than 200 mg/dL, blood pressure ≤120/80 mm Hg, no current smoking, no electrocardiographic (ECG) abnormalities, no history of diabetes, and no history of MI. Low-risk patients (4.0% men, 4.4% women) had significantly lower costs: $3,165 versus $4,780/yr (men), and $1,700 versus $3,585/yr (women).

Lipids, Cholesterol, and Diet

Review Articles and Meta-Analyses

3. **Smith GD**, et al. Cholesterol lowering and mortality: the importance of considering initial level of risk. *BMJ* 1993;306:1367–1373.

   This meta-analysis of 35 non-statin trials demonstrating a U-shaped mortality curve showed a significant 26% mortality reduction in patients with a high initial risk of CHD (>50 deaths/1,000 patient years). No significant effect was seen in patients with medium risk, whereas the low-risk group had a 22% higher mortality rate (<10 deaths/1,000 patient years). Absolute numbers: high-risk group, 16.5 lives saved/1,000 patient years; low-risk groups, 1.2 lives lost/1,000 patient years.

4. Cleeman JI, et al. National Cholesterol Education Program **(NCEP II)**. Summary of the second report of the NCEP expert panel on detection, evaluation, and treatment of high blood cholesterol in adults. *JAMA* 1993;269:3014–3023.

   NCEP recommendations for cholesterol management, which are based on consensus opinion of experts, are summarized in Table 1-1. The NCEP guidelines advocate universal TC testing in all adults at least once every 5 years and that measurement of HDL levels also be performed if accurate results are available. Approximately 7% of the U.S. adult population meet NCEP criteria for pharmacologic intervention.

5. **Levine GN**, et al. Cholesterol reduction in cardiovascular disease. *N Engl J Med* 1995;332:512–521.

This review discusses the important primary prevention, secondary prevention, and angiographic trials. The second part of the review focuses on the atherosclerotic process, with sections on plaque rupture and endothelial dysfunction.

6. **Garber AM**, et al. American College of Physicians (**ACP**) Guidelines. Part I: Guidelines for using serum cholesterol, high density lipoprotein cholesterol and triglyceride levels as screening tests for preventing coronary heart disease in adults; part II: cholesterol screening in asymptomatic adults, revisited. *Ann Intern Med* 1996;124:515–517; 518–531.

These evidence-based guidelines include several controversial recommendations. Screening for TC levels is not recommended for men under 35 years of age or women under 45 years of age unless the history or physical examination suggests a familial lipid disorder or two cardiac risk factors. The basis for this recommendation is the extremely low incidence of CHD-related deaths in these age groups; thus, the potential hazards of initiating therapy could outweigh the benefits. Also, the cost-effectiveness ratio is 1 million/ year life saved in these young age groups. Screening is considered appropriate but not mandatory for primary prevention in men 35 to 65 years of age and women 45 to 65 years of age; such screening should consist of only TC levels. Screening is not recommended for men and women over 75 years of age because of a lack of data from large trials in these age groups. All patients with known CHD or at high risk for CHD (e.g., history of stroke, claudication) should undergo lipid analysis. A rebuttal article in the same issue (pp. 505–508) argued that cholesterol levels should be tested earlier in life because cholesterol levels in young men are directly and linearly related to coronary risk later in life and that waiting until evidence of CHD manifests is ill-advised because 25% experience sudden cardiac death as the first manifestation of CHD. The argument was also made that older patients should be tested, citing subgroup analyses from several trials that show that benefits in persons over 65 years of age are almost identical to those in younger persons.

7. **Grundy SM**, et al. American Heart Association Task Force. When to start cholesterol-lowering therapy in patients with coronary heart disease. A statement for Healthcare Professionals from the AHA Task Force on Risk Reduction. *Circulation* 1997;95:1683–5 (editorials pp. 1642–1653).

This article endorses NCEP II recommendations and discusses drug(s) available to reduce lipid levels to target levels. One accompanying editorial defends the controversial American College of Physicians (ACP) guidelines, whereas two other editorials provide support of the more stringent NCEP screening guidelines. Three assertions from the latter editorials deserve mention: (a) the ACP concern that universal screening will lead to overprescribing cholesterol-leading medications is unfounded—only 0.2% and 1% of adults 25 to 34 and 35 to 44 years of age, respectively, are on such medications, whereas 61% and 76% have been tested; (b) the pessimistic ACP attitude toward dietary measures is not justified—if followed, the NCEP level I diet leads to a ~10% reduction in LDL cholesterol levels, and even if universal screening and subsequent dietary measures led to only a 2% reduction in the general population's TC levels, $2 billion/yr would be saved in health-care costs (see *Circulation* 1997;95:24); and (c) the elderly should be screened because they are at greatest absolute risk, and data show that statins also significantly reduce stroke rates.

8. **Hebert PR**, et al. Cholesterol lowering with statin drugs, risk of stroke and total mortality. *JAMA* 1997;278:313–321.

    This meta-analysis of 16 trials included ~29,000 patients with an average follow-up of 3.3 years. The use of statins was associated with 22% lower TC and 30% lower LDL levels. Statin-treated patients also had a 22% lower overall mortality rate [95% CI 12%–31%], 28% lower cardiovascular mortality [95% CI 16%–37%], and 29% fewer strokes [95% CI 14%–41%]. No increase in deaths were attributable to noncardiovascular causes or cancer.

9. **Bucher HC**, et al. Systematic review of the risk and benefit of different cholesterol-lowering interventions. *Arterioscler Thromb Vasc Biol* 1999;19:187–195.

    This analysis of 59 randomized, controlled trials with 85,431 participants, included 13 statin trials, 12 fibrate trials, 8 bile resin trials, 8 hormone trials, 2 niacin trials, 3 n-3 fatty acid trials, and 16 dietary intervention studies. Only statins showed a significant reduction in CHD-related mortality (RRR 0.66, 95% CI 0.54–0.79) and all-cause mortality rates (RRR 0.75, 95% CI 0.65–0.86). A meta-regression analysis showed that the variability of results across trials was largely explained by the magnitude of cholesterol reduction.

10. **Knopp, RH**. Drug treatment of lipid disorders. *N Engl J Med* 1999;341:498–511.

    This review discusses the major classes of lipid-lowering agents: statins, bile resins, nicotinic acid, and fibrates. The most extensive section is devoted to the statins; mechanism of action, indications, lipid-lowering effects, comparison of available agents, and adverse effects are concisely described.

Epidemiology

11. **Martin MJ**, et al. Multiple Risk Factor Intervention Trial (**MRFIT**). Serum cholesterol, blood pressure and mortality: implications from a cohort of 361,662 men. *Lancet* 1986;2:933–939.

    This analysis of 6-year follow-up data showed that cardiovascular mortality correlated with cholesterol levels. Increased cardiovascular mortality risk was seen with TC levels as low as 181 mg/dL. Relative risk was 3.8 for cholesterol levels above the 85th percentile (>253 mg/dL).

12. **Pekkanen J**, et al. Ten-year mortality from cardiovascular disease in relation to cholesterol level among men with and without preexisting cardiovascular disease. *N Engl J Med* 1990;322: 1700–1707.

    The study population was composed of 2,541 white males, 17% with cardiovascular disease at baseline. At an average follow-up of 10 years, cardiovascular mortality was significantly lower in patients with desirable (<200 mg/dL) versus high (>240) cholesterol levels: in patients with baseline cardiovascular disease, 3.8% versus 19.6%; in patients without baseline disease, 1.7% versus 4.9%. Other strong predictors of cardiovascular mortality were LDL (>160 mg/dL vs. <130 mg/dL; RR 5.9) and HDL levels (>45 mg/dL vs. <35 mg/dL: RR 6.0).

13. **Klag MJ**, et al. Serum cholesterol in young men and subsequent cardiovascular disease. *N Engl J Med* 1993;328:313–318.

    The study population was composed of 1,017 patients with extensive follow-up (range 27–42 years). A difference in baseline cholesterol level of 36 mg/dL (difference between 25th and 75th percentiles) was associated with a significantly increased risk of cardiovascular disease (RR 1.7), cardiovascular mortality rate (RR 2.0), and all-cause mortality rate before 50 years of age (RR 1.64) and at all ages (RR 1.2; 95% CI 0.93–1.58).

14. **Law MR**, et al. By how much and how quickly does reduction in serum cholesterol concentration lower the risk of ischaemic heart disease. *BMJ* 1994;308:367–373.

    This overview includes 10 prospective studies (~500,000 men with ~18,000 events), 28 randomized trials (~45,000 patients with ~4,000 events), and three international studies. Prospective cohort study data shows a 54% reduction in risk at age 40, decreasing to 20% at age 70. Randomized data show that the full effect is seen by 5 years (25% vs. 7% in first 2 years).

15. **Krumholz HM**, et al. Lack of association between cholesterol and coronary heart disease mortality, morbidity and all-cause mortality in persons older than 70 years. *JAMA* 1994;272:1335–1340.

    This prospective, 4-year cohort study included 997 older patients. An elevated serum TC level, low HDL, and high total serum to HDL ratio were not associated with higher mortality or morbidity. Adjusted odds ratios for all-cause mortality were 0.99 (>240 mg/dL vs. <200 mg/dL), 1.00 (lowest vs. highest HDL tertiles), and 1.03 (low vs. high tertiles for total serum/HDL).

16. **Verschuren WMM**, et al. Serum total cholesterol and long-term coronary heart disease mortality in different cultures. *JAMA* 1995;274:131–136.

    This was an analysis of 25-year follow-up data on 12,647 men in the observational Seven Countries Study (five European countries, the United States, and Japan). The RRs for the highest versus lowest quartiles of TC ranged from 1.5 to 2.3 (except for Japan, at 1.1). A 20 mg/dL increase in TC corresponded to an increase in CHD mortality risk of 12%.

17. **Iribarren C**, et al. Low serum cholesterol and mortality: which is the cause and which is the effect? *Circulation* 1995;92:2396–2403 (editorial pp. 2365–2366).

    This study included 5,941 Japanese men 45–68 years of age without prior CAD, stroke, or cancer, only 1%–2% of whom were on cholesterol-lowering drugs. At follow-up (16 years), a decline from a middle (180–239 mg/dL) to low (<180 mg/dL) total cholesterol level was associated with a 30% *higher* risk factor adjusted mortality. This finding is likely attributable to the increased cancer prevalence in this subgroup of men. Of note, data from the large MRFIT trial showed that cancer patients had TC levels that were 23% lower in the year prior to death.

18. **Haq IU**, et al. Sheffield risk and treatment table for cholesterol lowering for primary prevention of coronary artery disease. *Lancet* 1995;346: 1467–1471.

    The table provides numerous combinations of established coronary heart disease risk factors (e.g. hypertension, smoking, diabetes, age) that are associated with a ≥1.5% per year risk of coronary death in patients 52–70 years of age.

Primary Prevention

19. World Health Organization (**WHO**) Study. Committee of Principal Investigators. A cooperative trial in the primary prevention of ischgemic heart disease using clofibrate. *Br Heart J* 1978; 40:1069–1118.

    Design: Prospective, randomized, placebo-controlled, multicenter study; average follow-up 5.3 years.

    Purpose: To evaluate the effects of clofibrate on cholesterol levels and the incidence of major cardiovascular events.

    Population: 10,627 men 30–59 years of age with high TC levels (upper one third of distribution).

    Treatment: Clofibrate 1.6 g/day or placebo.

    Results: Clofibrate group had 8% lower TC and 20% fewer MIs.

20. Lipid Research Clinics Coronary Primary Prevention Trial (**LRC-CPPT**) results. Reduction in incidence of CHD. *JAMA* 1984; 251:351–364.

    Design: Prospective, randomized, double-blind, placebo-controlled, multicenter study. Primary end point was CHD-related death and nonfatal MI. The average follow-up was 7.4 years.

    Purpose: To evaluate the effects of cholestyramine on cholesterol levels and major cardiac events in hypercholesterolemic men at high risk of CHD events.

    Population: 3,806 men 35–59 years of age with TC >265 mg/dL and LDL >190 mg/dL.

    Exclusion Criteria: Triglycerides >300 mg/dL, history of MI, angina, or congestive heart failure.

    Treatment: Cholestyramine (24 g/day) or placebo.

    Results: Cholestyramine use was associated with 9% lower TC and 13% lower LDL cholesterol. Cholestyramine group had a 19% reduction in CHD-related death and MI (8.1% vs. 9.8%).

21. **Frick MH**, et al. Helsinki Heart Study: primary-prevention trial with gemfibrozil in middle-aged men with dyslipidemia. *N Engl J Med* 1987;317:1237–1245.

    Design: Prospective, randomized, double-blind, placebo-controlled, multicenter study. Primary end point was cardiac death and MI. The follow-up period was 5 years.

    Purpose: To investigate the effect of gemfibrozil on the incidence of CHD in asymptomatic middle-aged men at high risk because of elevated lipid levels.

    Population: 4,081 men 40 to 55 years of age with a non-HDL cholesterol level of ≥200 mg/dL.

    Exclusion Criteria: ECG abnormalities and congestive heart failure.

    Treatment: Gemfibrozil 600 mg twice daily or placebo.

    Results: Gemfibrozil initially increased HDL levels by >10%, followed by a small decline over time. TC and LDL levels were initially decreased by 11% and 10%, respectively, and remained consistent throughout the trial. The gemfibrozil group had 34% fewer cardiac events (7.3 vs. 41.4/1,000; $p < 0.02$); the decline in incidence became evident in the second year; no significant mortality difference was detected between groups (2.19% vs. 2.07%).

    Comments: A subsequent subgroup analysis showed that patients with triglyceride >200 mg/dL and an LDL:HDL ratio of >5:1 had a 3.8 times higher risk of cardiac events and that risk was reduced a substantial 71% with gemfibrozil (see *Circulation* 1992;85:37).

22. **Shepherd J**, et al. West of Scotland Coronary Prevention Study Group (**WOSCOPS**). Prevention of coronary heart disease with pravastatin in men with hypercholesterolemia. *N Engl J Med* 1995; 333:1301–1307 (editorial pp. 1350–1351).

    Design: Prospective, randomized, double-blind, multicenter trial. Primary end point was death from CHD and nonfatal MI. The average follow-up period was 4.9 years.

    Purpose: To evaluate the effectiveness of an HMG-CoA reductase inhibitor in preventing events in men with moderate hypercholesterolemia and no history of MI.

    Population: 6,544 men 45–64 years of age with TC ≥252 mg/dL (mean 272) and no history of MI.

    Treatment: Pravastatin 40 mg once daily or placebo.

    Results: Pravastatin group had 20% lower TC, 26% lower LDL, 31% fewer coronary events (nonfatal MI, death from CHD; $p < 0.001$), 32% lower cardiovascular mortality ($p = 0.033$), and nearly significant 22% overall mortality reduction ($p = 0.051$).

    Comments: Reduction in coronary events was independent of baseline cholesterol level (as in 4S trial); ~25% of U.S. population meets inclusion criteria.

23. **Downs JR**, et al. for the Air Force/Texas Coronary Atherosclerosis Prevention Study (**AFCAPS/TexCAPS**) Research Group. Primary prevention of acute coronary events with lovastatin in men and women with average cholesterol levels. *JAMA* 1998; 279:1615–1622.

    Design: Prospective, randomized, double-blind, multicenter study. Composite primary end point was fatal or nonfatal MI, unstable angina, and sudden cardiac death. Average follow-up period was 5.2 years.

    Purpose: To compare lovastatin with placebo for the prevention of first major coronary events in those without clinically evident atherosclerosis and with average TC and LDL and below average HDL levels.

    Population: 5,608 men 45–73 years of age and 997 postmenopausal women 55–73 years of age with TC 180–264 mg/dL, LDL 130–190 mg/dL, and HDL ≤45 mg/dL (men) or ≤47 mg/dL (women).

    Exclusion Criteria: Diabetes managed by insulin or associated with hemoglobin a1c 10%, and significant obesity (>50% ideal weight).

    Treatment: Lovastatin 20–40 mg once daily or placebo.

    Results: Lovastatin was associated with an RRR of 37% in first acute major coronary events (3.51% vs. 5.54%; $p < 0.001$). Several secondary end points occurred less frequently in the lovastatin group: (a) MI, RRR of 40% ($p = 0.002$); (b) unstable angina, RRR of 32% ($p = 0.02$); (c) coronary revascularization procedures, RRR of 33% ($p = 0.001$); (d) coronary events, RRR of 25% ($p = 0.006$); (e) cardiovascular events, RRR of 25% ($p = 0.003$). Lovastatin reduced LDL levels by 25% and increased HDL levels by 6%; no significant differences in adverse events was detected.

    Comments: Differences between the two groups appeared after 1 year (23 vs. 40 events). Only 17% of trial participants would have met NCEP guidelines for drug therapy, suggesting benefit of this agent extends to a wide population of hypercholesterolemic patients.

Secondary Prevention

24. **Coronary Drug Project**. Coronary Drug Project Research Group. Clofibrate and niacin in coronary heart disease. *JAMA* 1975;231: 360–381.
    Design: Prospective, randomized, multicenter study. Primary end point was all-cause mortality. Mean follow-up was 74 months.
    Purpose: To evaluate the effects of clofibrate and niacin on cholesterol levels and major cardiac events.
    Population: 8,341 men 30–64 years of age with ECG-documented prior MI.
    Treatment: Clofibrate 1.8 g/day or niacin 3 g/day.
    Results: Clofibrate group had a nonsignificant 6% decrease in TC and 7% fewer MIs; niacin group had a 10% decrease in TC, 26% lower triglycerides, and significant decrease in nonfatal MIs (but not fatal MIs).
    Comments: At 15-year follow-up (*see J Am Coll Cardiol* 1986; 8:1245), the niacin group had a significant 11% mortality reduction compared with placebo (52.0% vs. 58.2%, $p = 0.0004$).

25. **Buchwald H**, et al. Program on the Surgical Control of Hyperlipidemia (**POSCH**). Changes in sequential coronary arteriograms and subsequent coronary events. *JAMA* 1992;268:1429–1433 (see also *Am J Cardiol* 1990;66:1293).
    Design: Prospective, randomized, open label, multicenter study. Mean follow-up period was 9.7 years.
    Purpose: To evaluate if cholesterol lowering induced by partial ileal bypass surgery would reduce mortality and morbidity due to CHD.
    Population: 838 patients with an MI in the prior 6–60 months and TC ≥ 220mg/dL or LDL ≥ 140mg/dL after 6 weeks of dietary therapy.
    Exclusion Criteria: Obesity, hypertension, and diabetes.
    Treatment: Partial ileal bypass of distal 200 cm or one third of small intestine (whichever was greater); all patients were on the AHA phase II diet.
    Results: Surgical group had lower TC and LDL cholesterol levels (4.71 vs. 6.14 mM; 2.68 vs. 4.30 mM); surgical group had 35% reduction in incidence of cardiovascular death and MI at 5 years (82 vs. 125 events; $p < 0.001$); surgical group had significantly less angiographic progression ($p < 0.001$ at 5 and 7 years). Fewer surgical patients underwent coronary artery bypass surgery ($p < 0.0001$) and angioplasty ($p = 0.005$).

26. Scandinavian Simvastatin Survival Study Group (**4S**). Randomised trial of cholesterol lowering in 4444 patients with coronary heart disease: the 4S. *Lancet* 1994;344:1383–1389.
    Design: Prospective, randomized, double-blind, placebo-controlled, multicenter study. Primary end point was all-cause mortality. Median follow-up period was 5.4 years.
    Purpose: To evaluate whether simvastatin would improve survival of patients with CHD.
    Population: 4,444 patients 35–70 years of age with angina pectoris or previous MI (≥6 months earlier) and serum cholesterol 5.5–8.0 mM.
    Exclusion Criteria: Unstable angina, secondary hypercholesterolemia, planned coronary artery bypass surgery, or angioplasty.

Treatment: Simvastatin 20–40 mg once daily or placebo.

Results: Simvastatin group had 25% lower TC (TC), 35% lower LDL, and 8% higher HDL levels; simvastatin patients had significant 30% RRR in overall mortality (8.2% vs. 11.5%; $p = 0.0003$), as well as 39% fewer nonfatal MIs (7.4% vs. 12.1%), 41% fewer ischemic heart disease deaths (5.0% vs. 8.5%), and 34% fewer myocardial revascularization procedures (11.3% vs. 17.2%); of note, there was a 35% risk reduction among patients in the lowest quartile of baseline LDL (see *Lancet* 1995:345:1274).

Comments: Cost analysis showed that simvastatin-treated patients had 34% fewer cardiovascular-related hospital days and that there was $3,872 savings/patient, reducing the effective drug cost by 88% to 28 cents/day (see *Circulation* 1996;93:1796). A subsequent analysis showed the annual cost of life gained (all costs, including lost wages) ranged from $3,800 (70-year-old man with a TC level of 309 mg/dL) to $27,400 (35-year-old woman with a TC level of 213 mg/dL).

27. **Sacks FM**, et al. Cholesterol and Recurrent Events (**CARE**). The effect of pravastatin on coronary events after MI in patients with average cholesterol levels. *N Engl J Med* 1996;335:1001–1009.

Design: Prospective, randomized, double-blind, placebo-controlled, multicenter study. Primary end point was CHD death and nonfatal MI. Median follow-up period was 5.0 years.

Purpose: To study the effectiveness in a typical population of lowering LDL cholesterol levels to prevent coronary events after MI.

Population: 4,159 patients with MI within the prior 3–20 months and TC <240 mg/dL (mean 209) and LDL 115–174 mg/dL (mean 139).

Exclusion Criteria: Ejection fraction <25%, fasting glucose 220 mg/dL, and symptomatic heart failure.

Treatment: Pravastatin 40 mg once daily or placebo.

Results: Pravastatin group had 24% fewer cardiac deaths and nonfatal MIs (10.2% vs. 13.2%; $p = 0.003$), 26% lower rate of CABG surgery (7.5% vs. 10%; $p = 0.005$), 23% lower rate of balloon angioplasty (8.3% vs. 10. 5%), 31% fewer strokes ($p = 0.03$) and nonsignificant 20% mortality reduction ($p = 0.10$). The reduction in primary events was restricted to those with a baseline LDL ≥125 mg/dL (>150 to 175 mg/dL: 35% reduction, 125–150 mg/dL: 26% reduction, <125 mg/dL: 3% *increase*). Subsequent analysis found pravastatin use associated with a 32% reduction in stroke ($p = 0.03$) and 27% reduction in stroke or transient ischemic attack ($p = 0.02$) (*see Circulation* 1999;99:216). Another analysis of 1,283 patients 65–75 years of age showed a 32% RRR in major coronary events (19.7% vs. 28.1%), 45% RRR in coronary death (5.8% vs. 10. 3%), and 40% RRR in stroke (4.5% vs. 7.3%) (*see Ann Intern Med* 1998; 129:681).

28. The Long-term Intervention with Pravastatin in Ischaemic Disease (**LIPID**) Study Group. Prevention of cardiovascular events and death with pravastatin in patients with coronary heart disease and a broad range of initial cholesterol levels. *N Engl J Med* 1998;339:1349–1357.

Design: Prospective, randomized, double-blind, placebo-controlled, multicenter study. Primary end point was cardiovascular mortality. Mean follow-up period was 6.1 years.

Purpose: To evaluate the effects of lipid-lowering therapy on overall mortality in patients with a history of CAD and average cholesterol levels.

Population: 9,014 patients 31–75 years of age with MI or unstable angina within 3–36 months prior to study entry and an initial TC of 155–271 mg/dL.

Exclusion Criteria: Renal or hepatic disease, use of cholesterol-lowering medications, and significant medical or surgical event in prior 3 months.

Treatment: Pravastatin 40 mg daily or placebo.

Results: Pravastatin group had significant reduction in death from coronary heart disease, 6.4% versus 8.3% (RRR 24%; $p < 0.001$); pravastatin patients also had a lower overall mortality rate (11.0% vs. 14.1%, RRR 22%; $p < 0.001$), fewer MIs (7.4% vs. 10.3%, RRR 29%; $p < 0.001$), fewer strokes (3.7% vs. 4.5%, RRR 19%; $p = 0.048$), and less revascularization (13% vs. 15.7%, RRR 20%; $p < 0.001$); no significant adverse effects were associated with pravastatin.

29. **Pitt B**, et al. Atorvastatin Versus Revascularization Treatment (**AVERT**) Investigators. Aggressive lipid-lowering therapy compared with angioplasty in stable coronary artery disease. *N Engl J Med* 1999;341:70–76.

Design: Prospective randomized, open-label, multicenter study. Primary endpoint was 18 month incidence ischemic events consisting of cardiac death, resuscitation after cardiac arrest, nonfatal MI, cerebrovascular accident, CABG, angioplasty, and worsening angina resulting in hospitalization.

Purpose: To compare percutaneous coronary revascularization with lipid-lowering treatment for reducing ischemic events in patients with ischemic heart disease and stable angina pectoris.

Population: 341 patients with stable one- or two-vessel CAD, relatively normal left ventricular function, and a LDL ≥115 mg/dL who were referred for percutaneous revascularization.

Exclusion Criteria: Included left main or triple vessel disease, unstable angina or MI in prior 2 weeks, and left ventricular ejection fraction <40%.

Treatment: Atorvastatin 80 mg once daily or balloon angioplasty followed by usual care, which could include lipid-lowering treatment.

Results: Atorvastatin group had a 46% reduction in LDL levels (72 mg/dL) compared with an 18% reduction (to 199 mg/dL) in the angioplasty group. Incidence of ischemic events was 36% lower in the atorvastatin group (13% vs 21%; $p = 0.048$ [but not significant after adjustment for interim analyses]). In particular, the atorvastatin group had a lower incidence of coronary artery bypass surgery (1.2% vs 5.1%) and less frequent hospitalization for worsening angina (6.7% vs 14.1%).

30. **Rubins HB**, et al. Veterans Affairs HDL Cholesterol Intervention Trial (**VA-HIT**) Study Group. Gemfibrozil for the secondary prevention of coronary heart disease in men with low levels of high-density lipoprotein cholesterol. *N Engl J Med* 1999;341: 410–418.

Design: Prospective, randomized, placebo-controlled, double-blind, multicenter study. Primary outcome was a combined incidence of coronary heart disease death or nonfatal MI. Mean follow-up was 5.1 years.

Purpose: To evaluate if raising HDL cholesterol levels and lowering triglyceride levels would reduce major cardiac events in men with low HDL and LDL cholesterol.

Population: 2,531 men, 74 years of age, with CHD, HDL ≤40 mg/dL, LDL ≤140 mg/dL, and triglycerides ≤300 mg/dL.

Treatment: Gemfibrozil 1,200 mg once daily or placebo.

Results: Gemfibrozil therapy did not significantly reduce LDL levels, but did increase HDL by 6% at 1 year and decrease TG levels by 31% at 1 year. The gemfibrozil group had a significant reduction in CHD-related death or MI (17.3% vs 21.7%, relative risk reduction 22%, $p = 0.006$). There was a nonsignificant 10% reduction in all-cause mortality (15.7% vs 17.4%, $p = 0.23$).

Angiographic Analyses

31. **Brensike JF**, et al. National Heart, Lung, and Blood Institute (**NHLBI**). Effects of therapy with cholestyramine on progression of coronary atherosclerosis: results of the NHLBI Type II Coronary Intervention Study. *Circulation* 1984;69:313—324.

    This nonrandomized study included 143 patients 21–55 years of age with high LDL cholesterol (mean TC 323 mg/dL) and CAD by angiography. At follow-up (5 years), TC levels decreased by 11%, LDL was 19% lower, and HDL was 5% higher. Angiography showed no significant changes.

32. **Blankenhorn DH**, et al. Cholesterol-Lowering Atherosclerosis Study (**CLAS-I**). Beneficial effects of combined colestipol-niacin therapy on coronary atherosclerosis and coronary venous bypass grafts. *JAMA* 1987;257:3233–3240.

    Design: Prospective, randomized, placebo-controlled, partially blinded, multicenter study. Follow-up period was 2 years.

    Purpose: To evaluate whether combined therapy with colestipol and niacin will affect atherosclerosis and coronary venous bypass graft disease.

    Population: 162 nonsmoking men 40–59 years of age who had undergone prior coronary bypass graft surgery; average TC level was 245 mg/dL.

    Exclusion Criteria: Diabetes, hypertension (DBP >115 mm Hg), and congestive heart failure.

    Treatment: Colestipol 15 g twice daily and niacin 3–12 g/day or placebo.

    Results: Drug group had 26% lower TC, 43% lower LDL, and 37% higher HDL; as well as higher atherosclerosis regression rate (16.2% vs. 2.4%, $p = 0.002$) and fewer new lesions or adverse changes in bypass grafts ($p < 0.04$ and $p < 0.03$, respectively).

33. **Brown G**, et al. Familial Atherosclerosis Treatment Study (**FATS**). Regression of coronary artery disease as a result of intensive lipid-lowering therapy in men with high levels of apolipoprotein B. *N Engl J Med* 1990;323:1289–1298.

    Design: Prospective, randomized, double-blind, placebo-controlled (or colestipol-controlled), multicenter study. Follow-up period was 2.5 years.

    Purpose: To assess the effect of intensive lipid-lowering therapy on coronary atherosclerosis among high-risk men.

    Population: 146 men ≤62 years of age with documented CAD (at least one lesion with 50% stenosis, at least three lesions with 30% stenosis) and positive family history of CAD.

    Exclusion Criteria: Scheduled revascularization.

Treatment: Three groups: (a) lovastatin 20 mg twice daily and colestipol 5 mg three times daily for 10 days initially, then increased to 20 g three times daily; (b) niacin 125 mg twice daily initially, gradually increased to 1 g four times daily at 2 months, and colestipol; or (c) placebo lovastatin and colestipol (although colestipol is given if LDL is elevated).

Results: Conventional therapy group had minimal changes in LDL and HDL (−7% and +5%, respectively), whereas the changes were substantial in the treatment groups: colestipol and lovastatin, −46% and +15%; niacin and colestipol, −32% and +43%. Lesion progression in one of nine proximal coronary segments was seen in 46% of conventional therapy patients, compared with 21% and 25% in the two treatment groups, respectively. Lesion regression was more frequently observed in the treatment groups (32% and 39% vs. 11%). Clinical events (death, MI, revascularization for worsening symptoms) occurred significantly less often in treatment groups (6.5% and 4.2% vs. 19.2%). Nine patients withdrew due to side effects.

34. **Blankenhorn DH**, et al. Monitored Atherosclerosis Regression Study (**MARS**). Coronary angiographic changes with lovastatin therapy. *Ann Intern Med* 1993;119:969–976.

    Design: Prospective, randomized, placebo-controlled study. Primary end point was average change from baseline in percentage diameter stenosis of all lesions with ≥20% stenosis baseline. Mean follow-up period was 2.2 years.

    Purpose: To evaluate the effects of lovastatin on the progression of atherosclerosis coronary angiographic findings in patients with documented CAD.

    Population: 270 patients 37–67 years of age with TC 190–295 mg/dL and angiographically documented CAD.

    Exclusion Criteria: Use of lipid-lowering drugs in prior 2 months and candidates for CABG surgery.

    Treatment: Lovastatin 80 mg/day or placebo; all patients were put on a cholesterol-lowering diet.

    Results: Lovastatin group had 38% lower TC, 38% lower LDL, 8.5% higher HDL, and 0.9% regression of stenoses >50% (vs. +4.1% in placebo group; $p = 0.005$). Mean percentage diameter of stenosis increased by 2.2% in patients receiving placebo and 1.6% in lovastatin patients ($p > 0.20$).

35. **Waters D**, et al. Canadian Coronary Atherosclerosis Intervention Trial (**CCAIT**). Effects of monotherapy with an HMG-CoA reductase inhibitor on the progression of coronary atherosclerosis as assessed by serial quantitative angiography: the Canadian Coronary Atherosclerosis Intervention Trial. *Circulation* 1994;89: 959–968.

    Design: Prospective, randomized, double-blind, placebo-controlled study. Primary end point was a coronary score, defined as per patient mean of minimum luminal diameter changes. Follow-up period was 2 years.

    Purpose: To evaluate the effect of lovastatin on the progression of atherosclerosis.

    Population: 331 patients 21–50 years of age with documented atherosclerosis (on angiography in prior 12 weeks) and fasting serum TC 220–300 mg/dL.

Exclusion Criteria: Angioplasty within 6 months of qualifying angiogram, prior CABG surgery, scheduled angioplasty or CABG, and MI or unstable angina in prior 6 weeks.

Treatment: Lovastatin 20 mg/day, titrated to 40–80 mg/day over 16 weeks to achieve LDL ≤130 mg/dL, or placebo.

Results: Lovastatin reduced total and LDL levels by 21% and 29%, respectively, and slowed progression of lesions [–0.09 mm vs +0.05 mm; $p = 0.01$]. Lesion progression with no regression at other sites occurred less frequently in the lovastatin group (33% vs. 50%; $p = 0.003$). The lovastatin group also had fewer new coronary lesions ($p = 0.001$). In a subgroup of enrolled women on lovastatin, TC and LDL decreased by 24% and 32%, respectively, angiographic progression was reduced (28% vs. 59%), and fewer new lesions were observed (4% vs. 45%) (*see Circulation* 1995;92:2404).

36. **Haskell WL**, et al. Stanford Coronary Risk Intervention Project (**SCRIP**). Effects of intensive multiple risk factor reduction on coronary atherosclerosis and clinical events in men and women with coronary artery disease. *Circulation* 1994;89:975–990.

Design: Prospective, randomized, open, multicenter study. Primary end point was angiographic change in minimal artery diameter in segments with visible disease at baseline. Follow-up period was 4 years.

Purpose: To determine the effect of a program of intensive multifactorial risk reduction on the progression of coronary atherosclerosis.

Population: 300 patients (86% men) <75 years of age with angiographically documented coronary atherosclerosis.

Treatment: Risk reduction composed of low-fat and -cholesterol diet, exercise, no smoking, and antilipid drugs, or usual care.

Results: Risk reduction group had 22% lower LDL and apolipoprotein B, 20% lower triglycerides, 12% higher HDL, 20% increase in exercise capacity, and 39% fewer hospitalizations secondary to cardiac events (17.2% vs. 28.4%; $p = 0.05$). Risk reduction group showed a 47% reduction in narrowing of diseased segments (change in diameter –0.024 mm/yr vs. –0.045 mm/yr; $p < 0.02$).

37. **Oliver MF**, et al. Multicentre Anti-Atheroma Study (**MAAS**). Effect of simvastatin on coronary atheroma: the MAAS. *Lancet* 1994; 344:633–638.

Design: Prospective, randomized, double-blind, placebo-controlled, multicenter study. Follow-up period was 4 years.

Purpose: To study the effects on coronary atheroma of reducing lipoprotein concentrations with simvastatin in patients with known coronary disease.

Population: 270 patients with TC 190–295 mg/dL and angiographically documented CAD.

Exclusion Criteria: Use of lipid-lowering medications in prior 6 weeks, MI or unstable angina in prior 6 weeks, and prior coronary artery bypass surgery.

Treatment: Diet and simvastatin 20 mg once daily, or placebo.

Results: Compared with placebo group, simvastatin patients had 23% lower serum cholesterol, 31% lower LDL, and 9% higher HDL. Simvastatin group had a 2.6% reduction in the mean diameter stenosis, whereas the placebo group had a 3.6% increase. Simvastatin group also had less disease progression (41 vs 54 patients) and more frequent lesion regression (33 vs. 20 patients). No significant differences were seen in clinical event rates.

38. **Pitt B**, et al. Pravastatin Limitation of Atherosclerosis in Coronary arteries (**PLAC I**). PLAC I: reduction in atherosclerosis progression and clinical events. *J Am Coll Cardiol* 1995;26: 1133–1139.
Design: Prospective, randomized, blinded, placebo-controlled, multicenter study. Follow-up was 3 years.
Purpose: To evaluate the effect of diet and pravastatin on progression of coronary atherosclerosis in patients with mild to moderate hypercholesterolemia and CAD.
Population: 408 patients (mean age 57 years) with LDL cholesterol 130–190 mg/dL despite diet and at least one stenosis ≥50% in major coronary vessel.
Treatment: Pravastatin 40 mg once daily or placebo.
Results: At 3 years, pravastatin patients had 19% lower cholesterol, 28% lower LDL, and 7% higher HDL ($p \leq 0.001$). Progression of atherosclerosis was reduced by 40% ($p = 0.04$) in the pravastatin group, and they had fewer new lesions and 60% fewer MIs.
Comments: Results were achieved despite only 14% reaching NCEP goal of LDL ≤100 mg/dL.

39. **Jukema JW**, et al. Regression Growth Evaluation Statin Study (**REGRESS**). Effects of lipid lowering by pravastatin on progression and regression of coronary artery disease in symptomatic men with normal to moderately elevated serum cholesterol levels. *Circulation* 1995;91:2528–2540.
Design: Prospective, randomized, double-blind, placebo-controlled, multicenter study. Primary end point was change in average mean segment diameter and change in average minimum obstruction diameter.
Purpose: To determine the effect of 2 years of treatment with an HMG-CoA reductase inhibitor on coronary atherosclerosis.
Population: 885 patients with proven myocardial ischemia and TC 155–310 mg/dL (4–8 mmol/L) with angiographically documented coronary disease.
Treatment: Pravastatin 40 mg once daily or placebo.
Results: 88% had an evaluable angiogram. At 2 years, the pravastatin group had less progression of mean segment diameter and median minimum obstruction (−0.06 vs. −0.10 mm, $p = 0.019$; −0.03 vs. −0.09 mm, $p = 0.001$) and fewer new cardiovascular events (11% vs. 19%; $p = 0.002$). The pravastatin group had lower lipid levels (TC −20%, LDL −29%).
Comments: A substudy of 768 patients showed pravastatin was associated with less transient myocardial ischemia on 48-hour ambulatory monitoring [28% (baseline) to 19% vs. 20% to 23% (placebo); odds ratio 0.62] (*see Circulation* 1996;94:1503).

40. **Post-CABG** Trial Investigators. The effect of aggressive lowering of LDL cholesterol levels and low-dose anticoagulation on obstructive changes in saphenous venous coronary artery bypass grafts. *N Engl J Med* 1997;336:153–162 (editorial pp. 212–213).
Design: Prospective, randomized, 2 × 2 factorial, multicenter study. Primary end point was substantial progression of graft atherosclerosis (defined as new lesions, progression of lesions present at baseline, new occlusions). Angiography was performed at an average of 4.3 years.

Purpose: To (a) determine if aggressive lowering of LDL cholesterol in patients with saphenous venous CABGs is more effective than moderate lowering in delayed progression of graft atherosclerosis and (b) evaluate whether low-dose anticoagulation reduces bypass graft obstruction.

Population: 1,351 patients 21–74 years of age with LDL cholesterol 130–175 mg/dL who had undergone coronary artery bypass surgery in prior 1–11 years and had one patent graft.

Exclusion Criteria: Likelihood of revascularization or death within 5 years, ejection fraction <30%, and unstable angina or MI within prior 6 months.

Treatment: Aggressive lipid-lowering therapy with lovastatin 40–80 mg/day [goal LDL <85 (actual 93–97)] or moderate therapy with lovastatin 2.5—5.0 mg/day [LDL goal <140 (actual 132–136)]. Cholestyramine added if necessary. Second randomization to low-dose warfarin (mean international normalized ratio 1.4), or placebo.

Results: Aggressive therapy group had less atherosclerotic progression (≥0.6 mm diameter decrease), 27% vs. 39% (*p* < 0.001) and 29% less revascularization (6.5% vs. 9.2%; *p* = 0.03). No difference was detected between warfarin and placebo groups.

Comments: 7.5-year follow-up data showed low-dose anticoagulation patients with 31% lower incidence of death and MI. Death rates were as follows: aggressive LDL-lowering therapy plus warfarin, 11%; aggressive therapy plus placebo, 13%; moderate LDL-lowering therapy plus warfarin, 10%; moderate therapy plus placebo, 19%. Death plus MI rates were 18%, 21%, 18%, and 28% for the same groups, respectively.

41. **Herd JA**, et al. Lipoprotein and Coronary Atherosclerosis Study (**LCAS**). Effects of fluvastatin on coronary atherosclerosis in patients with mild to moderate cholesterol elevations (LCAS). *Am J Cardiol* 1997;80:278–286.

    Design: Prospective, randomized, double-blind, placebo-controlled study. Follow-up period was 2.5 years.

    Purpose: To evaluate if fluvastatin would favorable influence coronary atherosclerosis in patients with mildly to moderately elevated LDL cholesterol.

    Population: 429 CAD patients (19% female) 35–75 years of age and with LDL cholesterol 115–190 mg/dL.

    Exclusion Criteria: Coronary revascularization or MI in prior 6 months.

    Treatment: Fluvastatin 20 mg twice daily or placebo; 25% with LDL 160 mg/dL received open-label cholestyramine (maximum 12 g/day).

    Results: Fluvastatin only subgroup had 22.5% lower LDL (LDL in all fluvastatin patients was reduced by 23.9%). Angiograms at 2.5 years (340 patients) showed that the fluvastatin group had less progression vs. placebo (mean lumen diameter –0.028 vs. –0.100 mm; *p* < 0.01) and a nonsignificant 24% reduction in cardiovascular events (14.5% vs. 19.1%). A subsequent analysis showed that patients with low HDL levels (<35 mg/dL) had the greatest angiographic and clinical benefit (*see Circulation* 1999;99:736).

42. **Sacks FM**, et al. Harvard Atherosclerosis Reversibility Project (**HARP**). Effect on coronary atherosclerosis of decrease in plasma

cholesterol concentration in normocholesterolaemic patients. *Lancet* 1994;344:1182–1186.

This study randomized 79 nonsmokers to diet and placebo or pravastatin, nicotinic acid, cholestyramine, and gemfibrozil stepwise to reach a TC target of <165 mg/dL. Angiography performed at baseline and 2.5 years showed lower serum lipids (e.g., –28% TC) but no difference in minimal luminal diameter. No cases of myositis was seen with the combination of pravastatin and gemfibrozil.

43. Simvastatin/Enalapril Coronary Atherosclerosis Trial (**SCAT**). Preliminary results presented at the 48th American College of Cardiology (ACC) Scientific Session in New Orleans, LA, March 1999.

Prospective, randomized, placebo-controlled, double-blind, 2 × 2 factorial trial of 460 patients with documented CAD (70% also with a history of MI). Patients underwent a 1-month dietary run-in period, followed by a 1-month medication run-in. Patients received simvastatin 10–40 mg once daily or enalapril 2.5–10 mg twice daily. At follow-up (average 4 years), TC and LDL cholesterol decreased by 20.7% and 30.9%, respectively, in simvastatin patients, whereas they increased by 3.4% and 3.5% in placebo patients; enalapril had no significant effect on lipid levels. The simvastatin group had superior angiographic outcomes: smaller decrease in mean coronary diameter [0.06 vs. 0.12 mm (placebo); $p = 0.006$] and mean luminal diameter (0.08 vs. 0.15 mm; $p = 0.0002$) less progress in maximal percent stenosis (1.6% vs. 3.7%; $p = 0.0004$). Enalapril had no significant impact on these primary angiographic end points. However, the incidence of death, MI, and stroke was lower with enalapril compared with placebo (7% vs. 13%; $p = 0.043$). The simvastatin group did not display a similar significant reduction in this combined clinical end point, but simvastatin patients did undergo less frequent revascularization (6% vs. 12%; $p = 0.021$).

Triglycerides and Lipoprotein (a)

Review Articles and Meta-Analyses

44. **Austin MA**, et al. Hypertriglyceridemia as a cardiovascular risk factor. *Am J Cardiol* 1999;81:7B–12B.

This analysis of 17 studies enrolled 46,413 men and 10,864 women. Average follow-up period was 8.4 years. Elevated triglyceride levels were associated with a 32% increased cardiovascular risk in men and 76% in women. After adjustment for HDL and other risk factors, these increased risks were attenuated but remained statistically significant (men 14%, women 37%).

45. **Sprecher DL**. Triglycerides as a risk factor for coronary artery disease. *Am J Cardiol* 1998;82:49U–56U.

This review discusses data on triglyceride levels from case-control, epidemiologic, and randomized studies. It also examines the role of very low density lipoprotein (VLDL)-associated apo C-III, which is transported from HDL to VLDL or chylomicrons and then back to LDL when lipolysis occurs, and appears to contribute significantly to progression of atherosclerosis.

46. **Marcovina SM**, Koschinsky ML. Lipoprotein(a) as a risk factor for coronary artery disease. *Am J Cardiol* 1998;82:57U–66U.

This review has sections on the structure, measurement, and potential mechanisms of pathogenicity of Lp(a), as well as a summary of the limited case-control and prospective trial data suggesting a link between Lp(a) and the development of CAD.

Studies

47. **Ridker PM**, Hennekens CH, et al. A prospective study of lipoprotein(a) and the risk of MI. *JAMA* 1993;270:2195–9 (editorial 2224–2225).

    This nested case-control study of 296 Physician Health Study participants who subsequently developed MI and 296 controls, matched for smoking status and age, showed no evidence of an association between Lp(a) levels and the future MI risk. There were no significant differences between groups in median Lp(a) levels [103.0 mg/L (cases) vs. 102.5 mg/L; $p = 0.73$]. After adjustment for age and smoking status and even further adjustment for both lipid and nonlipid cardiovascular risk factors, there was no significant increased MI risk with higher Lp(a) levels.

48. **Criqui MH**, et al. Plasma triglyceride level and mortality from coronary heart disease. *N Engl J Med* 1993;328:1220–5.

    This study analyzed 7,505 patients in the Lipid Research Clinics Follow-up trial. The 12-year incidence of coronary death in both men and women increased with triglyceride levels. However, after adjustment for potential covariates, this association was no longer statistically significant.

49. **Schaefer EJ**, et al. Lipid Research Clinics Coronary Primary Prevention Trial (**LRC-CPPT**). Lipoprotein(a) levels and risk of coronary heart disease in men. *JAMA* 1994;271:999–1003 (editorial pp. 1025–1026).

    This study enrolled 3,806 men 35–59 years of age with TC >265 mg/dL and LDL >190 mg/dL. Patients were randomized to cholestyramine or placebo. Lp(a) was measured in serum obtained (and frozen) before randomization from 233 patients who manifested CHD (CHD) during the study (7–10 years), as well as from 390 CHD-free controls. Lp(a) levels were 21% higher in CHD cases (adjusted $p < 0.01$).

50. **Bostom AG**, et al. A prospective investigation of elevated lipoprotein(a) detected by electrophoresis and cardiovascular disease in women: the Framingham Heart Study. *Circulation* 1994;90:1688–1695.

    A total of 3,103 female Framingham Heart Study participants had Lp(a) indirectly measured at baseline by paper electrophoresis. A positive test result was defined as the presence of a detectable sinking pre-beta lipoprotein band; band presence was 51% sensitive and 95% specific for detecting plasma lipoprotein levels >30 mg/dL (threshold value associated with increased cardiovascular risk in men). At follow-up (mean 12 years), multivariate adjusted RR estimates were as follows: MI, 2.37 (1.48–3.81), total CHD, 1.61 (1.13–2.29), total cardiovascular disease, 1.44 (1.09–1.91).

51. **Assmann G**, et al. Hypertriglyceridemia and elevated lipoprotein(a) are risk factors for major coronary events in middle-aged men. *Am J Cardiol* 1996;77:1179–1184.

    Analysis of 8-year follow-up data of 4,849 Prospective Cardiovascular Munster (PROCAM) study patients, consisting of men

40–65 years of age who showed that elevated triglyceride levels were independently associated with an increased risk of major coronary events ($p < 0.001$ in a multivariate analysis). In the small subset (4.3%) of patients with TG >200 mg/dL and LDL: HDL > 5.0, risk was elevated by 6-fold.

52. **Bostom AG**, et al. Elevated plasma lipoprotein(a) and coronary heart disease in men <55 years old. *JAMA* 1996;276:544–548.

   The study population was composed of 2,191 Framingham Study patients. At follow-up (15 years), an elevated Lp(a) level (>30 mg/dL) was associated with CHD (MI, angina, sudden death): RR 1.9 (vs. TC >240 mg/dL, 1.8; vs. HDL <35 mg/dL, 1.8; vs. smoking, 3.6; vs. glucose intolerance, 2.7).

53. **Kinlay S**, et al. Risk of primary and recurrent acute MI from lipoprotein(a) in men and women. *J Am Coll Cardiol* 1996;28:870–875.

   This population-based case-control study was composed of 893 patients. The highest quintile of Lp(a) levels (>550 mg/L) was associated with a significantly higher risk of recurrent MI (odds ratio 1.77, 95% CI 1.03–3.03).

54. **Orth-Gomer K**, et al. Lipoprotein(a) as a determinant of coronary heart disease in young women. *Circulation* 1997;95:329–334 (editorial pp. 295–296).

   Retrospective analysis of 292 consecutive patients ≤ years of age with acute CHD events (110 MIs, 182 angina pectoris), and 292 controls. Comparing highest versus lowest quartiles, the age-adjusted odds ratio was 2.3 [2.9 after multiple risk factor adjustment (smoking, education, body mass index, SBP, TC, triglycerides, HDL)]. Premenopausal patients were at higher risk (odds ratio 5.1 vs. 2.4). The accompanying editorial stresses the need for large, prospective studies that use measurement methods unaffected by apo(a) size heterogeneity and that Lp(a) loses its predictive power when LDL is aggressively lowered.

55. **Nguyen TT**, et al. Predictive value of electrophoretically detected lipoprotein(a) for coronary heart disease and cerebrovascular disease in a community-based cohort of 9936 men and women. *Circulation* 1997;96:1390–1397.

   This prospective cohort study was composed of 9,935 people who had undergone lipoprotein analysis between 1968 and 1982. At follow-up (mean 13.2 years), semiquantitative levels were measured based on electrophoresis band pattern (0 = absent, 1 = trace, 2 = small increase, 3 = increase). A level of 3.0 (by enzyme-linked immunosorbent assay, mean 55.3 mg/dL) was associated with an increased risk of CAD [adjusted hazard ratios were 1.9 for women (95% CI 1.3–2.9) and 1.6 for men (95% CI 1.0–2.5)].

56. **Gaziano JM**, et al. Fasting triglycerides, HDL and risk of MI. *Circulation* 1997;96:2520–2525.

   This case-control study of 340 MI survivors ≤75 years of age and 340 age-, smoking-, and community-matched controls. After adjustment for age and gender, the risk of MI was 6.8 times higher in those with the highest triglyceride (TG) levels, and the risk was even higher (16-fold) in those with the highest triglyceride to HDL ratio.

57. **Jeppensen J**, et al. Triglyceride concentration and ischemic heart disease. *Circulation* 1998;97:1029–1036 (editorial pp. 1027–1028).

   This study of 2,906 Copenhagen Male Study participants initially free of cardiovascular disease found that high fasting triglyceride level is an independent risk factor for ischemic heart disease (IHD). At 8-year follow-up, the risk factor adjusted RRs of IHD were 1.5 (95% CI 1.0–2.3, $p = 0.05$) and 2.2 (95% CI 1.4–3.4; $p < 0.001$) for middle and higher thirds of triglyceride levels. Of note, a clear gradient of risk was found with increasing triglyceride levels within each level of HDL, including high HDL. The accompanying editorial recommends that triglycerides be checked as a part of a screening fasting lipid profile.

Antioxidants

General Articles and Meta-Analyses

58. **Diaz MN**, et al. Antioxidants and atherosclerotic heart disease. *N Engl J Med* 1997;337:408–416.

    This review article begins with a brief review of the major studies examining the relationship between antioxidants and CAD. Table 1-1 summarizes several descriptive, case-control, and prospective studies, as well as three randomized, double-blind, placebo-controlled trials (ATBC, CHAOS, Physicians Health Study). The remainder of the review focuses on the potential mechanism(s) of action of antioxidants, including reduced plaque rupture, platelet adhesion, and vasospasm.

59. **Jha P**, et al. The antioxidant vitamins and cardiovascular disease. *Ann Intern Med* 1995;123:860–872.

    This analysis of prospective and randomized trials enrolling 100 or more patients. Epidemiologic cohort studies show increased vitamin E intake associated with less cardiovascular disease (95% CI –31% to –65%), nonsignificant reductions with beta carotene (+12% to –46%), and vitamin C (+25% to –51%). Although the randomized trials showed no clear reductions with any agents, the authors assert that vitamin E doses used were probably suboptimal.

Studies

60. **Enstrom JE**, et al. Vitamin C intake and mortality among a sample of the U.S. population. *Epidemiology* 1992;3:194–202.

    This analysis of the first National Health and Nutrition Examination Survey (NHANES I) Epidemiologic Follow-up Study cohort was composed of 11,348 subjects 25–74 years of age. An index of vitamin C intake was established from detailed dietary measurements and use of vitamin supplements. At a median follow-up of 10 years, men with the highest vitamin C intake (>50 mg/day plus regular supplements) had significantly lower all-cause mortality and cardiovascular mortality rates [standardized mortality ratios 0.65 (0.52–0.80) and 0.58 (0.41–0.78)]. Among women, there was a nonsignificant mortality reduction [standardized mortality ratio 0.90 (0.74–1.09)], whereas cardiovascular deaths were significantly less frequent.

61. **Stampfer MJ**, et al. Vitamin E consumption and the risk of coronary disease in women. *N Engl J Med* 1993;328:1444–1449.

    This analysis focused on 87,245 Nurses Health Study subjects, who all completed diet questionnaires. Eight year follow-up data showed that the top quintile of intake compared with the lowest quintile had 34% less major CAD (95% CI 13%–50%). Most of this risk reduction was attributable to supplements (41% reduction with 2 years of use).

62. Cambridge Heart Antioxidant Study (**CHAOS**). Randomised controlled trial of Vitamin E in patients with coronary artery disease: CHAOS. *Lancet* 1996;347:781–786.

Design: Prospective, randomized, double-blind, placebo-controlled, single center study. Primary end point was nonfatal MI and cardiovascular death plus nonfatal MI. The median follow-up period was 510 days.

Purpose: To evaluate whether high-dose α-tocopherol would reduce subsequent risk of MI and cardiovascular death in patients with known CAD.

Population: 2,002 patients with angiographically proven coronary atherosclerosis.

Exclusion Criteria: Prior use of vitamin supplements containing vitamin E.

Treatment: Vitamin E 400 IU/day or 800 IU/day, or placebo.

Results: Treatment group had significant reduction in cardiovascular death and nonfatal MI (RR 0.53, 95% CI 0.34–0.083; $p = 0.005$). The beneficial effects on this composite end point were due to the 66% fewer nonfatal MIs (14 vs. 41 patients; $p = 0.005$); no difference in cardiovascular deaths was detected (27 vs. 23 patients; $p = 0.61$).

63. **Hennekens CH**, et al. **Physicians Health Study**. Lack of effect of long-term supplementation with beta carotene on the incidence of malignant neoplasms and cardiovascular disease. *N Engl J Med* 1996;334:1145–1149 (editorial pp. 1189–1190).

Design: Prospective, randomized, double-blind, placebo-controlled study. Average follow-up period was 12 years.

Purpose: To evaluate the effect of long-term supplementation of beta carotene on the incidence of cardiovascular disease and malignant neoplasms.

Population: 22,071 male physicians 40–84 years of age (in 1982).

Exclusion Criteria: History of cancer, MI, stroke, or transient cerebral ischemia.

Treatment: Placebo or beta carotene 50 mg every other day.

Results: A 78% rate of compliance was observed. No significant difference in malignant neoplasms (1,273 vs. 1,293 patients), lung cancer (82 vs. 88 patients), overall mortality (979 vs. 968 patients), cardiovascular-related deaths (338 vs. 313 patients), MIs (468 vs. 489 patients), or strokes (967 vs. 972 strokes) was observed between groups.

64. **Omenn GS**, et al. Beta-Carotene and Retinol Efficacy Trial (**CARET**). Effects of a combination of beta carotene and vitamin A on lung cancer and cardiovascular disease. *N Engl J Med* 1996;334:1150–1155 (editorial pp. 1189–1190).

Design: Prospective, randomized, double-blind, placebo-controlled, multicenter study. Mean follow-up period was 4 years.

Purpose: To evaluate the effects of a combination of beta carotene and vitamin A on the incidence of lung cancer and cardiovascular-related deaths.

Population: 18,314 smokers, former smokers, and workers exposed to asbestos.

Treatment: Beta carotene 30 mg and vitamin A 25,000 IU, or placebo, once daily.

Results: Trial was stopped 21 months early. Treatment group had increased RRs of lung cancer (1.28, 95% CI 1.04–1.57; $p = 0.02$), lung cancer death (RR 1.46, 95% CI 1.47—2.0), all-cause mortality (RR 1.17, 95% CI 1.03–1.33), and cardiovascular death (RR 1.26, 95% CI 0.99–1.61).

65. **Kushi LH**, et al. Dietary antioxidant vitamins and death from coronary heart disease in postmenopausal women. *N Engl J Med* 1996;334: 1156–1162.
Design: Prospective cohort study. Follow-up period was 7 years.
Purpose: To examine whether the dietary intake of antioxidants is related to mortality from CHD.
Population: 34,486 women without cardiovascular disease who completed a diet questionnaire in 1986.
Treatment: Vitamin A, E, and C intake as assessed by questionnaire.
Results: Vitamin E intake correlated with fewer CHD deaths; this association was strongest among non–vitamin users: RRs 0.42 in two highest quintiles of vitamin E intake (vs. lowest quintile). Vitamin E from supplements was not shown to be beneficial, although high doses and duration of use were not definitively addressed. Vitamin A and C intake did not have significant associations with the risk of death from CHD.

66. **Rapola JM**, et al. Alpha-Tocopherol Beta-Carotene Cancer Prevention Study (**ATBC**). Randomised trial of alpha-tocopherol and beta-carotene supplements on incidence of major coronary events in men with previous MI. *Lancet* 1997;349:1715–1720 (editorial pp. 1710–1711).
Design: Prospective, randomized, double-blind, placebo-controlled study. Primary end point was cardiac death and MI. Follow-up period was 5.3 years.
Purpose: To evaluate the effects of α-tocopherol and beta carotene supplements on the frequency of major coronary events.
Population: 1,862 male smokers 50–69 years of age with a history of MI.
Exclusion Criteria: Malignant disease, severe angina, and significant use of vitamins A, E, or beta carotene supplements.
Treatment: α-tocopherol 50 mg/day, beta carotene 20 mg/day, both, or placebo.
Results: No difference was detected between groups in incidence of cardiac death and MI, but the beta carotene and beta carotene plus α-tocopherol groups had more cardiac deaths (RRs 1.75 and 1.58; $p= 0.007$, $p = 0.03$). α-Tocopherol group had fewer nonfatal MIs [adjusted RR 0.62 (0.41–0.96)]. Authors speculate this to be due to more fatal MIs.
Comments: 24% of events occurred off therapy. Beta carotene serum levels were 19 times normal. Editorial points out that α-tocopherol dose used was 1/10th that of CHAOS [serum levels similar (45 vs. 51), but these correlate poorly with fat distribution] and synthetic form used (CHAOS: natural form).

67. **GISSI-Prevenzione** Investigators. Dietary supplementation with n-3 polyunsaturated fatty acids and vitamin E after myocardial infarction: results of the GISSI-Prevenzione trial. *Lancet* 1999;354:447–455 (editorial pp. 441–442).
Design: Prospective, randomized, open-label, multicenter study. Primary endpoint was death, nonfatal MI, and stroke. Average follow-up was 3.5 years.
Purpose: To evaluate the independent and combined effects of n-3 polyunsaturated fatty acids (PUFA) and vitamin E on morbidity and mortality after MI.

Population: 11,324 patients with a MI in previous 3 months.
Treatment: n-3 PUFA (1 g daily), vitamin E (300 mg/day), both, or none.
Results: n-3 PUFA group had a significant reduction in death, MI, and stroke (12.3% vs 14.6% [control], *p* = 0.023). All-cause mortality was 20% lower in the n-3 PUFA group (8.3% vs 10.4%). The vitamin E group had a nonsignificant reduction in death, MI, and stroke (13.1% vs 14.4%). Vitamin E use was associated with a significant 20% reduction in cardiovascular deaths.

Special Diets

68. **HOPE** (Heart Outcome Prevention Evaluation). Preliminary results presented at the European Society of Cardiology meeting in Barcelona, Spain, August, 1999. 9,541 patients over 55 years of age at high risk of cardiac events and with an ejection fraction ≥40% were randomized to vitamin E, 400 lv/day, vamipril 10 mg/day, both, or none (placebo). Vitamin E use was not beneficial (incidence of cardiovascular death, MI, and stroke was 16.0% vs 15.4% [placebo]. The Ramipril group had more than a 20% reduction in primary composite endpoint (13.9% vs 17.5% [placebo], *p* < 0.001).

69. **de Lorgeril M**, et al. A Mediterranean diet reduced mortality after MI. *Lancet* 1994;343:1454–1459.

    This prospective study was composed of 605 patients (91% men). The diet group underwent a 1-hour educational session. At 8 weeks and annually, a diet survey and counseling were administered. At follow-up (average 27 months), the Mediterranean diet group had a 73% lower incidence of death and nonfatal MI (2.7% vs. 11%; *p* = 0.001). Of note, this type of diet includes more bread, fruit, and margarine, and less meat, butter, and cream. A subsequent report with a mean follow-up of 46 months showed persistent benefits: 14 vs. 44 major events (cardiac death or nonfatal MI; *p* = 0.0001) (*see Circulation* 1999;99:779).

70. **Ascherio A**, et al. Dietary intake of marine n-3 fatty acids, fish intake and the risk of coronary disease among men. *N Engl J Med* 1995;332: 977–982 (editorial pp. 1024–1025).

    This analysis was performed on 44,895 Health Professionals Follow-up Study participants who completed detailed and validated dietary questionnaires. At 6-year follow-up, no significant associations were observed between dietary intake of n-3 fatty acids or fish intake and risk of coronary disease. The multivariate risk of CHD was 1.12 among men in the top quintile of n-3 fatty acid intake compared with men from the bottom quintile (95% CI 0.96–1.31). Of note, the risk of CHD death was 0.74 among men who ate any amount of fish compared with those who ate no fish; this finding was significant (95% CI 0.44–1. 23), but the risk did not decrease as fish consumption increased. The accompanying editorial concludes that a little fish may still do some good, but more fish is not necessarily better.

71. **Rimm EB**, et al. Vegetable, fruit and cereal fiber intake and risk of coronary heart disease among men. *JAMA* 1996;275:447–451 (editorial pp. 486–487).

    This observational study included 43,757 male physicians who filled out diet questionnaires. At 6-year follow-up, there were 41% fewer MIs in the highest fiber quintile. The greatest risk reduction was associated with cereal fiber: RR 0.71 for each 10-g increase. The editorial points out that the beneficial effect was confined to the highest quintile, probably the result of a healthy life-style (only 3.8% smokers, higher vitamin intake, etc.). We recommend a daily fiber intake of 25 g.

72. **Pietinen P**, et al. Intake of dietary fiber and risk of coronary heart disease in a cohort of Finnish men. *Circulation* 1996;94: 2720–2727 (editorial pp. 2696–2698).

   This analysis focused on 21,930 ATBC patients (all male smokers 50–69 years of age). At follow-up (average 6.1 years), MI and CHD deaths were found to be inversely associated with fiber intake. The highest quintile (34.8 g/day) versus lowest quintile (16.1 g/day) showed an RR of coronary death of 0.69 (*p* < .001 for trend). The same effect was evident after adjustment for cardiac risk factors and intake of beta carotene and vitamins C and E. The strongest association was seen with water-soluble and cereal (vs. vegetable fruit) fibers.

73. **Wolk A**, et al. Long-term intake of dietary fiber and decreased risk of coronary heart disease among women. *JAMA* 1999;281: 1998–2004.

   This analysis was performed on dietary data collected on Nurses Health Study participants in 1984, 1986, and 1990 (semiquantitative food frequency questionnaire). The response rate among the 68,782 women was 80%–90% during the 10-year follow-up period. Women in the highest quintile of total dietary fiber intake (median 22.9 g/day) had nearly a 50% lower incidence of major CHD events (age-adjusted RR 0.53; 95% CI 0.40–0.69) compared with women in the lowest quintile (median 11.5 g/day). This effect was attenuated after controlling for age, cardiovascular risk factors, dietary factors, and multivitamin supplement use (RR 0.77; 95% 0.57–1.04). The multivariate model found that a 10 g/day increase in total dietary intake resulted in a 19% RRR (95% CI 1%–34%). Among different sources of fiber (e.g., cereal, fruit, vegetables), only cereal fiber was associated with a significant reduction in CHD risk (multivariate RR 0.63 for each 5 g/day increase).

Smoking

74. **Willett WC**, et al. Cigarette smoking and non-fatal MI in women. *Am J Epidemiol* 1981;113:575–582.

   This retrospective case-control study was composed of 121,964 nurses 30–55 years of age who responded to a mail questionnaire. In logistic regression analysis, current smoking was associated with an RR of MI of 3.1 (95% CI 2.3–4.3).

75. **Friedman GD**, et al. Mortality in cigarette smokers and quitters. *N Engl J Med* 1981;304:1407–1410.

   This longitudinal study was composed of 26,187 persons with an average follow-up of 7.5 years. Study showed the substantial adverse effects associated with smoking. After adjustment for age, sex, and race, persistent smokers had a nearly twofold higher incidence of all-cause mortality and death CHD compared with persistent quitters and never smokers.

76. **Rosenberg L**, et al. The risk of MI after quitting smoking in men under 55 years of age. *N Engl J Med* 1985;313:1511–1514.

   This prospective case-control study was composed of 1,873 patients with first MI and 2,775 controls. Among current smokers, defined as smoking within the prior 12 months versus never, the age-adjusted RR of MI was 2.9 (95% CI 2.4–3.4). Among those who had quit smoking 12–23 months earlier versus never smokers the RR of MI was 2.0 (95% CI 1.1–3.8). Those who had quit 2 earlier had a risk similar to that of never smokers (RR 1.0).

77. **Willett WC**, et al. Relative and excess risks of coronary heart disease among women who smoke cigarettes. *N Engl J Med* 1987; 317:1303–1309.

This analysis focused on 119,404 Nurses Health Study participants with 6 years of follow-up; 30% were smokers. The number of cigarettes smoked per day was found to be associated with an increased risk of fatal CHD (in multivariate analysis, RR 5.4 for 25 cigarettes/day), MI (RR 6.3), and angina pectoris (RR 2.3). If 1–14 cigarettes/day, RRs (in multivariate analysis) were 1.8–2.5; 15–24 cigarettes/day, RRs 1.5–4.7; 45 cigarettes/day, RR of death and MI was 10.8. Overall, smoking was responsible for ~50% of events. The greatest absolute risks were seen with smoking in combination with other risk factors: smoking and hypertension, RR 22.2; smoking and hypercholesterolemia, RR 18.9; smoking and diabetes, RR 22.3.

78. **Rosenberg L**, et al. Decline in the risk of MI among women who stop smoking. *N Engl J Med* 1990;322:213–217.

This case-control study was composed of 910 patients with a first MI and 2,375 controls (all 25–64 years of age). Comparing current smokers to never smokers, the RR of MI was 3.6 (95% CI 3.0–4.4). The difference was less substantial when comparing exsmokers with never smokers (overall RR 1.2; 95% CI 1.0–1.7). However, the risk was higher in those who had quit 2 years earlier (RR 2.6; 95% CI 1.8–3.8), whereas there was no significant increased risk in those who had quit >3 years earlier.

79. **Kawachi I**, et al. Smoking cessation and time course of decreased risks of coronary heart disease in middle-aged women. *Arch Intern Med* 1994;154:169—175.

This prospective cohort study was composed of 117,006 nurses free of CHD in 1976. The average follow-up period was 11.7 years. In a multivariate analysis, among current smokers versus never smokers, the RR was 4.23 (95% CI 3.60–4.96); among those who started smoking before 15 years of age, RR 9.25; among former smokers, RR 1.48 (95% CI 1.22–1.79). After quitting, one third of the excess risk was gone at 3 years, and normal risk was attained after 10–14 years.

80. **Steenland K**, et al. Environmental tobacco smoke and coronary heart disease in the **ACS CPS-II** cohort. *Circulation* 1996; 94: 622–628 (editorial pp. 596–599).

This prospective study was composed of 353,180 women and 126,500 male nonsmokers. A 22% higher CHD mortality rate (95% CI) was observed among men married to current smokers; the corresponding RR for women married to current smokers was 1.1 (95% CI 0.96–1.22). The accompanying editorial provides analysis of data from 14 studies that shows an ~20% increased risk of CHD death in nonsmokers married to smokers.

81. **Kawachi I**, et al. A prospective study of passive smoking and coronary heart disease. *Circulation* 1997;95:2374–2379.

This analysis focused on 32,046 Nurses Health Study participants who did not smoke and were free of CHD in 1982. Of note, exposure was assessed by self-report and only at baseline. At 10-year follow-up, the adjusted CHD risk (nonfatal MI and cardiac death) was significantly higher among those with frequent smoke exposure (RR 1.91; 95% CI 1.11–3.28) and there was a trend of increased risk with occasional exposure (RR 1.58; 95% CI 0.93–2.68). There was no association between duration of living with a smoker and the incidence of CHD.

82. **He J**, et al. Passive smoking and the risk of coronary heart disease—a meta-analysis of epidemiologic studies. *N Engl J Med* 1999;340:920–926.

This analysis of 10 cohort and 8 case-control studies showed that nonsmokers exposed to environmental smoke had an RR of CHD of 1.25 (95% CI 1.17–1.32) compared with nonsmokers with no such exposure. This association was significant in both men and women and present in those exposed at home or in the workplace. A significant dose-response relationship was demonstrated: RR of CHD 1.23 in those exposed to smoke of 1–19 cigarettes/day versus RR of 1.31 in those exposed to 20 cigarettes/day ($p = 0.006$ for linear trend).

Diabetes

83. **Kannel WB**. Lipids, diabetes, and coronary heart disease: insights from the Framingham Heart Study. *Am Heart J* 1985;110: 1100–1107.

After risk factor adjustment, 26-year follow-up data showed that men with diabetes had a 70% increased risk of developing CHD, whereas the risk was 200% higher in women. High HDL levels (~85 mg/dL) were found markedly protective with an RR of CHD at 4 years of only 0.1–0.3. The combination of high LDL and low HDL resulted in the greatest risk of CHD: If LDL was 220 mg/dL and HDL 25 mg/dL, RR was 2.9.

84. **Barrett-Connor EL**, et al. Why is diabetes mellitus a stronger risk factor for fatal ischemic heart disease in women than in men? The Rancho Bernardo Study. *JAMA* 1991;265:627.

This prospective epidemiologic study was composed of 207 men and 127 women with diabetes at baseline and 2,137 adults with fasting euglycemia and no family history of diabetes. After adjusting for age, the relative hazard of ischemic heart disease death in diabetics versus nondiabetics was 1.8 in men and 3.3 in women. After other adjustments (SBP, TC, body mass index, smoking), the hazard ratios were similar (1.9 and 3.3). Thus, it appears that diabetes has a serious impact on women that appears to override their natural favorable survival advantage over men.

85. **Jonas M**, et al. Usefulness of beta-blocker therapy in patients with non-insulin dependent diabetes mellitus and coronary artery disease. *Am J Cardiol* 1996;77:1273–1277.

This analysis of 2,723 post-MI patients from the Bezafibrate Infarct Study showed that β-blockers are effective in individuals with NIDDM. The group of patients on β-blockers (33%) had a 44% lower 3-year mortality rate (7.8% vs. 14%). Most of this benefit was seen in the elderly, those with a history of MI, and those with poor functional capacity.

86. **Haffner SM**, et al. Mortality from coronary heart disease in subjects with type 2 diabetes and in nondiabetic subjects with and without prior MI. *N Engl J Med* 1998;339:229–234.

This Finnish-based population study found that diabetic subjects (n = 1,059) without a prior MI had a similar risk of subsequent MI compared with nondiabetic subjects (n = 1,373) with a prior MI. The 7-year incidence rates of MI among diabetics with and without a prior MI were 45.0% and 22%, compared with 18.8% and 3.5% in nondiabetics. The risk factor adjusted hazard ratio for death from CHD for diabetics without prior MI as compared with nondiabetics with a prior MI was 1.2 (95% CI 0.6–2.4).

87. **Gu K**, et al. Diabetes and decline in heart disease mortality in US adults. *JAMA* 1999;281:1291–1297.

This analysis of data from the First National Health and Nutrition Examination Survey (NHANES I; 1971–1975) and NHANES I Epidemiologic Follow-up Survey (1982–1984) showed that the declines in heart disease mortality seen in the general population have not occurred in diabetics. The two cohorts were followed up for mortality at an average of 8 to 9 years. Comparing the 1982–1984 period with the 1971–1975 period, nondiabetic men had a 36.4% decline in age-adjusted heart disease mortality compared with only a 13% decline for men with diabetes. Among women, nondiabetics had a 27% decline, whereas there was actually a 23% increase in diabetics. A similar pattern was found for all-cause mortality.

Hypertension

Review Articles/Miscellaneous

88. **Setaro JF,** Black HR. Current concepts: refractory hypertension. *N Engl J Med* 1992;327:543–547.

This review focuses on the evaluation of individuals whose blood pressure is not adequately controlled by a two-drug regimen. The differential of secondary hypertension is discussed, including renovascular hypertension, thyroid disease, sleep apnea, pheochromocytoma, primary aldosteronism, and coarctation of the aorta. There is a section on refractory hypertension due to exogenous substances (e.g., NSAIDs, oral contraceptives, anabolic steroids, alcohol, and tricyclic antidepressants). The final sections discuss the high incidence of suboptimal drug regimens and noncompliance (40% and 50%, respectively).

89. **JNC VI**. The sixth report of the Joint National Committee on prevention, detection, evaluation, and treatment of high blood pressure. *Arch Intern Med* 1997;157:2413–2446.

JNC VI defines hypertension as SBP >140 mm Hg and DBP >90 mm Hg, or taking hypertensive medication(s). Hypertensive individuals are assigned to one of three risk categories: Risk group A has no clinical cardiovascular disease, target organ damage, or other cardiac risk factors; risk group B has at least one risk factor, not including diabetes and no target organ damage or clinical cardiovascular disease; and risk group C has target organ damage and clinical cardiovascular disease and/or diabetes, with or without other risk factors. Initiation of drug therapy is indicated in all risk group C patients with elevated blood pressure, and risk group A and B patients with stage 2 or 3 hypertension (SBP ≥160 mm Hg, DBP ≥100 mm Hg) (*see* Table 1-2 for more details). When pharmacologic intervention is indicated, JNC VI advocates the use of diuretics and β-blockers as first-line agents in most patients. However, in a change from the

JNC V guidelines, other therapies are also recommended for individuals with specific characteristics. Examples include calcium-channel antagonists (long-acting dihydropyridines) for elderly patients with isolated systolic hypertension and ACE inhibitors in those with diabetes, congestive heart failure with LV dysfunction, or MI complicated by systolic dysfunction.

Epidemiology and Risk Factors

90. **Sagie A**, et al. The natural history of borderline isolated systolic hypertension. *N Engl J Med* 1993;329:1912–1917.

    This analysis focused on 2,767 of the original participants in the Framingham Heart Study. At 20-year follow-up, 80% with borderline isolated systolic hypertension (140–159 mm Hg) had progression to definite hypertension (SBP ≥160 mm Hg and DBP ≥90 mm Hg), compared with 45% of normotensive individuals ($p < 0.001$). After adjustment for multiple risk factors, borderline hypertension was associated with an excess long-term risk of cardiovascular disease (hazard ratio 1.47; 95% CI 1.24–1.74) and cardiovascular death (hazard ratio 1.57; 95% CI 1.24–2.00).

91. **Marmot MG**, et al. Alcohol and blood pressure: the **INTERSALT** study. *BMJ* 1994;308:1263–1267.

    This multicenter study was composed of 9,281 men and women 20–59 years of age. After adjustment for confounders, men who drank 300–499 mL alcohol/wk had 2. 7 and 1.6 mm Hg higher SBPs and DBPs, respectively, than nondrinkers; and men who consumed 500 mL alcohol/wk had pressures 4.6 and 3.0 mm Hg higher. Among women, heavy drinking (≥ 300 mL/wk) was associated with 3.9 and 3.1 mm Hg higher SBPs and DBPs, respectively.

92. **Psaty BM**, et al. The risk of MI associated with antihypertensive drug therapies. *JAMA* 1995;274:620–625.

    This controversial case-control study was composed of 623 cases and 2,032 controls followed from 1986 to 1993. Among patients initially free of cardiovascular disease, there was a 60% increased risk of MI with calcium-channel blockers with or without diuretics. Among patients on either calcium-channel blockers or β-blockers there was a 57% increased RR with calcium-channel blockade. Also, high doses of β-blockers were associated with a decreased risk, whereas high dose calcium-channel blockade was associated with increased risk. The accompanying editorial suggests that selection bias is likely; thus, patients prescribed calcium-channel blockers were significantly different (e.g., no control for LV dysfunction).

93. **Kannel WB**. Blood pressure as a cardiovascular risk factor. *JAMA* 1996; 275:1571–1576.

    This analysis of 36-year follow-data from the Framingham Heart Study shows that from age 30 to 65 years, the average increases in SBP and DBP are 20 and 10 mm Hg, respectively. There was no evidence of a change in the prevalence of hypertension over the past four decades. Hypertension occurs alone in only 20% (i.e., no diabetes, obesity, dyslipidemia). Hypertensive patients had increased RRs (M/F) of CAD (2.0/2.2), stroke (3.8/2.6), peripheral arterial disease (2. 0/3.7), and congestive heart failure (4.0/3.0). See Fig. 1-1 for estimated rates of CHD over 10 years according to different combinations of risk factors in men and women.

94. **O'Donnell CJ**, et al. Hypertension and borderline isolated systolic hypertension increase risks of cardiovascular disease and mortality in male physicians. *Circulation* 1997; 95:1132–1137.

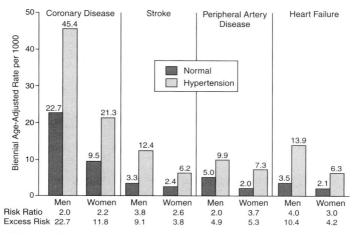

FIG. 1-1. Risk of cardiovascular events by hypertensive status in subjects aged 35 to 64 years, Framingham Study, 36-year follow-up. Coronary disease includes clinical manifestations such as myocardial infarction, angina pectoris, sudden death, other coronary deaths, and coronary insufficiency syndrome; peripheral artery disease is manifested as intermittent claudication. (From Kannel WB [93], with permission.)

This prospective cohort analysis focused on 18,682 Physicians Health Study participants, with a mean follow-up of 11.7 years. Isolated SBP (140–159 mm Hg) was associated with higher rates of stroke (RR 1.42) and cardiovascular death (RR 1.56), as well as a 22% higher all-cause mortality rate and nonsignificant increase in MI rate (RR 1.26).

95. **Moster d'A**, et al. Trends in the prevalence of hypertension, antihypertensive therapy, and left ventricular hypertrophy from 1950 to 1989. *N Engl J Med* 1999;340:1221–1227.

This analysis focused on 10,333 Framingham Heart Study participants. From 1950 to 1989, the age-adjusted prevalence of SBP 160 mm Hg or DBP 100 mm Hg declined from 18.5% to 9.2% among men and from 28.0% to 7.7% among women. There was also a decline in ECG evidence of LV hypertrophy: 4.5% to 2.5% and 3.6% to 1.1%.

Meta-Analyses

96. **Johnson AG**, et al. Do non-steroidal anti-inflammatory drugs affect blood pressure? A meta-analysis. *Ann Intern Med* 1994; 121:289–300.

This analysis was performed on data from 38 randomized, placebo-controlled trials and 12 randomized but not placebo-controlled trials (comparing two NSAIDs). NSAID use was associated with a 5.0 mm Hg higher elevated supine mean blood pressure. NSAIDs also antagonized the anti-hypertensive effect of β-blockers (blood pressure elevation 6.2 mm Hg). Sulindac and aspirin were found to have the least hypertensive effect.

97. **Schmieder RE**, et al. Reversal of left ventricular hypertrophy in essential hypertension: a meta-analysis of randomized double-blind studies. *JAMA* 1996;275:1507–1513 (editorial pp. 1517–1518).

This meta-analysis of 39 trials showed that a decrease in LV mass correlated significantly with a decrease in SBP ($r = 0.46$; $p < 0.001$) and a longer duration of anti-hypertensive therapy ($r = 0.38$; $p < 0.01$). ACE inhibitors achieved a greater reduction in LV mass than β-blockers and diuretics (-13% vs. -6%, $p < 0.05$; -13% vs. -7%, $p = 0.08$).

98. **Midgley JP**, et al. Effect of reduced dietary sodium on blood pressure. A meta-analysis of randomized controlled trials. *JAMA* 1996;275:1590–1597.

    This analysis was performed on 56 trials that met inclusion criteria; however, the heterogeneity of these studies was significant and publication bias was evident. A 100 mg/day reduction in daily urinary sodium excretion was associated with decreases in SBP of 3.7 mm Hg ($p < 0.001$) and DBP of only 0.9 mm Hg ($p = 0.09$). Of note, the authors do not recommend universal dietary sodium restriction.

99. **Psaty BM**, et al. Health outcomes associated with antihypertensive therapies used as first-line agents. *JAMA* 1997;277:739–745.

    Meta-analysis of 18 randomized, placebo-controlled trials with 48,220 patients. The use of β-blockers and high and low-dose diuretics were associated with fewer strokes (RRs of 0.71, 0.49, and 0.66, respectively) and less congestive heart failure (RRs of 0.58, 0.17, and 0.58). Low-dose diuretics were also associated with less CAD (RR 0.72) and lower all-cause mortality (RR 0.90; 95% CI 0.81–0. 99). Calcium-channel blockers and ACE inhibitors are associated with lower blood pressure, but major event and mortality data were limited.

100. **Gueyffier F**, et al. Antihypertensive drugs in very old people: a subgroup meta-analysis of randomised controlled trials. *Lancet* 1999;353;793–796.

    This analysis focused on 874 actively treated patients ≥ 80 years of age and 796 controls. Treated patients had a 34% lower stroke rate, 22% fewer cardiovascular events, and 39% lower incidence of congestive heart failure. However, cardiovascular and all-cause mortality rates were similar between the groups. The authors conclude that large-scale, adequately powered trial(s) are needed in very elderly patients to address the impact on mortality of anti-hypertensive agents.

Treatment

101. Metoprolol Atherosclerosis Prevention in Hypertension (**MAPHY**). Primary prevention with metoprolol in patients with hypertension: mortality results from the MAPHY study. *JAMA* 1988; 259:1976–1982.

    Design: Prospective, randomized, multicenter, open study. Median follow-up period was 4.2 years.

    Purpose: To investigate whether metoprolol lowers cardiovascular complications of high blood pressure to a greater extent than thiazide diuretics.

    Population: 3,234 white men 40–64 years of age.

    Treatment: Metoprolol (mean dosage 174 mg/day) or thiazide [hydrochlorothiazide (mean dosage 46 mg/day) or bendroflumethiazide (mean dosage 4.4 mg/day)].

    Results: Metoprolol group had 48% lower all-cause mortality (4.8 vs. 9.3 deaths/1,000 patient years) and 58% lower cardiovascular mortality (2.6 vs. 6.2 deaths/1,000 patient years).

102. Systolic HTN in Elderly Program (**SHEP**). Prevention of stroke by antihypertensive drug therapy in older persons with isolated systolic hypertension. *JAMA* 1991;265:3255–3264.
Design: Prospective, randomized, multicenter, double-blind, placebo-controlled study. Primary outcome was nonfatal and fatal (total) stroke. Average follow-up period was 4.5 years.
Purpose: To assess the ability of anti-hypertensive drug therapy to decrease the risk of stroke in individuals with isolated systolic hypertension.
Population: 4,736 patients ≥60 years of age (14% black, 57% women) with SBP 160–219 mm Hg and DBP <90 mm Hg; 3,161 patients were on anti-hypertensive drug(s).
Treatment: Step 1, chlorthalidone 12.5 mg/day, dose 2 25 mg/day; step 2, atenolol 25 mg/day, then 50 mg/day.
Results: At 5 years, 36% fewer strokes (5.2 vs. 8.2/1,000; $p = 0.0003$), lower SBP (143 vs. 155 mm Hg), and 27% decrease in nonfatal MI and coronary death were observed.

103. **Dahlof B**, et al. Swedish Trial in Old Patients with Hypertension (**STOP-HTN**). Morbidity and mortality in the STOP-HTN. *Lancet* 1991;338:1281–1285.
Design: Prospective, randomized, double-blind, placebo-controlled, multicenter study. Primary end point was stroke, MI, and other cardiovascular death.
Purpose: To evaluate the effects of several different anti-hypertensive agents on the incidence of major vascular events in older patients.
Population: 1,627 patients 70–84 years of age with SBP 180–230 mm Hg and DBP ≥ 90 mm Hg (or DBP 105–120 mm Hg).
Exclusion Criteria: MI or stroke within prior 12 months, isolated systolic hypertension (SBP >180 mm Hg and DBP <90 mm Hg).
Treatment: Atenolol (50 mg once daily), hydrochlorothiazide (HCTZ) (25 mg once daily) plus amiloride (2.5 mg once daily), metoprolol (100 mg once daily), pindolol (5 mg once daily), or placebo.
Results: At 25 months, treated patients had a significant 43% RRR in the incidence of all primary outcome measures (3.35%/yr vs. 5.55%/yr; $p = 0.0031$), 47% RRR in strokes (1.68%/yr vs. 3.13%/yr), 13% RRR in all MIs (1.44%/yr vs. 1.65%/yr), 70% RRR in other cardiovascular deaths (0. 25%/yr vs. 0.77%/yr), 50% RRR in vascular mortality (0.17%/yr vs. 0.34%/yr), and 43% RRR in total mortality (2.02%/yr vs. 3.54%/yr, $p = 0.0079$).

104. **Meade TW**, et al. Medical Research Council (**MRC**). MRC trial of treatment of hypertension in older adults: principal results. *BMJ* 1992;304:405–412.
Design: Prospective, randomized, single-blind, placebo-controlled study. Average follow-up period was 5.8 years.
Purpose: To determine if anti-hypertensive therapy in men and women 65–74 years of age reduces mortality and morbidity due to stroke and CHD.
Population: 4,396 patients not on any anti-hypertensive agents and with SBP 160–209 mm Hg and DBP <115 mm Hg.
Exclusion Criteria: Stroke or MI in prior 3 months, diabetes, and asthma.
Treatment: Hydrochlorothiazide (25–50 mg/day), amiloride (2.5–5. 0 mg/day), atenolol (50 mg/day), or placebo.
Results: Treated patients had 25% fewer strokes ($p = 0. 04$) and 19% fewer coronary events ($p = 0.08$). β-blockers induced non-

significant reduction; diuretics induced 31% fewer strokes and 44% fewer coronary events.

105. **Neaton JD**, et al. Treatment of mild hypertension study (**TOMHS**): final results. *JAMA* 1993;270:713–724 (editorial pp. 757–759).

Design: Prospective, randomized, multicenter, double-blind, placebo-controlled study. Average follow-up period was 4.4 years.

Purpose: To compare five drug treatments with placebo for long-term management of mild hypertension.

Population: 902 patients 45–69 years of age and not taking any anti-hypertensive medications at initial screening with DBP 90–99 mm Hg (at two visits).

Exclusion Criteria: History or evidence of cardiovascular disease or LV hypertrophy (based on ECG).

Treatment: Chlorthalidone 15 mg/day (diuretic), acebutolol 400 mg/day (β-blocker), doxazosin 1 mg/day (alpha-1 agonist), amlodipine 5 mg/day, enalapril 5 mg/day, or placebo (all a.m. dosing). All patients received nutritional-hygienic advice (low weight, low sodium, low alcohol, increased exercise).

Results: Drug therapy reductions were sizable in all six groups (DBP decreased by 8.6 to 12.3 mm Hg). Drug groups had a nonsignificant reduction in death and major cardiovascular events (5.1% vs. 7.3%; $p = 0.21$). Drug therapy also was associated with better quality of life and decreased resting ECG abnormalities; there were no differences seen between the five drug groups in LV mass, lipid levels, and other outcome measures.

106. **Materson BJ**, et al. **VA Cooperative Study**. Single-drug therapy for hypertension in men: a comparison of 6 antihypertensive agents with placebo. *N Engl J Med* 1993;328:914–921.

Design: Prospective, randomized, double-blind, placebo-controlled, multicenter study. Primary end point was DBP < 95 mm Hg. Follow-up period was 1 year.

Purpose: To compare the effectiveness of several different classes of anti-hypertensive therapies as monotherapy based on age and race.

Population: 1,292 men ≥21 years of age with DBP 95–109 mm Hg.

Treatment: Hydrochlorothiazide 12.5–50 mg/day, atenolol 25–100 mg/day, clonidine 0.2–0.6 mg/day, captopril 25–100 mg/day, prazosin 4–20 mg/day, sustained-release diltiazem 120–360 mg/day, or placebo.

Results: Overall success rates (DBP <95 mm Hg over 1 year) were as follows: diltiazem, 59%; atenolol, 51%; clonidine, 50%; hydrochlorothiazide, 46%; captopril, 42%; prazosin, 42%; and placebo, 25%. Certain drugs appeared to be more effective in particular subgroups of patients: in blacks (young and old), diltiazem best; young whites, captopril best; and older whites, atenolol best. Subsequent 1-year follow-up showed a significant reduction in LV hypertrophy in those receiving hydrochlorothiazide, captopril, and atenolol (−42.9, −38.7, and −28.1 g) (*see Circulation* 1997;95:2007).

Comments: One possible explanation for these findings is that blacks and older patients may be less responsive to ACE inhibition and more responsive to diuretics and calcium-channel blockade because of a higher prevalence of low-renin hypertension.

107. **Staessen JA**, et al. **Syst-Eur**. Randomised double-blind comparison of placebo and active treatment for older patients with isolated systolic hypertension. *Lancet* 1997;350:757–764.

Design: Prospective, randomized, double-blind, placebo-controlled, multicenter study. Primary end point was fatal and nonfatal stroke. Median follow-up period was 2 years.

Purpose: To investigate whether treatment of isolated systolic hypertension could reduce stroke and cardiovascular complications.

Population: 4,695 patients ≥60 years of age with average sitting SBP 160–219 mm Hg and DBP <95 mm Hg.

Exclusion Criteria: CHF, creatinine 180 μ*M,* and MI in prior year.

Treatment: Nitrendipine 10–40 mg/day with the possible addition of enalapril 5–20 mg /day and hydrochlorothiazide 12.5–25 mg/day, or matching placebos.

Results: At 2 years, treated patients had 42% fewer total strokes (7.9 vs. 13.7 per 1,000 patient years; p = 0.003) and 31% fewer fatal and nonfatal cardiac end points (p = 0.03). Treated patients had significantly lower SBPs and DBPs than placebo patients (−10.1 mm Hg and −4.5 mm Hg). There was a trend toward lower cardiovascular mortality with active treatment (−27%; p = 0.07), but all-cause mortality was not influenced (−14%; p = 0.22).

108. **Hansson L**, et al. for the Hypertension Optimal Treatment (**HOT**) study. Effects of intensive blood pressure lowering and low dose aspirin in patients with hypertension. Principal results of the Hypertension Optimal Treatment (HOT) randomized trial. *Lancet* 1998;351:1755–1762.

Design: Prospective, randomized, partially open, partially blinded (aspirin arm), multicenter study. Mean follow-up period was 3.8 years.

Purpose: To (a) assess the association between major cardiovascular events and three different target blood pressures as well as the actual DBP achieved during treatment; and (b) evaluate whether the addition of low-dose aspirin to anti-hypertensive treatment reduces major cardiovascular events.

Population: 18,790 patients 50–80 years of age (mean 61.5 years) with DBP 100–115 mm Hg.

Treatment: Target DBP levels of ≤90 mm Hg, ≤85 mm Hg, or ≤80 mm Hg. A five-step approach was used: step 1, felodipine 5 mg/day; step 2, addition of low-dose ACE inhibitor or β-blocker; step 3, felopidine increased to 10 mg/day; step 4, dose of ACE inhibitor or β-blocker increased; and step 5, addition of low-dose alternative agent or hydrochlorothiazide. All patients were randomized in double-blinded fashion to aspirin 75 mg/day or placebo.

Results: At 2 years, target DBP was achieved in 85%, 67%, and 75%. Mean DBPs were closely grouped: 85.2, 83.2, and 81.1 mm Hg. Incidence of primary composite end point did not significantly differ between the three groups, but there were significantly fewer cardiovascular events and deaths among diabetic patients assigned to a target DBP of ≤80 mm Hg compared with ≤90 mm Hg (p = 0.005, p = 0.016). There were no differences in blood pressure between aspirin- and placebo-treated patients. Aspirin use was associated with 15% fewer major events (p = 0.03), 36% reduction in fatal or nonfatal MI (p = 0.002), and similar rate of hemorrhagic and ischemic stroke. A subsequent substudy of 922 patients showed substantial quality of life improvement in the ≤80 mm Hg group (*see Blood Pressure* 1997;6:357).

Comments: Study was underpowered for two reasons: (a) actual mean DBPs were ~2 mm Hg apart instead of 5 mm Hg apart and (b) only 724 major cardiovascular events occurred over 3.8 years versus projected 1,100 over 2.5 years.

109. Captopril Prevention Project (**CAPPP**). Effect of angiotensin-converting-enzyme inhibition compared with conventional therapy on cardiovascular morbidity and mortality in hypertension: the Captopril Prevention Project (CAPPP) randomised trial. *Lancet* 1999;353:611–616 (editorial pp. 604–605).

Design: Prospective, randomized, multicenter, open study. Primary composite end points were fatal and nonfatal MI, stroke, and other cardiovascular deaths. Mean follow-up period was 6.1 years.

Purpose: To compare the effectiveness of captopril with a conventional anti-hypertensive regimen of diuretics or β-blockers on cardiovascular morbidity and mortality.

Population: 10,985 patients 25–66 years of age with DBP ≥100 mm Hg on two occasions.

Exclusion Criteria: Secondary hypertension and serum creatinine >150 μM.

Treatment: Captopril 50 mg once or twice daily, β-blockers (most common: metoprolol and atenolol), or diuretics (most common: hydrochlorothiazide and bendrofluazide).

Results: Two groups had a similar incidence of composite end point (11.1 and 10.2 events per 1,000 patient years in captopril and conventional therapy groups); captopril group had a trend toward lower cardiovascular mortality (RR 0.77; $p = 0.092$) but a higher incidence of fatal and nonfatal stroke (RR 1.15; $p = 0.044$); MI rates were similar.

Comments: Lower stroke risk in conventional group probably was due to lower initial blood pressure (−2 mm Hg).

110. **LaPalio L**, et al. Safety and efficacy of metoprolol in the treatment of hypertension in the elderly. *J Am Geriatr Soc* 1992;40:354–358.

This prospective, open label, observational study was composed of 21,692 patients 50–75 years of age with hypertension [SBP ≤200 mm Hg and DBP 90–104 mm Hg (no prior therapy) or ≤95 mm Hg (prior therapy)]. Exclusion criteria included use of β-blockers for angina, congestive heart failure, and heart block. Patients received metoprolol 100 mg/day. If DBP was still >90 mm Hg at 4 weeks, hydrochlorothiazide 25 mg/day was added. At 4 weeks, mean blood pressure was reduced from 162/95 to 149/87 mm Hg ($p < 0.001$), and at 8 weeks to 143/84 mm Hg. At the end of the study, 50% remained on metoprolol as monotherapy, whereas 27% needed combination therapy.

111. **Levy D**, et al. Hypertension And Lipid Trial (**HALT**). Principal results of the HALT: a multicenter study of doxazosin in patients with hypertension. *Am Heart J* 1996;131:966–973.

Open, noncomparative trial of 851 clinic patients. At 16 weeks, sitting and standing SBP and DBP were significantly lowered by doxazosin (range 12.5–16.1 mm Hg). There was no significant effect on heart rate. TC was lowered by 2.7% and LDL by 2.4%. The 5-year coronary disease risk was decreased by 14.7% in patients without prior anti-hypertensive therapy ($p < 0.0001$) and only 1.7% in patients with prior anti-hypertensive therapy ($p < 0.05$).

112. **Gong L**, et al. Shanghai trial of nifedipine in the elderly (**STONE**). *J Hypertens* 1996;14:1237–1245.

This prospective, randomized, single-blind, multicenter trial was composed of 1,632 patients 60–79 years of age with blood pressure ≥160/90 mm Hg. Patients received slow-release nifedipine (10–60 mg twice daily) or placebo; captopril or dihydrochlorothiazide was added if blood pressure remained elevated. At a mean follow-up of 30 months, the nifedipine group had experienced significantly fewer clinical end points, including MI, sudden death, congestive heart failure, and stroke (3.9% vs. 7.4%). Specifically, there was a 59% RRR in stroke or severe arrhythmia.

113. **Appel LJ**, et al. for the Dietary Approaches to Stop Hypertension (**DASH**) Research Group: a clinical trial of the effects of dietary patterns on blood pressure. *N Engl J Med* 1997;336:1117–1124.

This prospective, randomized study was composed of 459 adults with SBP <160 mm Hg and DBP 80–95 mm Hg. For 3 weeks, all participants were fed a control diet that was low in fruits, vegetables, and dairy products. They were then randomized to the control diet or a diet rich in fruits and vegetables or a combination diet rich in fruits, vegetables, and low-fat dairy products and with reduced saturated fat and total fat. Body weight and sodium intake were not modified. The combination diet resulted in significant reduction in systolic and diastolic blood pressure compared to control diet (11.4 mmHg and 5.5 mmHg, respectively; both $p < 0.001$).

114. **Krum H**, et al. The effect of an endothelin-receptor antagonist, bosentan, on blood pressure in patients with essential hypertension. *N Engl J Med* 1998;338:784–790.

This prospective, randomized trial was composed of 293 patients with mild to moderate hypertension. After a placebo run-in period of 4–6 weeks, patients were randomized to one of four doses of bosentan (100, 500, or 1,000 mg, 2,000 mg once daily), enalapril (20 mg once daily), or placebo. Compared with placebo, the bosentan 500-mg and 2,000-mg groups and enalapril group had similar significant reductions in DBP (−5.7 mm Hg vs. −5.8 mm Hg). Bosentan had no significant effect on heart rate, plasma levels of norepinephrine, plasma renin activity, and angiotensin II levels.

115. **Whelton PK**, et al. Trial of Nonpharmacologic Interventions in the Elderly (**TONE**). Sodium reduction and weight loss in the treatment of hypertension in older persons. *JAMA* 1998;279:839–846.

Prospective, randomized study of 875 individuals 60–80 years of age with SBP <145 mm Hg and DBP <85 mm Hg on a single anti-hypertensive medication. Obese patients (n = 585) were randomized to reduced sodium intake (≤1 g/day), weight loss, both, or usual care, whereas nonobese patients (n = 390) received reduced sodium or usual care. After 3 months of intervention, withdrawal of the anti-hypertensive medication was attempted. At a median follow-up of 29 months, reduced sodium intake compared with no reduction in sodium intake was associated with a significant reduction in the incidence of cardiovascular events (MI, heart failure, bypass surgery, angioplasty), recurrent hypertension, or reinitiation of anti-hypertensive therapy (relative hazard ratio 0.69, 95% CI 0.59–0.81; $p < 0.001$). Obese patients assigned to weight loss also had a lower incidence of the combined outcome measures compared with those not assigned to weight loss (relative hazard ratio 0.70, 95% CI 0.57–0.87; $p <$ 0.001). Overall, weight loss (average 3.5 kg) and sodium restriction resulted in an ~30% decrease in the need for anti-hypertensive medication. There were no differences in the frequency of cardiovascular differences between any groups, but it should be noted that the study was underpowered for this purpose.

Obesity and Weight

116. **Lissner L**, et al. Variability of body weight and health outcomes in the Framingham population. *N Engl J Med* 1991;324:1839–1844.

    Patients were asked to recall their weight at 25 years of age. Measured weight at first biennial examinations was analyzed, and end point after the 10th examination was tabulated. Highly variable weight was associated with increased mortality ($p = 0.005$ [men], $p = 0.01$), CHD mortality ($p = 0.0009$ [both]), and CHD morbidity ($p = 0.0009$, $p = 0.006$); RRs ranged from 1.27 to 1.93.

117. **Willett WC**, et al. Weight, weight change and coronary heart disease in women: risk within the normal weight range. *JAMA* 1995;273:461–465.

    This prospective cohort study was composed of 115,818 nurses 30–55 years of age with no history of CAD. Even modest weight gains after 18 years were associated with increased risk (end point was CHD death and nonfatal MI): RR 1.25 for 5- to 7.9-kg gain; RR 1.64 for 8- to 10.9 kg gain; 2.65 for 11- to 19-kg gain.

118. **Jousilahti P**, et al. Body weight, cardiovascular risk factors, and coronary mortality. *Circulation* 1996;93:1372–1379.

    This prospective cohort study was composed of Finnish men and women 30–59 years of age examined in either 1972 or 1977. CHD mortality was positively associated with body mass index. Among men, the body mass index–associated risk ratio of CHD, adjusted for age, study year, smoking, blood pressure, and cholesterol, was 1.03 per kg/m^2 ($p = 0.027$). Among women, the risk ratio was 1.05 ($p = 0.023$) when adjusted for only age and study year but was not statistically significant when the additional three variables were analyzed (1.03; $p = 0.15$).

119. **Rextrode KM**, et al. Abdominal adiposity and coronary heart disease in women. *JAMA* 1998;280:1843–1848.

    This analysis of 8-year follow-up data of 44,702 Nurses Health Study participants showed that a higher waist:hip ratio and greater waist circumference were associated with an increased risk of CHD. If waist:hip ratio was 0.88, the adjusted RR of CHD death or MI was 3.25 (vs. waist:hip ratio <0.72). A waist circumference of 38 inches was associated with an adjusted RR of CHD death and MI of 3.06. The independent predictive value of waist:hip ratio and waist circumference was also present in a subgroup with a body mass index of ≤25 kg/m^2.

120. **Bender R**, et al. Effect of age on excess mortality in obesity. *JAMA* 1999;281:1498–1504.

    This prospective cohort study was composed of 6,193 obese patients with a mean body mass index of 36.6 kg/m^2 and mean age of 40.4 years. At follow-up (median 14.8 years), standardized mortality ratios showed obesity was associated with significantly increased mortality (men, 1.67; women, 1.45). This increased risk associated with obesity decreased with advancing age among both men (18–29 years, 2.46; 30–39 years, 2.30; 40–49 years, 1.99;

50–74 years, 1.31) and women (18–29 years, 1.81; 30–39 years, 2.10; 40–49 years, 1.70; 50–74 years, 1.26) (trend test, $p < 0.001$)

Activity and Exercise

121. **Berlin JA,** Colditz GA. A meta-analysis of physical activity in the prevention of coronary heart disease. *Am J Epidemiol* 1990; 132:612–628.

This meta-analysis found a nearly twofold increased risk of death from CHD for individuals with sedentary compared with active occupations (RR 1.9; 95% CI 1.6–2.2).

122. **Leon AS,** Connett J. Physical activity and 10.5 year mortality in the Multiple Risk Factor Intervention Trial (**MRFIT**). *Int J Epidemiol* 1991;20:690–697.

This analysis focused on 12,138 male MRFIT subjects who had leisure time physical activity (LTPA) assessed by the Minnesota questionnaire. The level of LTPA was inversely related to all-cause mortality, CHD mortality, and cardiovascular mortality because those in the lowest LTPA tertile had excess mortality rates of 15%, 27%, and 22%, respectively, compared with men in the middle tertile. There was no significant further attenuation of risk with additional LTPA (tertile 3).

123. **Mittleman MA**, et al. Triggering of acute MI by heavy physical exertion. *N Engl J Med* 1993;329:1677–1683.

This analysis focused on interviews with 1,228 patients an average of 4 days after MI. Heavy exertion (≥6 metabolic equivalents) within 1 hour had occurred in 4.4%. The RR of acute MI in the 1 hour after exertion was 5.9; however, risk correlated with the frequency of exercise (less than once per week, RR 107; one to two times, RR 19.4; three to four times, RR 8.6; at least five times, RR 2.4.

124. **Willich SN**, et al. Physical exertion as a trigger of AMI. *N Engl J Med* 1993;329:1684–1690.

This analysis focused on interviews with 1,194 patients at 13 ± 6 days after MI. An increased risk of MI was associated with strenuous activity (≥6 metabolic equivalents; 7.1% of patients) at onset of acute MI (RR 2.1). The RR was also 2.1 for activity within 1 hour; infrequent exercise (less than four times per week) was associated with an RR of 6.9 (vs. 1.3).

125. **Blair SN**, et al. Influences of cardiorespiratory fitness and other precursors on cardiovascular disease and all-cause mortality in men and women. *JAMA* 1996;276:205–210.

This observational cohort study of 32,421 patients (78% men) demonstrated independent mortality predictors. Among men, low fitness (RR 1.52), smoking (1.65), abnormal ECG (1.64), increased TC (1.34), elevated SBP (1.34), and chronic illness (1.63) risks were defined. Among women, low fitness (2.1) and smoking (1.99) risks were defined. It is important to note that there is a fitness effect with any combination of smoking, TC, and blood pressure.

126. **Shephard RJ,** Balady GJ. Exercise as cardiovascular therapy. *Circulation* 1999;99:963–972.

This review discusses the biologic and physiologic effects of exercise and summarizes available data on its results in patients with documented CAD, hypertension, diabetes, obesity, dyslipidemia, and other conditions. There is also a section on exercise prescription that focuses on the recommended type(s), intensity, and frequency of exercise in various populations.

127. **Hakim AA**, et al. Effects of walking on coronary heart disease in elderly men. The Honolulu Heart Program. *Circulation* 1999; 100:9–13.

This study of 2,678 physically capable men aged 71 to 93 years who were observed over a 2 to 4 year follow-up period found that those who walked more than 1.5 miles a day had a lower incidence of developing coronary heart disease compared to those who walked less than one quarter mile a day (2.5 % vs 5.1%, $p <$ 0.01) and 0.25–1.5 miles a day (4.5%, $p < 0.01$). These findings were not altered by adjustment for age and other coronary heart disease risk factors.

Nonmodifiable Risk Factors

128. **Manson JE**, et al. A prospective study of walking as compared with vigorous exercise in the prevention of coronary heart disease in women. *N Engl J Med* 1999;341:650–658.

This prospective cohort study of 72,488 Nurses' Health Study participants found brisk walking, as assessed by a self-administered questionnaire, was associated with fewer coronary events. In multivariate analyses, women in the highest quintile group ($\geq$3 hours/wk at a brisk pace [$\geq$3 mph]), had a relative risk of 0.65 (95% CI 0.47–0.91) compared with those who walked infrequently. Regular vigorous exercise ($\geq$ 6 METs) was associated with similar risk reductions (30%–40%).

129. **Colditz GA**, et al. A prospective study of parental history of MI and coronary artery disease in men. *Am J Cardiol* 1991;67: 933–938.

This prospective study was composed of 45,317 male health professionals 40–75 years of age with no diagnosis of CAD. At a mean follow-up of 1.6 years, if a parent had an MI at <70 years of age, the RRs of cardiac death, MI, PTCA, or CABG were 2.2 (maternal factor) and 1.7 (paternal factor). The risk increased with lower parental age.

130. **Wei JY**. Age and the cardiovascular system. *N Engl J Med* 1992; 327:1735–1739.

This review discusses the impact of age on the myocardium, vasculature, cardiac output, diastolic function, blood pressure regulation, and effects of exercise training.

131. **Marenberg ME**, et al. Genetic susceptibility to death from coronary heart disease in a study of twins. *N Engl J Med* 1994; 330:1041–1046.

This analysis is composed of data taken from 21,004 Swedish twins in 1961 and 1963; average follow-up was 26 years. Among men, RRs (of death secondary to CHD) if the twin died of CHD at <55 years of age were 8.1 (monozygous) and 3. 8 (dizygous). Among women, RRs were 15.0 and 2.6, respectively; overall, RRs decreased with increased age.

132. **Ciruzzi M**, et al. Frequency of family history in patients with acute MI. *Am J Cardiol* 1997;80:122–127.

This case-control study was composed of 1,060 cases and 1,071 controls. Among cases with a twofold higher incidence of positive family history (more than one first-degree relative with a history of MI), the incidence of MI was 31% vs. 15% for controls. After risk factor adjustment (age, sex, cholesterol, smoking, diabetes, hypertension, body mass index, education, social class, exercise), the overall odds ratio was 2.18 (at least one relative, 2.04; two relatives, 3.18). If < 55 years of age with two relatives, the odds ratio was 4.42; ≥ 55 years of age with two relatives, odds ratio 3.00; family history plus TC 240 mg/dL, odds ratio 4.5; family history plus hypertension, odds ratio 4.5; family history plus current smoking, odds ratio 5.77.

Alcohol

133. **Regan TJ**. Alcohol and the cardiovascular system. *JAMA* 1990; 264:377–381.

   This review describes the adverse effects of alcohol, including subclinical LV dysfunction, heart failure, arrhythmias (e.g., atrial fibrillation), and stroke. There is also a section that discusses the epidemiologic data correlating low to moderate ethanol intake with a reduced risk of CAD.

134. **Hein HO**, et al. Alcohol consumption, serum LDL cholesterol concentration and risk of ischemic heart disease: 6 yr follow-up in the Copenhagen male study. *BMJ* 1996;312:736–741.

   This prospective study was composed of 2,826 patients without coronary artery disease. At 6 years, 6.1% had experienced a first ischemic event. The association between alcohol and ischemic heart disease was highly dependent on LDL. With an LDL level of 5.25 mM, among abstainers the incidence of ischemic heart disease is 16.4%; among those who have 1–21 drinks/wk, 8.7%; among those who have ≥22 drinks/wk, 4.4%. After risk factor adjustment, RRs were 0.4 ($p < 0.05$) and 0.2 ($p < 0.01$). If LDL level is <3.63 mM, no benefit is thought to be gained from any level of alcohol consumption.

135. **Pearson TA**. From the Nutrition Committee of AHA. Alcohol and heart disease. *Circulation* 1996;94:3023–3025.

   The Nutrition Committee of the AHA recommendations include consulting a physician to assess risks and benefits of alcohol consumption, with contraindications including family history of alcoholism, hypertriglyceridemia, liver disease, uncontrolled hypertension, and pregnancy. If no contraindications are present, one to two drinks/day are considered safe and probably beneficial (associated with 30%–50% decrease in risk of CAD in numerous prospective epidemiologic studies).

136. **Camargo CA Jr**. Moderate alcohol consumption and risk for angina pectoris or MI in U.S. male physicians. *Ann Intern Med* 1997;126:372–375.

   This prospective cohort study of 22,071 patients confirms the substantial body of data correlating moderate ethanol consumption with decreased CHD risk. One drink/day versus less than one drink/week confers an RR of angina of 0.69 (95% CI 0.59–0.81) and an RR of MI of 0.65 (95% CI 0.52–0.81).

137. **Muntwyler J**, et al. Mortality and light to moderate alcohol consumption after MI. *Lancet* 1998;352:1882–1885.

   This analysis is composed of 90,150 men in the Physicians Health Study, 5,358 with prior MI. At 5-year follow-up, there were 920 deaths. After adjustment for confounders, moderate intake was associated with a significant decrease in total mortality ($p = 0.016$). Mortality RRs were one to four drinks/mo, 0.85 (95% CI 0.69–1.05); two to four drinks/wk, 0.72 (95% CI 0.58–0.89); one drink/day, 0.79 (95% CI 0.64–9.96); and two drinks/day, 0.84 (95% CI 0.55–1.26).

Hormone Status and Hormonal Replacement

138. **Stampfer MJ**, et al. Postmenopausal estrogen therapy and cardiovascular disease. *N Engl J Med* 1991;325;756–762.

    This prospective cohort study was composed of 48,470 postmenopausal women without prior cardiovascular disease or cancer. The trial had excellent control and adjustment for risk factors. At an average follow-up of 7 years, estrogen patients had a significant 11% RRR in total mortality, 28% RRR in cardiovascular mortality, and 44% RRR in the incidence of major coronary disease. There was no significant difference in stroke rates. Based on these results and prior data, the following epidemiologic consensus was offered in the accompanying editorial: (a) CHD mortality decreased by 40%–50%, (b) up to 60% fewer hip fractures occurred, (c) breast cancer rates were ~30% higher, and (d) up to a sixfold higher incidence of endometrial cancer was observed with estrogen alone. It is important to note that the RRs and absolute risks are much different: Many more CHD deaths were avoided than endometrial deaths caused.

139. **Grodstein F**, et al. Postmenopausal estrogen and progestin use and the risk of cardiovascular disease. *N Engl J Med* 1996; 335:453–461.

    This prospective cohort analysis focused on 59,337 Nurses Health Study participants who were 30–55 years of age and free of known cardiovascular disease at baseline. At an average follow-up of 11.2 years, combined estrogen and progestin users had a lower incidence of major CHD (MI, death) compared with non-hormone and estrogen only users (adjusted RRs 0.39 and 0.60). Thus, the addition of progestin does not appear to attenuate the cardioprotective effects of postmenopausal estrogen therapy. Of note, there were no significant differences in stroke rates.

140. **Koh KK**, et al. Effects of hormone-replacement therapy on fibrinolysis in postmenopausal women. *N Engl J Med* 1997;336: 683–690.

    This randomized crossover study addressed estrogen 0.625 mg once daily in 20 patients and transdermal estradiol 0.1 mg daily in 20 patients, either alone or in combination with medroxyprogesterone 2.5 mg once daily for 1 month. Greater than 50% reduction in PAI-1 levels was seen with estrogen with or without medroxyprogesterone. These findings may explain part of the protective effect of hormone-replacement therapy on CAD.

141. **Grodstein F**, et al. Postmenopausal hormonal therapy and mortality. *N Engl J Med* 1997;336:1769–1775 (editorial pp. 1821–1822).

    This nested case-control study addressed 3,637 Nurses Health Study deaths (10 controls per death). To prevent drug discontinuation bias, hormone status used was from the last biennial questionnaire before death or diagnosis of fatal disease. Analysis showed that current hormone therapy users had a lower mortality risk: adjusted RR of death vs. never users was 0.63 (adjusted for body mass index, smoking, hypertension, TC, diabetes, positive family history of MI or breast cancer, parity, early menarche). This benefit decreased with time, mostly due to increased breast cancer mortality (+43%; RR 0.80 with >10 years use). Current users with cardiac risk factors (69%) had the largest mortality reduction (RR 0.51), whereas a low-risk group

(13%; never smoked, normal cholesterol, no hypertension or diabetes, body mass index <25) had a nonsignificant 11% RRR. The protective effect was lost 5 years after discontinuation of therapy. Of note, there was no increased breast cancer risk with a positive family history. Accompanying editorial asserts that the study design may not have adequately controlled for life-style differences between users and nonusers.

142. **Hulley S**, et al. Heart and Estrogen/progestin Replacement Study (**HERS**). Randomized trial of estrogen and progestin for secondary prevention of coronary heart disease in postmenopausal women. *JAMA* 1998;280:605–613 (editorial pp. 650–652).
Design: Prospective, randomized, blinded, placebo-controlled, multicenter study. Average follow-up period was 4.1 years.
Purpose: To determine if estrogen plus progestin alters the risk for CHD events in postmenopausal women with known coronary disease.
Population: 2,763 women <80 years of age (mean age 66.7 years).
Exclusion Criteria: CHD event in previous 6 months, sexual hormone use in previous 3 months, history of pulmonary embolism, deep venous thrombosis, breast cancer, and endometrial cancer.
Treatment: Conjugated equine estrogens (0.625 mg once daily) and medroxyprogesterone (one tablet once daily) or placebo.
Results: Compliance rates were 82% at 1 year and 75% at 3 years. No difference in primary outcome (MI plus cardiovascular death; relative hazard 0.99) was observed. Lack of effect was observed despite the hormone group having 11% lower LDL and 10% higher HDL (each $p < 0.001$). The hormone group had more events in year 1 and fewer in years 4 and 5. The hormone group had more venous thromboembolism (relative hazard 2.89; 95% CI 1.50–5.58) and gall bladder disease (relative hazard 1.38; 95% CI 1.00–1.92).
Comments: Accompanying editorial advocates that current users should not stop taking their medication (time effect). There are also other hormone benefits (e.g., bone and menopausal symptoms). Other ongoing studies include the Women's Health Initiative (results in 2005) and WELL-HART (angiographic end point).

143. **Sourander L**, et al. Cardiovascular mortality and cancer morbidity and mortality and sudden cardiac death in postmenopausal women on oestrogen replacement therapy (**ERT**). *Lancet* 1998;352:1965–1969.
This prospective cohort study is composed of 7,944 women, with an average follow-up of 6.7 years. Current estrogen replacement therapy was associated with lower rates of cardiovascular mortality [adjusted odds ratios 0.21 (95% CI 0.08–0.59) and 0.75 (95% CI 0.41–1.37) in current and former users, respectively]. Estrogen replacement therapy was not associated with a significant increase in incidence of breast cancer, whereas endometrial cancer was more common in current users (RR 5.06; 95% CI 2.47–10.41).

Other

Homocysteine

144. **Clarke R**, et al. Hyperhomocysteinemia: an independent risk factor for vascular disease. *N Engl J Med* 1991;324:1149–1155.

This study of 123 patients years of age showed that hyper-homocysteinemia (defined as >24 μM after methionine-loading) was present in 42% with cerebrovascular disease, 28% with peripheral vascular disease, and 30% with CAD (0% in 27 controls). After risk factor adjustment, RR of vascular disease was 3.2.

145. **Stampfer MJ**, et al. A prospective study of plasma homocysteine and risk of MI in U.S. physicians. *JAMA* 1992;268:877–891.

In this case-control study of Physicians Health Study participants, MI patients (n = 271) had higher plasma homocysteine levels than age- and smoking-matched controls (11.1 vs. 10.5 nM). RR of MI was 3.4 among those with homocysteine levels above the 95th percentile compared with those with levels at or below the 90th percentile.

146. **Boushney CJ**, et al. A quantitative assessment of plasma homocysteine as a risk factor for vascular disease. *JAMA* 1995;274: 1049–1057.

Meta-analysis of 27 nonrandomized studies showed the following odds ratios associated with a 5 μM increment in homocysteine levels for CAD (men, 1.6; women, 1.8) and cerebrovascular disease (1.5). Although increased folic acid intake (700 μg/day) decreased levels by ~4 μM, there are no good data on whether lowering high homocysteine levels with dietary supplementation significantly reduces the associated risk.

147. **Nygard O**, et al. Total plasma homocysteine and cardiovascular risk profile. *JAMA* 1995;274:1526–1533.

This analysis focused on 16,176 patients 40–67 years of age without prior hypertension, diabetes, CHD, or cerebrovascular disease. Homocysteine levels were higher in men and increased with age (40–42 years of age, 10.8 μM; 65–67 years of age, 12.2 μM). There was a strong positive correlation, especially among women, with number of cigarettes smoked per day (0 cigarettes, 1.5; ≤20 cigarettes, 11.7), TC (<155 mg/dL, 10. 3; ≥310 mg/dL, 11.2), DBP (>70 mm Hg, 10.3; >100 mm Hg, 11.2), and heart rate (<60 beats/min, 10.4; >100 beats/min, 11.6). An inverse relationship to physical activity was observed (none, 11.1; heavy, 10.4). The precise threshold for increased risk is still unclear.

148. **Morrison HI**, et al. Serum folate and the risk of fatal coronary heart disease. *JAMA* 1996;275:1893–1896 (editorial pp. 1929–1930).

This retrospective study of 5,056 patients showed that 15-year CHD mortality was correlated with serum folate levels (>6 ng/mL vs. <3 ng/mL meant a 69% increased risk). Accompanying editorial stresses the need for randomized trials to study whether folate (diet or supplements) would decrease cardiovascular disease [e. g. three arms, including placebo, folate (dosage 400–650 μg/day), and folate plus B$_{12}$].

149. **Schwartz SM**, et al. MI in young women in relation to plasma total homocysteine, folate and a common variant in the methylenetetrahydrofolate reductase gene. *Circulation* 1997;96:412–417.

This population-based case-control study was composed of 79 cases and 386 controls <45 years of age. MI patients had a higher mean plasma homocysteine level (13.4 vs. 11.1 μM, $p = 0.0004$) and lower mean folate (12.4 vs. 16.1 nM, $p = 0.018$). B$_{12}$ levels were similar. After risk factor adjustment, for homocysteine levels of 15.6 vs. <10 nM, the odds ratio was 2.3 (95% CI 0.94–5.64), and for folate levels of 8.39 vs. <5.27 nM, the odds ratio was 0.54 (95% CI 0.23–1.28).

150. **Nygard O**, et al. Plasma homocysteine levels and mortality in patients with coronary artery disease. *N Engl J Med* 1997; 337:230–236.

   Prospective study of 587 patients with CAD by angiography; 318 had undergone CABG surgery and 120 PTCA, and 149 were on medical therapy. At follow-up (median 4.6 years), the adjusted mortality ratios were as follows (reference group <9 μmol): (units = μmol) 9.0–14.9, 1.9; 15.0–19.9, 2.8; and 20, 4.5 (p trend 0.02). Cardiovascular mortality ratios were 3.3, 6.3, and 9.9 (p trend 0.01).

151. **Jacques PF**, et al. The effect of folic acid fortification on plasma folate and total homocysteine concentrations. *N Engl J Med* 1999;340:1449–1454.

   This study analyzed blood samples of Framingham Offspring Study participants taken from January 1991 to December 1994 and compared them with subsequent samples obtained prior to fortification of enriched grain with folic acid (January 1995 to September 1996; control group) and after fortification was implemented (September 1997 to March 1998; study group). Among study group subjects who did not use vitamin supplements, mean folate concentrations more than doubled from the baseline to follow-up visit (4.6–10.0 ng/mL; $p < 0.001$) and the prevalence of low folate levels (<3 ng/mL) markedly decreased from 22.0% to 1.7% ($p < 0.001$). The mean total homocysteine concentration decreased form 10.1 to 9.4 μM and the prevalence of high homocysteine levels (>13 μM) decreased from 18.7% to 9.8% ($p < 0.001$). There were no significant changes in folate or homocysteine concentrations in control group subjects.

152. **Ridker PM**, et al. Homocysteine and risk of cardiovascular disease among postmenopausal women. *JAMA* 1999;281:1817–1821.

   This prospective, nested case-control study was composed of 122 Women's Health Study participants who experienced cardiovascular disease and 244 age- and smoking-matched controls. At follow-up (mean 3 years), case subjects had higher baseline homocysteine levels (14.1 vs. 12.4 μM; $p = 0.02$). The RR of cardiovascular events with homocysteine levels in the 95th percentile (≥20.7 μM) was 2.6. The increased risk persisted after adjustment for other traditional risk factors. Of note, self-reported vitamin use at study entry was associated with lower homocysteine levels.

153. **Bostom AG**, et al. Nonfasting plasma total homocysteine levels and all-cause and cardiovascular disease mortality in elderly Framingham men and women. *Arch Intern Med* 1999;159: 1077–1080.

   Nonfasting plasma homocysteine levels were obtained in 1933 Framingham Study participants between 1979 and 1982; mean age was 70 years. At follow-up (median 10.0 years), proportional hazards modeling showed that homocysteine levels in the upper quartile (≥14.26 μM) compared with levels in the lower three quartiles were associated with RRs of all-cause and cardiovascular mortality of 2.18 and 2.17, respectively (95% CIs 1.86–2.56 and 1.68–2.82). These RR estimates remained significant [1.54 (95% CI 1.31–1.82), 1.52 (1.16–1.98)] after adjustment for age, sex, SBP, diabetes, smoking, TC, and HDL.

154. **Folsom AR**, et al. Atherosclerosis Risk in Communities (**ARIC**). Prospective study of coronary heart heart disease incidence in relation to fasting total homocysteine, related genetic polymorphisms, and B vitamins. *Circulation* 1998;98:204–210 (editorial pp. 196–199).

     This prospective analysis focused on 15,792 ARIC participants 45–64 years of age (at enrollment); average follow-up period was 3.3 years. Total plasma homocysteine was associated with increased age- and race-adjusted CHD incidence in women ($p <$ 0.05) but not men. CHD was associated negatively with plasma pyridoxal 5-phosphate and, in women only, plasma folate and vitamin supplementation. After adjusting for other risk factors, only plasma pyridoxal 5-phosphate was associated with CHD incidence [RR of highest vs. lowest quintile 0.28 (95% CI 0.1–0.7)]. The C677T mutation of the methylenetetrahydrofolate reductase gene and three mutations of cystathionine B-synthase gene were not associated with CHD incidence.

155. **Bots ML**, et al. Homocysteine and short-term risk of myocardial infarction and stroke in the elderly. *Arch Intern Med* 1999;159:38–44.

     This nested case-control study of 104 MI patients, 120 stroke patients, and 533 controls was drawn from 7,983 Rotterdam Study participants. The age- and sex-adjusted risk of stroke and MI increased 6%–7% for every 1 μM increase in total homocysteine. Only those in the highest quintile of homocysteine levels ($>$18.6 μM) had a significantly increased risk; odds ratios were 2.43 and 2.53 for MI and stroke, respectively.

Hematologic and Inflammatory Markers

156. **Ernst E, Resch KL**. Fibrinogen as a cardiovascular risk factor: a meta-analysis and review of the literature. *Ann Intern Med* 1993;118:956–963.

     This analysis of six prospective epidemiologic studies included a total of 92,147 person years. All studies showed that fibrinogen was associated with an increased risk of subsequent MI and stroke [summary odds ratio 2.3 (95% CI 1.9–2.8)]. After multivariate analysis, this significant association persisted.

157. **Thompson SG**, et al. Hemostatic factors and the risk of MI or sudden death in patients with angina pectoris. *N Engl J Med* 1995;332:635–641.

     This study addressed 3,043 patients who underwent angiography; follow-up angiography was performed at 2 years. A high rate of sudden death or MI was associated with high fibrinogen (3.28 vs. 3.00 g/L; $p = 0.01$), von Willebrand Factor antigen (138 vs. 125%; $p = 0.05$), and tissue plasminogen activator antigen (11.9 vs. 10.0; $p = 0.02$).

158. **Folsom AR**, et al. Atherosclerosis Risk in Communities (**ARIC**). Prospective study of hemostatic factors and incidence of coronary heart disease. *Circulation* 1997;96:1102–1108.

     This study was composed of 14,477 patients who were initially 45–64 years of age and free of CAD. During follow-up (5.2 years), cardiac events occurred in 1.6%. Increased fibrinogen was associated with a higher likelihood of CHD: RR 1.48 (men), 1.21 (women). Top versus lowest quintile RRs were 3.66 (men) and 3.50 (women). Multivariate analysis showed that four factors were associated with total mortality: fibrinogen [RRs 1.30 (men) and 1.37 (women)]; Factor VIII (RRs 1.28 and 1.37); von Willebrand factor (RRs 1.13 and 1.27); and white blood cell count (RRs 1.15 and 1.29).

159. **Ridker PM**, et al. Inflammation, aspirin, and the risk of cardiovascular disease in apparently healthy men. *N Engl J Med* 1997; 336:973–979.

Case control study of 543 Physicians' Health Study participants who had an MI, stroke, or venous thrombosis, and 543 participants who did not have a vascular event at a long-term follow-up (>8 years). Baseline c-reactive protein (CRP) concentrations were significantly higher in men who subsequently had an MI (1.51 vs 1.13 mg/L, $p < 0.001$) or ischemic stroke (1.38 vs 1.13 mg/L, $p = 0.02$), but not venous thrombosis (1.26 vs 1.13 mg/L, $p = 0.34$) than among men without vascular events. Men in the highest quartile of CRP values had, as compared to those in lowest quartile, an approximately 3-fold and 2-fold higher risk of MI and stroke, respectively (relative risk 2.9, $p < 0.001$; relative risk 1.9, $p = 0.02$). The use of aspirin was associated with a substantial (55.7%) reduction ($p = 0.02$) in MI among men in the highest CRP quartile, but only a nonsignificant (13.9%) reduction among those in the lowest quartile.

160. **Ridker PM**, et al. Prospective study of C-reactive protein and the risk of future cardiovascular events among apparently healthy women. *Circulation* 1998;98:731–733.

This nested case-control study was composed of 122 Women's Health Study participants with first cardiovascular event (MI, stroke, coronary angioplasty, coronary bypass surgery, or cardiovascular death) and 244 age- and smoking-matched controls free of cardiovascular disease for 3 years. Elevated CRP levels were strongly associated with increased events ($p = 0.001$); highest levels were associated with an approximately fivefold increase in risk of vascular event (RR 4.8; 95% CI 2.3–10.1; $p = 0.0004$), and sevenfold increase in MI and stroke (RR 7.3; 95% CI 2.7–19.9; $p = 0.001$). Risk estimates were independent of other risk factors, and CRP was predictive in both low- and high-risk patients.

161. **Danesh J**, et al. Association of fibrinogen, C-reactive protein, albumin, or leukocyte count with coronary heart disease. *JAMA* 1998;279:1477–1482.

These meta-analyses of prospective studies were derived from 18 fibrinogen studies with 4,018 CHD cases; seven CRP studies with 1,053 CHD cases; eight albumin studies with 3,770 CHD cases; and seven leukocyte count studies with 5, 337 CHD cases. In all cases, patients with levels in the top third were compared with those with the lowest third levels. Patients in the top third of fibrinogen, CRP, and leukocyte levels had elevated CHD risks [risk ratios 1.8 (95% CI 1.6–2.0), 1.7 (95% CI 1.4–2.1), and 1.4 (95% CI 1.3–1.5)], whereas patients in the lowest third of albumin levels had higher CHD risks (risk ratio 1.5; 95% CI 1.3–1.7).

162. **Ridker PM**, et al. Inflammation, pravastatin and the risk of coronary events after MI in patients with average cholesterol levels. *Circulation* 1998;98:839–844.

This nested case control study was composed of 391 CARE patients with MI or cardiovascular death and 391 age- and sex-matched controls. Cases had higher CRP ($p = 0.05$) and serum amyloid A (0.006) levels; the highest quintiles had ~3/4 higher risk of recurrent events [RRs 1.77 ($p = 0.02$), 1.74 ($p = 0.02$)]. Greatest risk was seen in placebo patients with elevated CRP and serum amyloid A (RR 2.81; $p = 0.007$). Overall, the risk association between inflammation and risk was attenuated and nonsignificant in pravastatin patients [RR 1.29 ($p = 0.5$) vs. RR 2.11 ($p = 0.048$) in placebo patients].

163. **Thogersen AM**, et al. High plasminogen activator inhibitor and tPA levels in plasma precede a first acute MI in both men and women. *Circulation* 1998;98:2241–2247.

    In this prospective nested case-control study, 78 cases and 156 controls were matched for age, sex, and sampling time. MI patients had significantly higher tissue plasminogen activator and PAI-1 levels. For tissue plasminogen activator, the ratio of quartile 4 to 1 was 5.9. For tissue plasminogen activator only, the increase was independent of smoking, body mass index, hypertension, diabetes, and cholesterol. Increased von Willebrand factor levels were only associated with acute MI in a univariate analysis.

164. **Koenig W**, et al. C-reactive protein, a sensitive marker of inflammation, predicts future risk of coronary heart disease in initially healthy middle-aged men. *Circulation* 1999;99:237–242.

    This analysis focused on 936 men enrolled in MONICA (Monitoring Trends and Determinants in Cardiovascular Disease), a general population cohort study. At 8-year follow-up, the hazard rate ratio of CHD events associated with a one standard deviation increase in the CRP level was 1.67 (95% CI 1.29–2.17), and after adjustment for age and smoking, 1.50 (95% CI 1.14–1.97).

165. **Ma J**, et al. A prospective study of fibrinogen and risk of MI in the Physicians Health Study. *J Am Coll Cardiol* 1999;33:1347–1352.

    Analysis of blood samples from 199 men with MI and 199 age- and smoking-matched control subjects free of cardiovascular disease. Cases had significantly higher baseline fibrinogen levels (245 vs. 262 mg/dL; $p = 0.02$). Individuals with fibrinogen levels above the 90th percentile ($\geq$343 mg/dL) had an approximately twofold increase in MI risk [age- and smoking-adjusted RR 2.09 (95% CI 1.15–3.78)] compared with those with fibrinogen <343 mg/dL. When lipids and other coronary risk factors were controlled, the results were similar. Also, there was no interaction between fibrinogen levels and aspirin treatment.

Infection

166. **Saikku P**, et al. Chronic *Chlamydia* pneumonia infection as a risk factor for coronary heart disease in the Helsinki Heart Study. *Ann Intern Med* 1992;116:273–278.

    This study was composed of 4,071 patients, with 5 years of follow-up. Logistic regression analysis demonstrated that increased immunoglobulin A and the presence of immune complexes were associated with an increased incidence of CHD [odds ratio 2.7, 2.1, 2.9 (both)]. After risk factor adjustment, the odds ratios were 2.3, 1.8, and 2.6.

167. **Davidson M**, et al. Confirmed previous infection with *Chlamydia pneumoniae* (**TWAR**) and its presence in early coronary atherosclerosis. *Circulation* 1998;98:628–633.

This retrospective study was derived from serum specimens obtained at a mean of 8.8 years prior to death and autopsy tissue from 60 indigenous Alaskans at low CHD risk. *C. pneumoniae* was tested via immunocytochemistry (ICC) and polymerase chain reaction (PCR) (tissue) and micro-immunofluorescence (serum). TWAR was identified by either PCR or ICC in raised coronary atheroma in 25% and early flat lesions in 11%. Odds ratio for TWAR in raised atheroma after IgG level 1:256 >8 years earlier was 6.1 (95% CI 1.1–9.4) and for all coronary tissues after adjustment for confounders was 9.4 (95% CI 2.6–33.8).

168. **Ridker PM**, et al. Prospective study of herpes simplex virus, cytomegalovirus, and the risk of future MI and stroke. *Circulation* 1998;98:2796–2799.

This prospective, nested case-control study was composed of 643 Physicians Health Study participants who developed a first MI or thromboembolic stroke and 643 age-and smoking-matched controls. At 12-year follow-up, the RRs for future MI and stroke were 0.94 (95% CI 0.7–1.2) for herpes simplex virus seropositivity and 0.72 (95% CI 0.6–0.9) for cytomegalovirus seropositivity. The authors postulate that the inverse relationship of cytomegalovirus with MI and stroke may be due to chance because the direction of the association contradicts proposed biological mechanisms and previous cross-sectional and retrospective data.

169. **Meier CR**, et al. Antibiotics and risk of subsequent first-time acute MI. *JAMA* 1999;281:427–431 (editorial pp. 461–462).

This population-based case-control analysis focused on 3,315 case patients ≤75 years of age with a first MI between 1992 and 1997 and 13,139 controls matched for age, sex, general practice attended, and calendar time. The study excluded patients with major cardiovascular risk factors. Cases were significantly less likely to have used tetracycline antibiotics or quinolones in the preceding 3 years [odds ratio 0.70 (95% CI 0.55–0.90) and 0.45 (0.21–0.95)]. No effect was seen for prior use of penicillins, cephalosporins, sulfonamides, and macrolides.

170. **Ridker PM**, et al. Prospective study of *Chlamydia pneumoniae* IgG seropositivity and risks of future MI. *Circulation* 1999; 99:1161–1164.

This nested case control study was composed of 343 Physicians Health Study participants who subsequently had a first MI and an equal number of age- and smoking-matched controls. Immunoglobulin G antibodies directed against *C. pneumoniae* were measured in baseline blood samples. There was no increased risk of future MI with increasing immunoglobulin G titers (RRs 1.1, 1.0, 1.1, 1.0, and 0.8 for immunoglobulin G titers 1:16, 1:32, 1:64, 1:128, and 1:256).

171. Azithromycin in Coronary Artery Disease: Elimination of Myocardial Infection with *Chlamydia* (**ACADEMIC**). Randomized secondary prevention trial of azithromycin in patients with coronary artery disease and serological evidence for *Chlamydia pneumoniae* infection. *Circulation* 1999;99:1540–1547 (editorial pp. 1538–1539).

This prospective, randomized trial was composed of 302 patients with CAD and *C. pneumoniae* titers 1:16. Patients received azithromycin (500 mg/day for 3 days, then 500 mg/wk for 3 months) or placebo. There was no significant difference between the two groups in the incidence of the 3-month composite primary end point of four inflammatory markers (CRP, interleukin-1, interleukin-6, tumor necrosis factor). At 6 months, the azithromycin group did have a lower global rank sum score of these four markers ($p = 0.011$); specifically, change score ranks were significantly lower for CRP ($p = 0.011$) and interleukin-6 ($p = 0.043$). Antibody titers were unchanged, and there was no difference in the incidence of cardiovascular events at 6 months [9 (azithromycin) vs. 7 patients]. Of note, these results contradict earlier nonrandomized data.

Psychologic and Personality Characteristics and Stress

172. **Jiang W**, et al. Mental stress-induced myocardial ischemia and cardiac events. *JAMA* 1996;275:1651–1656.

    This cohort study was composed of 126 CAD patients with exercise-induced ischemia. Mental stress was induced by five mental stress tasks: mental arithmetic, public speaking, mirror trace, reading, and type A structured interview. At 5-year follow-up, baseline mental stress ischemia was found to be associated with 2.8 times higher risk of cardiac events (independent of age, ejection fraction, and prior MI).

173. **Barefoot JC**, et al. Depression and long-term mortality risk in patients with coronary artery disease. *Am J Cardiol* 1996;78:613–617.

    This analysis focused on 1,250 patients assessed with the Zung Self-Rating Depression Scale. At a median follow-up of 15.2 years, patients with moderate to severe depression had a 69% and 78% greater odds of cardiac death and overall mortality, respectively.

174. **Kubzansky LD**, et al. Is worrying bad for your heart? A prospective study of worry and coronary heart disease in the Normative Aging Study. *Circulation* 1997;95:818–824.

    This study was composed of 1,759 men who completed a questionnaire in 1975 on social conditions, health, finances, self-definition, and aging. At 20-year follow-up, multivariate analysis showed worry about social conditions was associated with a higher incidence of nonfatal MI [RR 2.4 (95% CI 1.4–4.1)] and total CHD [RR 1.48 (95% CI 0.99–2.2)].

175. **Gullette ECD**, et al. Effects of mental stress on myocardial ischemia during daily life. *JAMA* 1997;277:1521–1526 (editorial pp. 1558–1559).

    In this prospective, case-crossover study, 58 of 132 outpatients with CAD had ischemia on 48-hour Holter monitoring ($\geq$ mm ST depression for 1 minute). The risk of ischemia was increased in the hour after the following negative emotions: tension [adjusted RR 2.2 ($p < 0.05$)] and frustration [adjusted RR 2.2 ($p < 0.05$)]. This study raises several questions, including whether there is a different prognosis for triggered versus nontriggered ischemia and whether there is a benefit to prevention (and if so, which medications are best)?

176. **Rozanski A**, et al. Impact of psychological factors on the pathogenesis of cardiovascular disease and implications for therapy. *Circulation* 1999;99:2192–2217.

    This thorough review examines the effects on the incidence of cardiovascular disease of several psychologic factors, including depression, anxiety, personality and character traits, social isolation, and stress (acute and chronic). The known and/or potential pathophysiologic mechanisms are described, and there is a concluding section on therapeutic implications.

Genetics and Miscellaneous

177. **Marenberg ME**, et al. Genetic susceptibility to death from coronary heart disease in a study of twins. *N Engl J Med* 1994; 330:1041–1046.

   This analysis focused on 21,004 Swedish twins, with 26-year follow-up data. The RRs of death due to CHD if one twin died of CHD at <55 years of age were 8.1 (monozygous) and 3.8 (dizygous). For women, the RRs were 15.0 and 2.6. Overall, the RRs decreased with increasing age.

178. **Samani NJ**, et al. A meta-analysis of the association of the deletion allele of the ACE gene with MI. *Circulation* 1996;94:708–712.

   This analysis focused on 15 studies with 3,394 MI cases and 5,479 controls. The incidence of genotypes was as follows: II, 22.7%; ID, 49%; and DD, 28.3%. The risk of MI was higher in the DD group versus the ID and II groups combined (odds ratio 1.26; $p < 0.001$). Pairwise odds ratios were 1.36 for DD and II, 124 for DD and ID, and 1.09 for ID and II (p = NS).

179. **Ridker PM**, et al. PlA1/A2 polymorphism of platelet glycoprotein IIIa and risks of myocardial infarction, stroke, and venous thrombosis. *Lancet* 1997;349:385–388.

   This nested case-control study of Physicians Health Study participants showed no significant association between the Pl allele and cardiovascular disease. There were a total of 704 cases, consisting of 374 men with a first MI, 209 with strokes, and 121 with venous thrombosis, as well as 704 matched controls. Mean follow-up was 8.6 years. The frequency of Pl allele was similar between cases (MI, 13.5%; stroke, 13.4%; venous thrombosis, 14.5%) and controls (14.8%).

180. **Laule M**, et al. A1/A2 polymorphism of glycoprotein IIIa and association with excess procedural risk for coronary catheter interventions. *Lancet* 1999;353:708–712 (commentary pp. 687–688).

   This study was composed of 1,000 consecutive patients with CAD (by angiography) and 1,000 age- and sex-matched controls; 653 case patients underwent interventions (angioplasty, n = 271; stenting, n = 280; directional atherectomy, n = 102). There was no evidence that the A2 allele was associated with an excess procedural risk, as assessed by a 30-day composite of death plus MI plus target vessel revascularization (RR 1.36; p = 0.37). Also, there was no association between the allele and the presence of CAD (odds ratio 0.99). Although these results contrast with the positive results seen in the smaller studies (*see N Engl J Med* 1996; 334:1090, *Lancet* 1996;348:485, and *Circulation* 1997;96:1424), they confirm those obtained from the larger Physicians Health Study and the ECTIM group (*see Thromb Haemost* 1997;77: 1170–1181).

181. **Doggen CJM**, et al. Interaction of coagulation defects and cardiovascular risk factors. Increased risk of myocardial infarction associated with Factor V Leiden or prothrombin 20210A. *Circulation* 1998;97:1037–1041.

   This case-control study was composed of 560 men with a first MI at <70 years of age and 646 controls. The frequency of the 20210 AG genotype in the two groups was 1.8% and 1.2%, respectively. The presence of this AG genotype was associated with a nonsignificantly increased risk of MI (odds ratio 1.5; 95% CI 0.6–3.8). Among carriers of the Factor V Leiden mutation, there was a similar nonsignificant increase in the risk of MI (odds ratio 1.4; 95% CI 0.8–2.2). When other cardiovascular risk factors were present, the associated odds ratios were significantly higher: hypercholesteremia (odds ratio 2.4; 95% CI 0.2–26.7), obesity (2.8; 95% CI 1.0–8.1), hypertension (3.3; 95% CI 1.2–7.4), diabetes (5.9; 95% CI 0.7–50.0), smoking (6.1; 95% CI 3.0–12.5).

Antiplatelet Drugs for Primary and Secondary Prevention

Review Articles and Meta-Analyses

182. **Antiplatelet Trialists Collaboration**. Collaborative overview of randomised trials of antiplatelet therapy. I: Prevention of death, myocardial infarction, and stroke by prolonged antiplatelet therapy in various categories of patients. *BMJ* 1994; 308:81–106.

     This analysis focused on 145 randomized trials of antiplatelet agents versus control (~70,000 high-risk and ~30,000 low-risk patients) and 29 randomized trials comparing different agents (~10,000 high-risk patients). High-risk patients were considered those with known vascular disease or other condition associated with increased risk of occlusive vascular disease. Among all high-risk patients, antiplatelet therapy was associated with reductions of ~⅓ in nonfatal MI, ~⅓ in nonfatal stroke, and ~⅙ in vascular death (all $p < 0.00001$). Aspirin for secondary prevention was observed to confer a significant additional benefit seen when used between years 1 and 3, suggesting that indefinite treatment is most effective. The use of aspirin for primary prevention was only a trend toward decreased vascular events (5-year benefit of ~4 per 1,000 patients treated, $p = 0.09$).

183. **Sharis PJ**, et al. The antiplatelet effects of ticlopidine and clopidogrel. *Ann Intern Med* 1998;129:394–405.

     This review describes the mechanism of action, clinical applications, and side effect profiles of these two thienopyridines. Particular attention is focused on the use of ticlopidine in patients undergoing coronary stent implantation and the effects of clopidogrel in the large CAPRIE trial.

184. **Hennekens CH**. Update on aspirin in the treatment and prevention of cardiovascular disease. *Am Heart J* 1999;137:S9–S13.

     This review summarizes the substantial data showing the significant benefits of aspirin in secondary prevention, including an ~15% reduction in total cardiovascular deaths and ~25% reduction in major vascular events. The inconclusive data from the only two major primary prevention trials is also discussed.

Studies

Primary Prevention

185. **Peto R**, et al. Randomized trial of prophylactic daily aspirin in British male doctors. *BMJ* 1988;296:313–316.

     A total of 5,139 apparently healthy male physicians were randomized in a 2:1 fashion to aspirin 500 mg/day or no treatment. At follow-up (average 5.5 years), the aspirin group had a nonsignificant 10% mortality reduction, whereas the incidence of confirmed nonfatal MI was similar in both groups (~0.43%/yr).

186. Physicians Health Study. Steering Committee of the Physicians Health Study Research Group. Final report on aspirin component of the ongoing Physicians' Health Study. *N Engl J Med* 1989; 321:129–135.
     Design: Prospective, randomized, double-blind, placebo-controlled study. Average follow-up period was 5 years.
     Purpose: To determine whether low-dose aspirin decreases cardiovascular mortality.
     Population: 22,071 male physicians 40–84 years of age.
     Treatment: 325 mg every other day or placebo.
     Results: Aspirin group had a 44% reduction in the risk of MI (0.255%/yr vs. 0.44%/yr, $p < 0.00001$). This benefit was restricted to those >50 years of age. The aspirin group also had a nonsignificant reduction in cardiovascular mortality (RR 0.96), as well as a nonsignificant increase in stroke rate (RR 2.1; $p = 0.06$). Among 333 patients with chronic stable angina, the risk of MI was reduced an astonishing 87% (*see Ann Intern Med* 1991;114:875).
     Comments: This study was stopped early because of the highly significant reduction in nonfatal MIs. However, as a result, the evidence regarding stroke and total cardiovascular deaths is inconclusive because of the very low event rates.

187. **Manson JE**, et al. A prospective study of aspirin use and primary prevention of cardiovascular disease in women. *JAMA* 1991; 266:521–527.
     This analysis of data on ~87,000 Nurses Health Study participants showed that consumption of one to six tablets of aspirin per week was associated with a 32% lower incidence of first MI ($p = 0.005$). This benefit was restricted to those >50 years of age and most substantial in smokers and those with hypertension and hypercholesterolemia.

188. **Juul-Moller S**, et al. Swedish Angina Pectoris Aspirin Trial (**SAPAT**). Double-blind trial of aspirin in primary prevention of MI in patients with stable chronic angina pectoris. *Lancet* 1992;340:1421–1425.
     Design: Prospective, randomized, double-blind, placebo-controlled study. Average follow-up period was 50 months.
     Purpose: To compare aspirin and placebo in patients with a history of chronic stable angina.
     Population: 2,035 chronic stable angina patients 30–80 years of age.
     Exclusion Criteria: Prior MI, NSAID use, and requirement for anticoagulation.
     Treatment: Aspirin 75 mg/day or placebo; all patients received sotalol (40–480 mg/day) for symptoms.
     Results: Aspirin group had 34% reduction in MI and sudden death (8.0% vs. 11.8%; $p = 0.003$). There was a nonsignificant excess of major bleeds in the aspirin group (20 vs. 13 patients).

Secondary Prevention

189. **Klimt CR**, et al. Persantine-Aspirin Reinfarction Study (**PARIS II**). PARIS II: secondary coronary prevention with persantine and aspirin. *J Am Coll Cardiol* 1986;7:251–269.
     Design: Prospective, randomized, placebo-controlled study. Average follow-up period was 23 months.

Purpose: To evaluate the effectiveness of the combination of aspirin and persantine on mortality in patients with a recent MI.
Population: 3,128 patients with an MI 4 weeks to 4 months earlier.
Treatment: Persantine 75 mg/day and aspirin 300 mg/day, or placebo.
Results: Aspirin and persantine group had 30% lower 1-year mortality (24% at end of study).

190. **Krumholz HM**, et al. Aspirin for secondary prevention after acute MI in the elderly: prescribed use and outcomes. *Ann Intern Med* 1996;124: 292–298 (editorial pp. 335–338).

This observational study was composed of 5,490 consecutive patients without contraindications to aspirin. Only 76% were given aspirin at hospital discharge. Aspirin use was associated with a 23% lower 6-month mortality rate. Risk factors for nonprescription were poor ejection fraction, diabetes, long stay, low albumin, and discharge to other than home.

191. **Gent M**, et al. Clopidogrel versus Aspirin in Patients at Risk of Ischaemic Events (**CAPRIE**). A randomised, blinded, trial of clopidogrel versus aspirin in patients at risk of ischaemic events (CAPRIE). *Lancet* 1996;348;1329–1339.

Design: Prospective, randomized, multicenter study. Primary end point was ischemic stroke, MI, and vascular death. Mean follow-up period was 1.9 years.
Purpose: To compare the effectiveness of clopidogrel to aspirin in preventing major vascular events.
Population: 19,185 patients with a history of recent ischemic stroke (1 week to 6 months earlier), MI ($\leq$35 days earlier), or symptomatic peripheral arterial disease.
Treatment: Clopidogrel 75 mg once daily or aspirin 325 mg/day.
Exclusion Criteria: Carotid endarterectomy or severe deficit after stroke, uncontrolled hypertension, and scheduled major surgery.
Results: Clopidogrel group had a 8.7% reduction in the primary composite end point (5.32 vs. 5.83%/yr; $p = 0.043$). The peripheral arterial disease subgroup had a significant 23.8% reduction in the primary end point ($p = 0.003$), whereas the stroke patients had a nonsignificant 7.3% reduction ($p = 0.26$) and MI patients had a nonsignificant 3.7% increase (7.4% reduction if any prior MI). A subsequent analysis of all 8,446 patients with any history of MI showed that clopidogrel was associated with a statistically insignificant 7.4% decrease in the combined end point. There was no difference in incidence of side effects, including neutropenia (clopidogrel, 0.1%; aspirin, 0.17%).
Comments: Further studies are needed to evaluate the effectiveness of clopidogrel in combination with aspirin and in the acute MI setting.

Invasive Procedures and Revascularization

CORONARY ANGIOGRAPHY

Indications

1. Unstable angina (*see* Chapter 3).
2. Recurrent angina after percutaneous coronary intervention (PCI) or after coronary artery bypass graft (CABG) surgery.
3. Incapacitating angina pectoris despite medical therapy.
4. Complicated myocardial infarction (MI) (e.g. recurrent ischemia, heart failure or hypotension, ventricular septal defect, mitral regurgitation, ventricular tachycardia at >48 hours, history of MI, failed thrombolysis).
5. Preoperative assessment (valve repair/replacement, other high-risk surgery).
6. Positive exercise treadmill test result.
7. Miscellaneous: aortic dissection, unexplained ventricular failure, suspected congenital heart disease, postcardiac transplantation, and pericardial tamponade or constriction.

Controversial indications:

1. After non–Q-wave MI. The Veteran Affairs Non–Q-wave Infarction Strategies in Hospital (VANQWISH) study and Organization to Assess Strategies for Ischemic Syndromes (OASIS) registry analysis both showed no significant difference between conservative (catheterization only if refractory/recurrent ischemia) and invasive therapy, but Fragmin during Instability in CAD (FRISC) II results showed benefit in the invasive group.

Flow Grade (see page 86)

The Thrombolysis in myocardial infarction (TIMI) flow grade system is typically used to assess flow:

Grade 0: no anterograde flow beyond the point of occlusion.
Grade 1: contrast goes beyond occlusion but fails to opacify the entire distal bed.
Grade 2: entire vessel opacified, but the rate of entry to and clearance from the distal bed of the contrast is slower than normal.
Grade 3: normal flow.

The TIMI corrected frame count is a more precise method and allows for quantitative assessment of flow as a continuous variable (2).

Stenosis Morphology (see page 87)

The American College of Cardiology (ACC) /American Heart Association (AHA) Classification (4) is enumerated as follows:

Type A: discrete, concentric, readily accessible, nonangulated segment, smooth contour, little or no calcification, nonostial, no major side branch involved, no thrombus present.

Type B: tubular, eccentric, moderate tortuosity, moderately angulated segment (45–90 degrees), irregular contour, moderate to heavy calcification, total occlusion for ≤3 months, ostial location, bifurcation lesion, thrombus present.

Type B1: one B characteristic.

Type B2: two B characteristics.

Type C: diffuse, excessive tortuosity, extremely angulated segment (>90 degrees), total occlusion for >3 months, inability to protect major side branch, degenerated vein graft lesion.

PERCUTANEOUS TRANSLUMINAL CORONARY ANGIOPLASTY

Procedural Details

Medications (see pages 100–120)

1. Aspirin 325 mg before and continued daily thereafter (112).
2. Heparin initial bolus 100U/kg. The target activated clotting time (ACT) is 250 to 300 seconds using a Hemotec device and 300 to 350 seconds using a Hemochrom device [low periprocedural ACT is associated with increased complications (101)]. Unless PCI is complicated (e.g., residual thrombus), prolonged heparin infusion is not necessary because it is does not decrease ischemic complications and results in more frequent bleeding (44,46) (see also *JACC* 1999;34:461). The use of low-molecular-weight heparins in this setting requires further evaluation; one small study showed no differences between enoxaparin and unfractionated heparin in ischemic complications, procedural success, and bleeding (48).
3. Glycoprotein IIb/IIIa inhibitor. If used, lower heparin dosage indicated (initial bolus 700/µg) with a target ACT of ~250 seconds. Use of standard ACT target in early trials resulted in increased bleeding.

Access (see page 91)

The right femoral artery is the most common arterial access site. If the patient has severe aortic or femoral vascular disease, radial or brachial artery access is often feasible (*see Am Heart J* 1995;129:1). A 6- to 8-French (F) catheter is used. [In one study, use of smaller 6F catheters showed less bleeding and similar procedural success compared to 7F and 8F catheters (19).] Use of femoral closure devices has resulted in less postsheath removal bleeding.

Contrast Agent (see pages 91, 92)

Some studies have shown low osmolar ionic contrast agents to result in fewer recurrent ischemic events than nonionic agents (18,22). However, a more recent study, in which more than 80% of patients underwent stent implantation, found no significant advantages with low ionic contrast use (20).

Balloon Inflation (see pages 90, 91)

Typically performed at 5 to 8 atmospheres, prolonged inflation (e.g., 5 minutes) has been shown in randomized studies to result in better procedural success but has no impact on major event rates or restenosis (15,17).

Efficacy (see pages 87–90)

Success rates of approximately 90% to 95% have been achieved in most institutions [vs. 64% success rate in first major report (15)]. Failures occur when the lesion cannot be crossed, inadequate balloon dilatation is achieved, and abrupt closure occurs.

Predictors of failure are listed as follows:

1. Chronic occlusion.
2. Stenoses that are long, angulated, eccentric, at an ostium or branch point, calcified, and/or associated with intraluminal thrombus (16).
3. Hospital with low volume (6,7).
4. Low operator volume (8,9).
5. Vein grafts (especially if >3 years old).
6. Female gender.
7. Advanced age.

Applications

Stable Angina (see pages 88, 89)

PTCA vs Medical Therapy

The Angioplasty Compared to Medicine (ACME) study (10) compared percutaneous transluminal coronary angioplasty (PTCA) with medical therapy in one-vessel disease. The PTCA group had increased exercise time and less use of antianginal medications but had a higher frequency of MI (4%) and emergent coronary artery bypass surgery (2%).

The Veterans Administration Angioplasty Compared to Medicine (VA ACME) study (11) also showed that PTCA in patients with one-vessel coronary artery disease (CAD) resulted in improved exercise time, less angina, and better quality of life score.

The Randomized Intervention Treatment of Angina (RITA-2) trial (12) showed that angioplasty was associated with less angina and longer treadmill time but with an increased incidence of death or MI due to procedure-related MI events.

PTCA vs CABG

See CABG section (p. 85).

Unstable Angina

Angioplasty was associated with a lower success rate (85%–90%) when used in patients with unstable angina, and abrupt closure and restenosis were more common (*see* Chapter 3).

Acute MI

In experienced centers with short door-to-balloon times, primary PTCA has been associated with lower mortality than thrombolytic therapy (*see* Chapter 4). However, the availability and institutional volume and experience are limiting factors.

After Thrombolytic Therapy

Studies performed in the 1980s found that routine immediate PTCA was harmful (TAMI I, TIMI IIA, and ECSG trials; *see* Chapter 4), whereas delayed PTCA (at 18–48 hours) was associated with similar outcomes (SWIFT and TIMI IIB; *see* Chapter 4).

PTCA is indicated in patients with high-risk features, such as cardiogenic shock, persistent pain or ischemia, and ventricular tachycardia or fibrillation. Of note, recent data suggest that it can be performed routinely and safely after reduced-dose thrombolysis (PACT and TIMI 14; *see* Chapter 4).

Complications (see pages 106–119)

1. Death (<0.1%).
2. MI (<5%). Retrospective analyses suggest that even small non–Q-wave MIs [often occurring in the absence of symptoms or electrocardiographic (ECG) changes and detected by routine creatine kinase (CK) and CK-MB measurement] result in increased incidence of ischemic complications and subsequent recurrent MI, revascularization, and death (90–92). One analysis showed that the relative risk (RR) of cardiac mortality increased by 1.05 per 100 U/L increase in CK levels (93).
3. Urgent coronary artery bypass surgery (<0.5%).
4. Severe dissection and abrupt closure (<1%). Closure results from extensive dissection, thrombosis, or vasospasm. It is more likely to occur if ACT is low (101). Aspirin has been proven to decrease its incidence, whereas abciximab use has resulted in a lower incidence of urgent revascularization (64–70). Treatment options include (a) conservative medical therapy (reasonable if collateralization is adequate or amount of jeopardized myocardium is small); (b) stent placement [restores flow in >90% of patients, but infarcts occur in up to 20% and reocclusion (over days to weeks) occurs in about 10%]; (c) repeat PTCA (50% success rate; perfusion catheter often is used, which allows balloon inflation for 10–30 minutes); or (d) emergent CABG (25%–50% still suffer a Q-wave MI).
5. Other acute complications. Pseudoaneurysm, in one study, required surgical repair in 7% of cases (102). Stroke is encountered in less than 0.1% of such surgeries, ischemic stroke being more common than hemorrhagic stroke. Another major risk factor is severe peripheral vascular disease.
6. Restenosis (104,105) usually occurs at 3 to 6 months, with an incidence of approximately 30% (50%–60% for chronic occlusion). Risk factors include may be categorized as clinical (diabetes, unstable angina, smoking, male, hypertension, end-stage renal disease, high cholesterol; anatomic [angiographically visible thrombus (97), proximal location, saphenous vein graft, left anterior descending (LAD) artery, chronic occlusion, stenosis > 5–10 mm long], or procedural (residual stenosis >30%).

Pharmacologic Prevention of Restenosis (see pages 119–125)

1. Probucol, an antioxidant agent, has shown promise in the Multivitamins and Probucol (MVP) trial and two smaller trials (107–109). Of note, MVP patients were elective PTCA patients who were pretreated with probucol for 1 month. Probucol appears to achieve its benefits via a primary effect on remodeling (*see Circulation* 1999;99:30).
2. Tranilast and pemirolast are antiallergic drugs that also inhibit the migration and proliferation of vascular smooth muscle cells. In small nonrandomized studies, patients who

received these oral agents for 3 to 4 months had substantially lower restenosis rates (110,111).

3. Cilostazol, a new antiplatelet agent that selectively blocks phosphodiesterase type III, was found to reduce restenosis and target lesion revascularization rates by >50% in one recent study of 211 patients (see *Circulation* 1999;100:21).

4. Numerous other therapies have shown no benefit in randomized trials, including aspirin (112), low-molecular-weight heparins (114,121,122,125), subcutaneous unfractionated heparin (119), hirudin (118), 3-hydroxy 3-methylglutaryl coenzyme A (HMG-CoA) reductase inhibitors (115,124), angiotensin-converting enzyme (ACE) inhibitors (117), calcium-channel blockers (126), n-3 fatty acids (127), platelet-derived growth factor antagonists (116), thromboxane antagonists (113,120), and nitric oxide donors (123).

Interventional Treatment of Restenosis (see pages 128, 129)

Second PTCA is performed only if recurrent symptoms emerge. It has a high initial success rate because restenosis is typically characterized by fibroproliferative tissue versus atherosclerotic plaque. However, recurrent restenosis still occurs in 25% to 35%.

Radiation has yielded promising results in initial studies, with restenosis rates typically less than 20%. Gamma radiation sources were used in the Scripps Coronary Radiation to Inhibit Proliferation Post-Stenting (SCRIPPS) trial, Washington Radiation for In-Stent Restenosis Trial (WRIST), and GAMMA-1 trial (135,137,139), whereas beta sources were used in the Beta Energy Restenosis Trial (BERT) and BETA-WRIST (136,138). No study has compared the two types of radiation.

STENTING

Advantages versus PTCA

1. Larger mean luminal diameter achieved.
2. Good angiographic outcome.
3. Lower restenosis rates (15%–30%) and fewer repeat interventions.

Disadvantages

1. Higher cost.
2. Difficulty treating restenosis when it occurs.
3. Thrombosis (incidence <1% with antiplatelet regimens but associated with high mortality).
4. Requirement for antiplatelet therapy (though typically for only 2–4 weeks).
5. Limitations to ≥2.5 mm diameter vessels.

Uses and Indications (see pages 112, 113)

1. Stable angina/CAD. See sections below on stenting versus PTCA and adjunctive glycoprotein IIb/IIIa inhibition.
2. Unstable angina (*see* Chapter 3 and section on glycoprotein IIb/IIIa.
3. Acute MI (*see* Chapter 4).
4. Stenoses in vessels larger than 3 mm [newer stents being tested for use in smaller (2.5 mm) lesions].
5. Abrupt closure after PTCA.

6. High-risk lesions (e.g., left main disease in patients unable to have CABG).
7. Saphenous vein grafts. Lower restenosis rates have been reported in two retrospective analyses (17% vs. ~50% with PTCA) (80,81), whereas the randomized Saphenous Vein *de novo* (SAVED) trial found a nonsignificant reduction in restenosis (37% vs. 46%) (82).
8. Chronic total occlusions. Restenosis rates were also better than with PTCA—32% vs. 74%, 32% vs. 68%, and 56% vs. 70% in the Stenting in Chronic Coronic Occlusion (SICCO), Gruppo Italiano di Studio sullo Stent nelle Occlusioni Coronariche (GISSOC), and TOSCA trials, respectively (76–78).

Stenting versus PTCA

Initial studies found stenting resulted in less restenosis but did not reduce the incidence of major cardiac events or death; recent studies have shown more favorable outcomes with stenting.

Major Trials (see pages 92–110)
1. In the Stent Restenosis Study (STRESS) (24), composed of 410 patients, stenting was associated with higher procedural success, less restenosis at 6 months (31% vs 46%, $p = 0.046$), and a trend toward less revascularization ($p = 0.06$), but there was no significant reduction in clinical events.
2. In the Benestent I study (27), composed of 520 patients, the stent group had lower revascularization but no difference in major clinical events.
3. In the Benestent II study (28), composed of 827 patients, the heparin-coated stent group had a nearly 50% lower restenosis rate vs PTCA (16% vs. 31%).
4. In the more recent EPISTENT study (69, 70), composed of 2,399 patients, the rates of target vessel revascularation (TVR) at 6 months for stent and stent plus abciximab were significantly lower than for PTCA and abciximab (10.6% and 8.7% vs 15.4%; $p = 0.005$, $p < 0.001$).

Primary Stenting versus PTCA with Provisional Stenting (see page 95)
1. In the Optimal Coronary Balloon Angioplasty with Provisional Stenting versus Primary Stent (OCBAS) study (31), composed of 116 patients, similar angiographic restenosis and TVR rates were observed.
2. In the Optimal PTCA and Provisional Stent versus Primary Stent (OPUS) trial (32), composed of 479 elective PCI patients randomized to PTCA with provisional stenting or primary stenting, the latter group had a significant reduction in the primary composite end point (death, MI, and TVR). Primary stenting also had higher initial costs but lower overall costs by 6 months due to a significantly lower reintervention rate.

Drug Regimen (see pages 101–120)
1. Aspirin 325 mg/day indefinitely (112).
2. Ticlopidine (250 mg twice daily for 2–4 weeks) is more effective than the anticoagulant regimen (e.g., intravenous heparin followed by warfarin). In three randomized studies—Intra-

coronary Stenting and Antithrombotic Regimen (ISAR), Full Anticoagulation versus Aspirin and Ticlopidine (FANTASTIC), and Stent Anticoagulation Restenosis Study (STARS) (49,50,53)—50% to 80% fewer cardiac end points were reached (Fig. 2–1). Aspirin and ticlopidine were also superior in high-risk patients. An approximately 50% reduction in major events was observed in the Multicenter Aspirin and Ticlopidine Trial after Intracoronary Stenting (MATTIS) (52). An aspirin-only regimen has not been shown consistently to be adequate in low-risk groups (55,57,59).

Ticlopidine 250 mg twice daily for 10 to 14 days (vs. 28 days) appears adequate (58). Most stent thrombosis occurs early, and the shorter course limits neutropenia risk. Pretreatment is likely beneficial. In one study, fewer non–Q-wave MIs occurred with 3 days of pretreatment versus less than 1 day of treatment (5% vs. 29%) (60).

3. Clopidogrel has been used as an alternative to ticlopidine (54, 62, 63). Results of the Clopidogrel Aspirin Stent International Cooperative Study (CLASSICS) showed clopidogrel (75 mg once daily for 4 weeks ± 300–375 mg loading dose) to be as effective as ticlopidine in preventing stent thrombosis and clinical events, but it is much better tolerated (54) (Fig. 2-1). More importantly, as shown in the large Clopidogrel versus Aspirin in Patients at Risk of Ischaemic Events (CAPRIE) trial (*see* Chapter 1, ref. 19), the risk of neutropenia with clopidogrel is very low (~0.1%). (Preliminary results of a recent study have shown 60% platelet inhibition [measured using 5 μmol adenosine diphosphate (ADP)] is achieved within approximately 4 hours versus 4 to 5 days with regular dosing and 6 to 7 days with ticlopidine 250 mg twice daily (66).

Complications (see pages 117–129)

Subacute stent thrombosis occurs in 1% to 2% of procedures [used to be >5% before high-pressure balloon inflation and anti-platelet regimens were introduced (95,97)], and typically results in MI or death. One study showed a 90% incidence of MI and 17% mortality rate (96).

Most cases of restenosis occur within the first 6 months, with an incidence of approximately 20% to 25% [higher rates in smaller vessels and diabetics (125)]. Promising results are being achieved with radiation. In the GAMMA-1 randomized trial, a 58% lower restenosis rate was seen in the radiation group (139).

ATHERECTOMY (see pages 96–99)

The Coronary Angioplasty versus Excisional Atherectomy Trial (CAVEAT) I and CAVEAT II (33,35) both showed that directional coronary atherectomy (DCA) achieved better initial success rates compared with balloon angioplasty within native vessel and saphenous vein graft lesions, respectively. However, the atherectomy groups did not have significantly lower higher restenosis rates, and the incidence of death and MI was higher. In the Canadian Coronary Atherectomy Trial (CCAT) (34), the atherectomy group did not have increased complications, but again the restenosis rate was similar. Two studies that employed a more

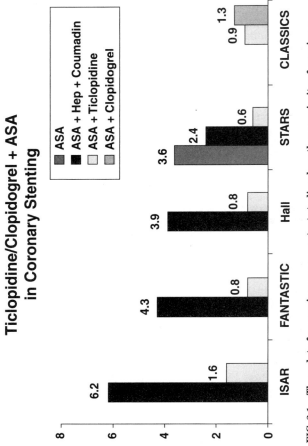

FIG. 2-1. These data from major coronary stent studies show the superiority of a regimen consisting of aspirin and/or ticlopidine or clopidogrel.

refined/optimal atherectomy technique—the Optimal Atherectomy Restenosis Study (OARS) and Balloon versus Optimal Atherectomy Trial (BOAT) (36,37)—showed lower restenosis rates with atherectomy and similar major complication rates. In the BOAT, directional atherectomy was performed with adjunctive PTCA if indicated. None of the trials mentioned above compared atherectomy to stenting. The Atherectomy before Multilink Improves Lumen Gain and Clinical Outcomes (AMIGO) trial will randomize 750 patients, including those with ostial and bifurcation stenoses and chronic total occlusions, to atherectomy and stenting versus stenting alone.

Rotational atherectomy was evaluated in the Excimer Laser, Rotational Atherectomy, and Balloon Angioplasty Comparison (ERBAC) trial (42) in patients with type B or C lesions, and the atherectomy group was found to have a better procedural success rate than the balloon angioplasty (PTCA) or excimer laser groups, but the 6-month restenosis rate was higher compared with that observed with PTCA (57% vs. 47%; $p < 0.05$). Since this trial was completed, there have been substantial technical improvements, so the multicenter Study to Determine Rotablator and Transluminal Angioplasty Strategy (STRATAS) (38) was undertaken. Patients were randomized to aggressive rotablator therapy (70%–90% burr-to-artery ratio) or standard rotablator (50%–70% burr-to-artery ratio), and at 6 months, there were no significant differences between the two groups in mean luminal diameter, restenosis, or clinical events.

EXCIMER LASER (see pages 98, 99)

The Amsterdam-Rotterdam (AMRO) trial (41) found that excimer laser compared with PTCA in patients with long lesions (>10 mm in length) achieved similar restenosis and clinical event rates. In the ERBAC trial (42), laser therapy was compared with rotational atherectomy and PTCA in patients with type B or C lesions, and PTCA was found to have a lower restenosis rate and less TVR than laser. Finally, the Laser Angioplasty versus Angioplasty (LAVA) trial (43) showed that laser-facilitated PTCA was associated with more complications and a major event rate similar to that found with PTCA alone. Based on these less than encouraging results, the use of laser treatment has remain limited. It is unclear if the use of laser therapy by very experienced operators in patients with complex lesions and chronic occlusions (see *JACC* 1999;34:25) can achieve better results.

PCI WITH ADJUNCTIVE GLYCOPROTEIN IIb/IIIa INHIBITION

Over the past several years, there has been increasing use of glycoprotein IIb/IIIa inhibitors in patients with acute coronary syndromes and those undergoing percutaneous transluminal intervention (i.e., PCI) (Fig. 2-2). Below is a review of the various agents that have been evaluated in PCI.

Abciximab (see pages 106–109)

This monoclonal antibody fragment binds tightly to the glycoprotein IIb/IIIa receptor and has shown the most impressive results in patients undergoing PCI.

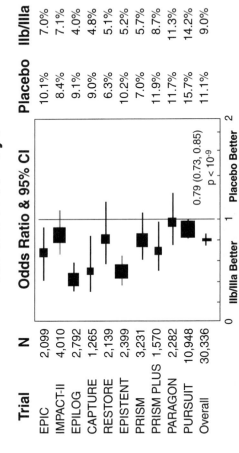

IIb/IIIa Inhibitors in PCI and ACS

Death/MI at 30 Days

Trial	N	Odds Ratio & 95% CI	Placebo	IIb/IIIa
EPIC	2,099		10.1%	7.0%
IMPACT-II	4,010		8.4%	7.1%
EPILOG	2,792		9.1%	4.0%
CAPTURE	1,265		9.0%	4.8%
RESTORE	2,139		6.3%	5.1%
EPISTENT	2,399		10.2%	5.2%
PRISM	3,231		7.0%	5.7%
PRISM PLUS	1,570		11.9%	8.7%
PARAGON	2,282		11.7%	11.3%
PURSUIT	10,948		15.7%	14.2%
Overall	30,336		11.1%	9.0%

0.79 (0.73, 0.85)
$p < 10^{-9}$

0   1   2

IIb/IIIa Better   Placebo Better

FIG. 2-2.   Glycoprotein IIb/IIIa inhibitors in PCI and acute coronary syndromes. (Adapted from Topal EJ, et al. *Lancet* 1999, with permission.)

In the Evaluation of 7E3 for the Prevention of Ischemic Complications (EPIC) trial (64), composed of 2,099 high-risk patients (acute MI, postinfarct angina with ECG changes, high-risk clinical or angiographic features), the group receiving abciximab 0.25 mg/kg intravenous bolus then 10 µg/min infusion for 12 hours had 35% fewer end points compared with the placebo group. At 3-year follow-up, this benefit was still present, and among the MI and unstable angina patients, there was an impressive 60% decrease in the all-cause mortality rate.

In the c7E3 Fab Antiplatelet Therapy in Unstable Refractory Refractory Angina (CAPTURE) trial (66), composed of 1,265 unstable angina patients, the abciximab group had a significant 29% reduction in primary composite end point at 30 days but not at 6 months. This loss of benefit is attributed to abciximab infusion being stopped 1 hour following PCI.

In the Evaluation in PTCA to Improve Long-term Outcome with Abciximab Glycoprotein IIb/IIIa Blockade (EPILOG) trial (67), composed of 2,792 nonacute coronary syndrome patients, abciximab showed a greater than 50% reduction in primary composite end point at 30 days, and the reduction remained significant at 6 months and 1 year.

In the Evaluation of Platelet IIb/IIIa Inhibitor for Stenting (EPISTENT) trial (69), composed of 2,399 CAD patients randomized to stent plus placebo, stent plus abciximab, or balloon angioplasty plus abciximab, the two abciximab groups had a significantly lower incidence of death, MI, and urgent revascularization at 30 days (5.3% and 6.9% vs. 10.8%). One year mortality was also lower (Fig. 2–3).

Eptifibatide (see page 107)

In the Integrelin to Minimise Platelet Aggregation and Coronary Thrombosis (IMPACT II) trial (65), composed of 4,010 patients randomized to eptifibatide 135 µg/kg bolus 10 to 60 minutes preprocedure then 0.50 to 0. 75 µg/kg/min for 20 to 24 hours or placebo, eptifibatide was associated with a nonsignificant 9.2% reduction in primary composite end point at 30 days and a significant 22% reduction in on-treatment analysis.

In the Platelet Glycoprotein IIb/IIIa in Unstable Angina Receptor Suppression Using Integrelin Therapy (PURSUIT) trial (*see* Chapter 3), a reduction in death or MI at 30 days of 31% was observed in patients undergoing PCI.

Tirofiban (see page 109)

Tirofiban is currently approved by the U.S. Food and Drug Administration for use in acute coronary syndromes with or without PCI, but not in elective PCI.

In the Randomized Efficacy Study of Tirofiban for Outcomes and Restenosis (RESTORE) (68), composed of 2,139 patients randomized to tirofiban 10 µg/kg bolus over 3 minutes then 0.15 µg/kg/min for 36 hours or placebo, the tirofiban group had significantly fewer events at 2 days and 7 days but not at 30 days.

In the Platelet Receptor Inhibition in Ischemic Syndrome Management in Patients Limited by Unstable Signs and Symptoms (PRISM-PLUS) trial (*see* Chapter 3), PCI patients showed a reduction in death or MI of approximately 35%.

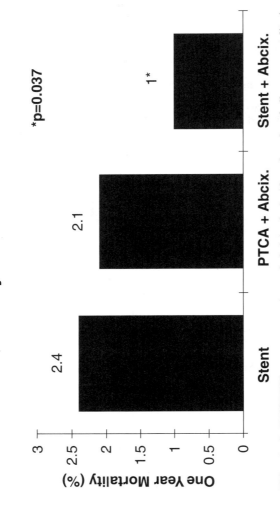

FIG. 2-3. In EPISTENT coronary stenting and abciximab significantly reduced all-cause mortality in comparison with stenting alone and PTCA plus abciximab. (Presented by Topal EJ at the 71st AHA Scientific Session in Dallas, November 1998.)

Xemilofiban (see page 110)

Used as an oral agent in the large Evaluation of Oral Xemilofiban in Controlling Thrombotic Events (EXCITE) trial (70), the xemilofiban 20 mg group had fewer events at 2 days, but there was no significant reduction in the 6-month primary composite end point.

CORONARY ARTERY BYPASS SURGERY

Risk factors for operative mortality include advanced age, female gender, smoking, and left ventricular dysfunction (*see J Thorac Cardiovasc Surg* 1994;108:73).

Saphenous Vein Grafts

Eight percent to 12% of saphenous vein grafts occlude in the early postoperative period (most due to technical factors), and 12% to 20% more occlude in first year (typically due to intimal proliferation and thrombosis), then 2% to 4% per year (overall 50% at 10 years). Results of the Post-CABG trial (*see* Chapter 1) showed a 30% to 40% slowing of graft atherosclerosis with very aggressive low-density lipoprotein (LDL)-lowering therapy (average achieved LDL 90 mg/dL).

Internal Mammary Artery (see pages 130, 136)

The patency rate for the internal mammary artery (IMA) is 85% to 95% at 10 years. Use is associated with improved long-term survival. A 27% lower mortality rate was observed in the Coronary Artery Surgery Study (CASS) registry analysis (145). In another analysis, IMA use was associated with a 40% lower 10-year mortality rate among three-vessel disease patients (160).

Coronary Artery Bypass Surgery versus Medical Therapy (see pages 131, 132)

Three major clinical trials—the European Coronary Surgery Study (ECSS), CASS, and Veterans Administration (VA) study—helped to define the groups of patients that benefit from bypass surgery (Table 2-1). Of note, these three studies were performed before the common use of the IMA for revascularization. The ECSS enrolled 768 men less than or equal to 65 years of age and found that surgery resulted in improved survival compared with medical therapy. The majority of the benefit was seen in patients with proximal LAD artery stenoses (146). The CASS enrolled 780 patients less than or equal to 65 years of age and found CABG to be associated with a trend toward lower mortality in patients with three-vessel disease and an ejection fraction of less than or equal to 50% (147). Long-term follow-up showed better survival with CABG in patients with left main equivalent disease (severe proximal LAD and left circumflex disease) and left ventricular dysfunction (*see Circulation* 1995;91:2335). The VA study found no significant mortality between groups at 11-year follow-up, but CABG was beneficial in certain patients subgroups: (a) three-vessel disease and left ventricular dysfunction and (b) clinically high-risk patients (at least two of following: resting ST depression, history of MI, or history of hypertension) (148).

Table 2-1. Major Trials Comparing CABG with Medical Therapy

Trial	No. of Patients Randomized		5-Year Mortality			7-Year Mortality			10-Year Mortality		
	CABG	Medical Treatment	CABG	Medical Treatment	Odds Ratio	CABG	Medical Treatment	Odds Ratio	CABG	Medical Treatment	Odds Ratio
VA	332	354	58	79	0.74	76	106	0.69	118	141	0.83
European	394	373	30	63	0.40	51	76	0.58	91	109	0.72
CASS	390	390	20	32	0.60	43	53	0.79	72	83	0.84
Texas	56	60	10	13	0.79	15	18	0.85	23	25	0.97
Oregon	51	49	4	8	0.44	7	11	0.55	14	14	0.94
New Zealand	51	49	5	7	0.65	7	13	0.43	15	16	0.94
New Zealand	50	50	8	8	1.00	10	11	0.90	17	16	1.15
Total	1,324	1,325	135 (10.2%)	210 (15.8%)	0.61 $p < 0.0001$	209 (15.8%)	288 (21.7%)	0.68 $p < 0.001$	350 (26.4%)	404 (30.5%)	0.83 $p = 0.03$

Data from these three major trials and 4 smaller studies show CABG is associated with significantly lower mortality than medical therapy. This benefit was most marked in patients with 3-vessel disease and left main disease. (Adapted from Yusuf S, et al., with permission (142).)

An overview of 2,649 patients from the above three trials and four smaller studies showed that CABG-compared initial medical management was associated with a significantly lower mortality rate at 5 years (odds ratio 0.61), 7 years (odds ratio 0.68), and 10 years (odds ratio 0.83) (142) (Table 2–1). The risk reduction was most marked in patients with left main disease and three-vessel disease (odds ratios 0.32 and 0.58). High-risk patients (defined as those with two of following: severe angina, history of hypertension, prior MI, and ST segment depression at rest) had a 29% mortality reduction with CABG at 10 years compared with a non-significant trend toward higher mortality in low-risk patients [none of first three risk factors (ST depression allowed)]. Overall, these results demonstrate that patients with more severe coronary disease, poor left ventricular dysfunction, and high-risk clinical characteristics derive a significant benefit from bypass surgery.

Coronary Artery Bypass Surgery versus PTCA (see pages 130–135)

The RITA, German Angioplasty Bypass Surgery Investigation (GABI), Emory Angioplasty versus Surgery Trial (EAST), Coronary Angioplasty versus Bypass Surgery Revascularization Investigation (CABRI), and Estudio Randomizado Argentino de Angioplastia versus Cirugia (ERACI) (150–153,156) all enrolled stable patients with one-to three-vessel CAD. Overall, they showed no mortality difference between CABG and PTCA groups. CABG patients did have longer hospitalizations, fewer repeat interventions, and better quality of life (e.g., less angina and better functional status) at follow-up. The Bypass Angioplasty Revascularization Investigation (BARI) study enrolled 1,829 patients (41% with three-vessel CAD); the CABG group had a 85% lower revascularization rate at 5 years, but there was no significant mortality reduction. Importantly, there was a 44% lower rate of mortality ($p = 0.003$) among diabetic patients who underwent bypass surgery versus PTCA (154).

A recent meta-analysis of eight trials with 3,371 patients (144) showed no significant mortality differences between CABG and PTCA. CABG patients did have 90% fewer interventions at 1 year. Of note, only a small proportion of patients screened for these trials (5%–10%) were actually randomized. Thus, these findings cannot be readily extrapolated to groups of patients with high-risk characteristics (e.g., left main disease, severe left ventricular dysfunction, chronically occluded vessels).

It is also important to note that these trials were completed prior to the frequent use of stenting. The preliminary results from the Arterial Revascularization Therapy Study (ARTS) (155), which compared stenting to bypass surgery in 1,200 patients with multivessel CAD, found similar rates of adverse outcomes at 30 days [6.8% (surgery) and 8.7% (stenting)] but a significantly lower incidence of repeat revascularization among bypass patients (0.8% vs. 3.7%). Further studies are warranted, but these results are similar to those seen in the numerous studies comparing balloon angioplasty with bypass surgery.

New Techniques

A minimally invasive thoracotomy approach (with or without cardiopulmonary bypass) can be used for bypass of isolated LAD artery disease. The procedure results in less postoperative patient discomfort and shorter hospital stays. However, no randomized studies have been published to date, and longer term follow-up data are not yet available (*see Ann Thorac Surg* 1996;62:1545).

TRANSMYOCARDIAL REVASCULARIZATION (see pages 137, 138)

Initial studies showed that surgical transmyocardial laser revascularization (TMR) provides symptomatic relief of severe angina (see *JACC* 1999;33:1021; *Circulation* 1998;II-73). The reduction in anginal symptoms is apparent within 48 hours. This may be due to temporary blood flow through the created channels to the subendocardial area. However, the channels soon close down (necropsy reports show dense fibrous scarring). It is postulated that persistent relief (164, 166) is attributable to angiogenesis with the creation of new collateral vessels. However, some investigators are concerned that the relief of angina is achieved by denervation and that continued diastolic dysfunction persists in the absence of angina. More importantly, the perioperative mortality rate is approximately 5%, and in unstable angina patients or those with an ejection fraction under 30%, this rate is twice as high. Preliminary results from studies using a percutaneous approach (laser channels created from within the heart) suggest similar angina relief can be achieved with lower rates of mortality and morbidity (167,168).

REFERENCES

General Review Articles and Miscellaneous

1. **Bittl JA.** Advances in coronary angioplasty. *N Engl J Med* 1996; 335:1290–1302.

   This review covers all major methods of PCI. A detailed section on stents reviews new design innovations, applications, subacute stent thrombosis, and restenosis. The next section discusses new antithrombotic therapies, focusing on glycoprotein IIb/IIIa inhibitors. The last major section reviews data comparing balloon angioplasty with medical therapy and other procedures, including bypass surgery.

2. **Gibson CM,** et al. TIMI frame count. *Circulation* 1996;93: 879–888.

   This article describes a new method that quantifies coronary artery flow as a continuous variable (vs. assignment to one of four flow grades (i.e., TIMI grade 0, 1, 2, or 3). A total of 393 patients (315 TIMI-4 acute MI patients and 78 subjects without MI) were analyzed. The method was found to be reproducible (difference between two injections, 4.7 ± 3.9). Among normal patients, the LAD artery took 1.7 times longer to completely fill than the right coronary artery and circumflex arteries (36.2 vs. 20.4, 22.2; both $p < 0.001$). After thrombolysis, mean corrected counts (LAD, divide by 1.7) were 39.2 at 90 minutes and 31.7 by 18 to 36 hours ($p < 0.001$), both were higher than patients without acute MI.

3. **Topol EJ,** Serruys PW. Frontiers in interventional cardiology. *Circulation* 1998;98:1802–1820.

This review article focuses on four areas of interventional cardiology with important advances: platelet inhibition, prevention of restenosis, stent evolution, and angiogenesis. The platelet section discusses the effectiveness of aspirin and ticlopidine at preventing stent thrombosis and reviews all the major clinical trials that have used glycoprotein IIb/IIIa inhibitors in conjunction with PCI.

4. **Zaacks SM**, et al. Value of the ACC/AHA Stenosis Morphology Classification for coronary interventions in the late 1990s. *Am J Cardiol* 1998;82:43–49.

This prospective analysis was derived from 957 consecutive interventions in 1,404 lesions from June 1994 to October 1996. The overall procedural success rate was 91.9%. There were no significant differences in success rates between type A, B1, and B2 lesions (96.3%, 95.5%, 95.1%), but all were better than type C (88.2%; $p < 0.003$, $p < 0.004$, $p = 0.0001$, respectively). Multiple regression analysis showed that total occlusion and vessel tortuosity were predictive of procedural failure. Lesion type did not predict device use or complications. Actual predictors of complications were bifurcation lesions ($p = 0.0045$), presence of thrombus ($p = 0.0001$), inability to protect a major side branch ($p = 0.0468$), and degenerated vein graft lesions ($p = 0.0283$).

5. **Scanlon PJ**, et al. ACC/AHA guidelines for coronary angiography: a report of the American College of Cardiology/American Heart Association Task Force on Practice Guidelines (Committee on Coronary Angiography). *J Am Coll Cardiol* 1999;33:1756–1824.

These extensive guidelines begin with a discussion of the utilization, costs, and morbidity and mortality associated with angiography. The majority of the guidelines focus on the use of angiography for specific conditions, including known or suspected CAD (e.g., stable angina, unstable angina, acute MI), and recurrence of symptoms after revascularization, congestive heart failure, valvular disease, and congenital heart disease.

Angioplasty

Relationship of Operator and Hospital Volume to Outcomes

6. **Jollis JG**, et al. The relation between the volume of coronary angioplasty procedures at hospitals treating Medicare beneficiaries and short-term mortality. *N Engl J Med* 1994;331: 1625–1629.

This analysis was conducted on 218,000 Medicare patients who underwent PTCA from 1987 to 1990. A significant mortality difference was found between the 10% treated at the highest and lowest (<50 procedures/yr) volume centers (2.5% vs. 3.9%). There was also a difference in the CABG surgery rate (2.8% vs. 5.3%).

7. **Kimmel SE**, et al. The relationship between coronary angioplasty procedure volume and major complications. *JAMA* 1995; 274:1137–1142 (editorial pp. 1169–1170).

This cohort study showed an association between low hospital volume and increased complications. The cohort consisted of 19,594 non-MI patients undergoing a first PTCA. Higher volume was associated with lower mortality ($p = 0.04$), emergency bypass surgery ($p < 0.001$), and major complications ($p < 0.001$). Multivariate analysis (adjusted for case mix) showed that the associations persisted, but the mortality difference was not significant. No difference was demonstrated in outcomes when comparing hospitals performing 200 versus >200 procedures. However, for hospitals performing 400–599 and 600 versus <200 procedures/yr, the adjusted odds ratios for major complications were 0.66 and 0.54 ($p = 0.03$, $p = 0.001$).

8. **Ellis SG**, et al. Relation of operator volume and experience to procedural outcome of percutaneous coronary revascularization at hospitals with high interventional volume. *Circulation* 1997;96:2479–2484 (editorial pp. 2467–2470).

   This retrospective analysis focused on 12,985 patients at five centers (1993–1994). The data examined were on 38 operators who had 30 cases/yr (mean 163) and who had practiced 8 ± 5 years. Adverse outcomes (death and death plus Q-wave MI plus emergency CABG were found to be related to the number of cases per year [best-fit with log caseload: $r= 0.37$ ($p = 0.01$); $r= 0.58$ ($p < 0.001$)]. There were 69% fewer complications among patients treated by operators performing >270 versus 670 cases/yr ($p < 0.001$). This effect was present even among low-risk patients (5.9% vs. 1.7%–2.4%) and those with only type A and B1 lesions. No effect was seen with years of experience. Importantly, these difference were not consistent for all operators, hence the controversy surrounding standards applied to all operators.

9. **Jollis JG**, et al. Relationship between physician and hospital coronary angioplasty volume and outcome in elderly patients. *Circulation* 1997;95:2485–2491 (editorial pp. 2467–2470).

   This analysis focused on 97,478 Medicare patients treated by 6,115 physicians at 984 hospitals in 1992. Median procedure volume was only 13 per operator; hospital median 98. After risk factor adjustment, low-volume operators were associated with an increased rate of bypass surgery (<25, 3.8%; 25–50, 3.4%; >50, 2.6%; $p < 0.001$) and low-volume hospitals were associated with higher bypass surgery and mortality rates (<100, 3.9%/2.9%; 100–200, 3.5%/2.5%; >200, 3.0%/2.3%; $p < 0.001$). Improved outcomes were seen with up to 75 and 200 Medicare cases/yr, respectively. The accompanying editorial points out that data were acquired in the early stent era and prior to the use of adjunctive glycoprotein IIb/IIIa inhibition.

Comparison of Angioplasty to Medical Therapy

10. **Parisi AF**, et al. Angioplasty Compared to Medicine (**ACME**). A comparison of angioplasty with medical therapy in the treatment of single-vessel coronary artery disease. *N Engl J Med* 1992;326:10–16.

    Design: Prospective, randomized, multicenter study. Primary end point was change in exercise tolerance, frequency of angina attacks, and nitroglycerin use.
    Purpose: To compare medical therapy with balloon angioplasty in patients with one significant coronary artery stenosis.
    Population: 212 patients with a single 70%–99% stenosis.
    Treatment: The drug therapy group included oral isosorbide dinitrate with sublingual glyceryl trinitrate and/or β-blockers and/or calcium antagonists. The balloon angioplasty group was given calcium antagonists before and for 1 month after the procedure, and heparin and glyceryl trinitrate during and until

12 hours after the procedure. All patients received aspirin 325 mg orally daily.

Results: Balloon angioplasty (PTCA) was successful in 80% and reduced stenoses from 76% to 36%. The PTCA group had less angina (64% vs. 46%; $p < 0.01$), better exercise performance [+2.1 minutes [6 months vs. baseline exercise test) vs. +0.5 minutes; $p < 0.0001$], and more improvement in quality of life score (+8.6 units vs. +2.4 units; $p = 0.03$). However, the PTCA group did have more complications [emergency bypass surgery in 2 patients, MIs in 5 (vs. 3), and repeat PTCA in 16).

11. **Folland ED**, et al. VA Angioplasty Compared to Medicine (**VA ACME**). Percutaneous transluminal coronary angioplasty vs medical therapy for stable angina pectoris. *J Am Coll Cardiol* 1997;29:1505–1511.

Design: Prospective, randomized, double-blind, multicenter study.

Purpose: To compare balloon angioplasty with medical therapy in patients with documented coronary disease and chronic stable angina.

Population: 328 patients with stable angina and positive exercise treadmill test; 101 patients had two-vessel disease (≥70% stenosis in proximal two thirds), and 227 had one-vessel disease.

Exclusion Criteria: Medically refractory unstable angina, prior coronary revascularization, ejection fraction ≤30%.

Treatment: Medical therapy or balloon angioplasty.

Results: Among two-vessel patients there were no significant changes between treatment groups in exercise treadmill test duration (performed at 2–3 years), or freedom from angina and quality of life. However, fewer angioplasty patients had improved perfusion imaging results (59% vs. 75%) and higher average stenosis of worst lesions (74% vs. 56%). Among one-vessel disease patients, the angioplasty group had more improvement in exercise time (+2.1 vs. +0.6 minutes; $p < 0.001$) and quality of life score (+7.1 vs. +1.5; $p = 0.01$), and were more angina free (63% vs. 48%; $p = 0.02$).

12. Randomized Intervention Treatment of Angina (**RITA-2**) Trial participants. Coronary angioplasty vs medical therapy for angina: the RITA-2 trial. *Lancet* 1997;350:461–468.

Design: Prospective, randomized, double-blind, multicenter study. Primary end point was death and nonfatal MI. Follow-up period was 2.7 years.

Purpose: To compare the effects of coronary angioplasty and conservative medical care in patients considered suitable for either treatment.

Population: 1,018 patients, 53% with grade 2 angina, 47% with prior MI, only 7% with three-vessel disease.

Exclusion Criteria: Unstable angina in prior 7 days, left main CAD, early revascularization necessary or planned.

Treatment: Medical therapy or balloon angioplasty (in the latter group. The procedure was performed in 93% at a median of 5 weeks).

Results: Angioplasty group had increased rates of death and MI (6.3% vs. 3.3%; $p = 0.02$). Benefit was mostly attributable to procedure-related events. However, the PTCA group had 7% less grade 2 angina at 2 years and longer exercise treadmill test time at 3 months (+35 seconds; $p < 0.001$).

13. **Dakik HA**, et al. Intensive medical therapy vs coronary angioplasty for suppression of myocardial ischemia in survivors of acute MI. *Circulation* 1998;98:2017–2023 (editorial pp. 1985–1986).

This prospective, randomized pilot study was composed of 44 stable MI survivors, with mean follow-up of 1 year. Ischemia was quantified with adenosine [210]Tl tomography at 4.5 ± 2.9 days and repeated at 43 ± 26 days. Total stress-induced left ventricular perfusion defect size was comparably reduced with medical therapy (isordil + metoprolol + diltiazem; 38% baseline to 26%, $p < 0.0001$) and balloon angioplasty (35% to 20%, $p < 0.0001$). Patients who remained clinically stable had greater reduction in ischemic perfusion defect size (–13% vs. –5%; $p < 0.02$). Event-free survival was best in the 24 patients with ≥9% reduction in perfusion defect size (96% vs. 65%; $p = 0.009$). These findings need to be confirmed in larger randomized trials. The 6,000-patient National Heart, Lung, and Blood Institute (NHLBI)-sponsored Study of Coronary Revascularization and Therapeutic Evaluations (SOCRATES) and the 3,260-patient VA-based (Clinical Outcomes Utilization Revascularization and Aggressive Drug Evaluation (COURAGE) trial will compare intensive medical therapy with revascularization over 5–7 years.

Technical Aspects

14. **Gruntzig AR**, et al. Nonoperative dilatation of coronary-artery stenosis. Percutaneous transluminal coronary angioplasty. *N Engl J Med* 1979;301:61–68.

In this first major report of balloon angioplasty, 50 patients with angina (mean duration 13 months) underwent angioplasty. All patients received aspirin 1 g/day for 3 days (starting 1 day before), heparin and dextran during the procedure, and warfarin through follow-up (6–9 months). The procedural success rate was 64%. Five patients required coronary artery bypass surgery and three experienced an MI.

15. **Ohman EM**, et al. A randomized comparison of the effects of gradual prolonged vs standard primary balloon inflation on early and late outcome. *Circulation* 1994;89:1118–1125.

This randomized study of 478 patients showed the benefits of prolonged balloon inflation. Patients underwent 15-minute inflation one to two times or 1-minute inflation two to four times. The prolonged inflation group had the higher procedural success (≤50% residual stenosis; 95% vs. 89%, $p = 0.016$) and less dissection (3% vs. 9%; $p = 0.003$). Follow-up angiography performed at an average 6 months in 77% of patients without in-hospital events showed no significant difference in restenosis rate (44%) or clinical events [death, MI, coronary artery bypass surgery, or repeat angioplasty]; 34% (15-minute group) vs. 26%, $p = 0.15$).

16. **Tan K**, Sowton E. Clinical and lesion morphology determinants of coronary angioplasty success and complications: current experience. *J Am Coll Cardiol* 1995;25:855–865.

This analysis focused on 729 patients who underwent angioplasty of 994 vessels and 1,248 lesions. The procedural success rates were 96% (type A), 93% (type B), and 80% (type C) (A vs.

B2, $p = 0.03$; B1 vs. B2, $p = 0.02$; B2 vs. C, $p < 0.001$). Abrupt closure occurred in 2.1%, 2.6%, and 5% (B1 vs. B2, $p = 0.01$; C1 vs. C2, $p = 0.04$). Predictors of procedural failure included presence of long lesions, calcified lesions, thrombus, and 80%–99% stenosis. Predictors of abrupt closure included presence of long lesions, calcified lesions, thrombus, and angulation.

17. **Eltchaninoff H**, et al. Effects of prolonged sequential balloon inflations on results of coronary angioplasty. *Am J Cardiol* 1996; 77:1062–1066.

This randomized study showed the short-term favorable results with prolonged balloon inflation. Two hundred eighty-nine patients were randomized to standard balloon inflation (three to five times for ≤1 minute) or prolonged inflation (three to five times for 3–5 minutes). Prolonged balloon inflation was associated with higher initial success (92% vs. 80%; $p < 0.002$) and decreased dissection rate (14% vs. 30%; $p < 0.001$), but no difference in restenosis at 4–6 months (46% vs. 42%).

18. **Grines CL**, et al. A randomized trial of low osmolar ionic vs nonionic contrast media in patients with MI or unstable angina undergoing percutaneous transluminal coronary angioplasty. *J Am Coll Cardiol* 1996;27:1381–1386 (editorial pp. 1387–1389).

This randomized study of 211 patients with acute MI or unstable angina showed that the use of ionic low osmolar contrast media reduced the risk of ischemic complications. Patients received nonionic or ionic low osmolar contrast media during coronary angiography. The ionic media group had fewer recurrent ischemic events requiring repeat catheterization (3.0% vs. 11.4%; $p = 0.02$) and repeat angioplasty during initial hospitalization (1.0% vs. 5.8%; $p = 0.06$). At 1 month, the ionic contrast group had a reduced need for bypass surgery (0% vs. 5.9%; $p = 0.04$) and reported fewer symptoms of any angina or angina at rest (8.5% vs. 20.0%, $p = 0.04$; 0% vs. 5.9%, $p = 0.04$).

19. **Metz D**, et al. Comparison of 6F with 7F and 8F guiding catheters for elective coronary angioplasty: results of a prospective, multicenter randomized trial. *Am Heart J* 1997;134:131–137.

This study showed that bleeding and procedural complications decreased with the use of 6-French (F) catheters. Four hundred sixty patients with an ejection fraction of 30% and target lesions that could accommodate a 6F catheter were enrolled. There were no differences in procedural success rates (87%, 6F; 88%, 7F and 8F) or stenting rates (21%, 6F; 25%, 7F and 8F). The 6F group had ~40% fewer femoral access site complications (13.8% vs. 23.5%; $p < 0.01$), had shorter procedure and fluoroscopy times, used less contrast, and had shorter post-sheath removal femoral compression times (11.7 vs. 14.1 minutes; $p < 0.01$).

20. **Chevalier B**, et al. Does nonionic contrast medium still modify angioplasty results in the stent era? *J Am Coll Cardiol* 1999; 33(suppl A):85A.

This analysis focused on 1,713 consecutive patients (3/96 to 2/97) undergoing coronary intervention with a low osmolarity ionic contrast medium (ICM) and 1,826 with a nonionic contrast medium (NICM; 3/97 to 2/98). Clinical and angiographic data were similar in both groups. The incidence of minor and major events, including distal embolization, side branch occlusion, stent thrombosis, Q-wave MI, and death, were similar in both groups. The authors suggest that the higher use of stenting in the current era (>80% in this study) has eliminated the benefits of NICM use.

21. **Schrader R**, et al. A randomized trial comparing the impact of nonionic (iomeprol) versus an ionic (ioxaglate) low osmolar contrast medium on abrupt vessel closure and ischemic complications after coronary angioplasty. *J Am Coll Cardiol* 1999;33:395–402.

    This prospective, randomized trial was composed of 2,000 patients undergoing PTCA. The frequency of reocclusions requiring repeat intervention was similar in both groups [in laboratory, 2.9% (iomeprol) and 3.0% (ioxaglate); out of laboratory, 3.1% and 4.1%]. Major ischemic complication rates were also similar (emergency CABG, 0.8% and 0.7%; MI, 1.8% and 2.0%; in-hospital cardiac death, 0. 2% and 0.2%). The iomeprol group had higher rates of dissection and stenting (31.6% vs. 25.7%, $p = 0.004$; 31.6% vs. 25.7%, $p = 0.004$), whereas allergic reactions requiring treatment occurred only in the ioxaglate group (0.9%; $p = 0.002$).

22. Contrast Media Utilization in High Risk Percutaneous Transluminal Coronary Angioplasty (**COURT**). Preliminary results presented at 71st AHA Scientific Session in Dallas, TX, November 1998.

    A total of 853 patients undergoing high-risk interventions were randomized to a nonionic isoosmolar contrast agent (iodixanol) or an ionic low-osmolar contrast agent (ioxaglate). Angiographic success was significantly better in the nonionic contrast patients (92.2% vs. 85.9%; $p = 0.004$). The nonionic contrast group had a significantly lower incidence of the primary composite end point of in-hospital MI, abrupt closure, recatheterization, or emergent revascularization (5.2% vs. 9.5%).

Stent Studies

Review Articles

23. **Eeckhout E**, et al. Stents for intracoronary placement: current status and future direction. *J Am Coll Cardiol* 1996;27:757–765.

    The review begins with a historical overview followed by a brief discussion of the major stent types (e.g. Wallstent, Flexstent, and Palmaz-Schatz stents). Indications for stenting are described.

24. **Pepine CJ**, et al. Coronary artery stents (ACC Expert Consensus Document). *J Am Coll Cardiol* 1996;28:782–794.

    The Cardiac Catheterization Committee recognized that stenting reduces the risk for restenosis and the need for repeat interventional procedures compared with PTCA alone in selected subsets of patients, but cautioned against generalizing these findings to other situations where data were limited or not available (e.g., saphenous vein graft lesions, restenotic lesions).

25. **Goy J-J**, Eeckhout E. Intracoronary stenting. *Lancet* 1998;351: 1943–1949.

    The focus of this review is on the indications for stenting, including elective stenting for primary and secondary prevention of restenosis, bail-out, saphenous vein graft disease, chronic total occlusion, and acute MI. Future directions are discussed, including randomized trials to compare stenting and bypass surgery, different types of stents, coated stents, and radiation therapy.

Studies Comparing Stenting with PTCA

26. **Fischman DL**, et al., Stent Restenosis Study (**STRESS**). A randomized comparison of coronary-stent placement and balloon angioplasty in the treatment of coronary artery disease. *N Engl J Med* 1994;331: 496–501.

    Design: Prospective, randomized, open label, multicenter study. Primary end point was angiographic restenosis.

    Purpose: To compare the results of elective balloon angioplasty with Palmaz-Schatz stent implantation on clinical outcomes and restenosis in patients with *de novo* coronary lesions.

    Population: 410 patients with *de novo* 70% stenotic lesions ≤15 mm long and in vessels with a diameter of ≥3 mm.

    Exclusion Criteria: MI in previous 7 days, ejection fraction <40%, diffuse coronary or left main artery disease, and angiographic evidence of thrombus.

    Treatment: Balloon angioplasty or Palmaz-Schatz stent. All patients received aspirin 325 mg daily. Stented patients received dextran (started 2 hours before the procedure), heparin 10,000–15,000 U before the procedure and infusion for 4–6 hours after sheath removal, dipyridamole 75 mg three times daily for 1 month, and warfarin for 1 month.

    Results: Stent group had better procedural success (96.1% vs. 89.6%; $p = 0.011$), greater increase in lumen diameter (1.7 vs. 1.2 mm, $p < 0.001$; at 6 months, 1.56 vs. 1.24 mm, $p < 0.01$), and a lower rate of restenosis at 6 months (31% vs. 42%; $p = 0.046$). No significant difference in early clinical events (days 0–14) was observed between the two groups (19.5% vs. 23.8%). The stent group did have a nonsignificant reduction in revascularization rate (10% vs. 15%; $p = 0.06$).

    Comments: 1-year cost analysis showed the cost of stenting to be $800 more per patient despite lower costs during follow-up (*see Circulation* 1995;92:2480).

27. **Benestent I.** Serruys PW, et al. A comparison of balloon-expandable stent implantation with balloon angioplasty in patients with coronary artery disease. *N Engl J Med* 1994;331:489–495.

    Design: Prospective, randomized, multicenter study. Primary end point was death, stroke, MI, CABG, or need for repeat percutaneous intervention during hospitalization.

    Purpose: To compare elective balloon angioplasty with Palmaz-Schatz stenting in patients with stable angina and *de novo* coronary lesions.

    Population: 520 patients 30–75 years of age with stable angina and one *de novo* coronary lesion <15 mm long and in vessel >3 mm in diameter.

    Treatment: Balloon angioplasty or Palmaz-Schatz stenting. All patients received aspirin 250–500 mg/day and dipyridamole 75 mg three times daily (started 1 day prior to procedure and continued for >6 months); heparin 10,000 U was given before the procedure. Stented patients received dextran 1,000 mL over 6–8 hours and then warfarin for 3 months (target international normalized ratio 2.5–3.5).

    Results: No differences were observed between groups in incidence of death, stroke, MI, or subsequent revascularization during index hospitalization, and no differences were observed in composite end point of in-hospital clinical events (6.2% and 6.9%).

At 7 months, the stent group did have a significant reduction in primary composite end point (20.1% vs. 29.6%, $p = 0.02$), with the majority of this difference attributed to fewer second angioplasties (10% vs. 20.6%; $p = 0.001$). The stent group had more vascular complications (13.5% vs. 3.1%; $p < 0.001$) and longer hospital stays (8.5 vs. 3.1 days; $p = 0.001$). The 1-year follow-up data showed similar rates of death, MI, and CABG, but the stent group had 26% fewer primary end points (23% vs. 31%; $p = 0.04$), primarily due to ~50% fewer repeat PTCAs (10% vs. 21%; $p = 0.001$) (*see J Am Coll Cardiol* 1996;27:255).

Comments: Results suggest that stenting reduces the need for repeat interventions but does not reduce the incidence of major clinical events. Longer hospital stay with stenting was attributable to the aggressive antithrombotic regimen. Of note, intimal hyperplasia was not decreased by stenting.

28. **Benestent II.** Serruys PW, et al. for the Benestent Study Group. Randomised comparison of heparin-coated stents with balloon angioplasty in selected patients with coronary artery disease (Benestent II). *Lancet* 1998;352:673–681.

Design: Prospective, randomized, double-blind, multicenter study. Primary end point was death, MI, and need for revascularization at 6 months.

Purpose: To compare elective balloon angioplasty with heparin-coated Palmaz-Schatz stents in patients with *de novo* coronary artery lesions.

Population: 827 patients with stable angina or stabilized unstable angina with one or more *de novo* lesions >18 mm long and in vessels ≥3 mm in diameter.

Exclusion Criteria: Left main disease, lesion at bifurcation with side branch diameter >2.0 mm, ejection fraction <30%, and MI in prior 7 days.

Treatment: Heparin-coated stents (10, 15, or 20 mm) or balloon angioplasty, and 1:1 subrandomization to clinical or angiographic follow-up. Stent patients received ticlopidine 250 mg twice daily for 1 month.

Results: Stent group had an approximately one-third lower incidence of primary end point (12.8% vs. 19.3%; $p = 0.013$). The 30-day stent thrombosis rate was only 0.2%. In the subgroup undergoing angiographic follow-up, stented patients had a larger mean lumen diameter (1.89 vs. 1.66 mm; $p = 0.0002$) and less restenosis (16% vs. 31%; $p = 0.0008$). In the group assigned to clinical follow-up, the stent group had superior 1 year event-free survival [89% vs. 79%, $p = 0.004$ (RRs: cardiac events, 0.66; TVR, 0.60)]. Of note, the stent group patients with angiographic follow-up underwent 2.5 times more interventions (13.5% vs. 5.4%) than clinical follow-up patients, whereas this ratio was only 1.5 among balloon angioplasty patients (18.7% vs. 12.4%).

29. **Versaci F**, et al. A comparison of coronary artery stenting with angioplasty for isolated stenosis of the proximal left anterior descending coronary artery. *N Engl J Med* 1997;336:817–822.

This randomized trial was composed of 120 patients with an ejection fraction ≥40%, no MI within the previous month, and isolated stenoses of the LAD artery. Patients underwent stenting (using high-pressure inflation and warfarin for 3 months) or balloon angioplasty (PTCA). All patients received aspirin and diltiazem (first doses given 1 day prior to the procedure) and intravenous heparin during the procedure. Procedural success rates were similar (stent, 95%; PTCA, 93%). The stent group had superior outcomes: lower 1-year event-free survival (no recurrent angina, MI, death; 87% vs. 70%, $p = 0.04$) and over 50% reduction in restenosis (19% vs. 40%; $p = 0.02$). Stented patients did have a longer hospital stay (6.5 vs. 5.0 days; $p = 0.04$), but this was likely due to warfarin use, which is now been supplanted by aggressive antiplatelet regimens. The authors emphasize the need for a study comparing CABG with stenting.

Provisional Stenting

30. **Sigwart U**, et al. Intravascular stenting to prevent occlusion and restenosis after transluminal angioplasty. *N Engl J Med* 1987; 316: 701–706.

   In this first major report of coronary stenting, 24 stents were placed in 19 patients who presented with restenosis (n = 17) or abrupt closure (n = 4) after PTCA or saphenous graft disease (n = 3). Three patients had stent thrombosis (one death), and 0 of 12 had restenosis at 3- to 6-month angiography.

31. **Rodriguez R**, et al. on behalf of the OCBAS Investigators. Optimal coronary balloon angioplasty with provisional stenting versus primary stent (**OCBAS**). *J Am Coll Cardiol* 1998;32: 1351–1357.

   Design: Prospective, randomized, multicenter study. Primary end point was angiographic restenosis and target vessel revascularization at 6 months.

   Purpose: To determine any significant difference in restenosis rates between lesions treated with primary elective stenting versus those treated with optimal balloon angioplasty.

   Population: 116 patients with symptomatic CAD undergoing successful balloon angioplasty (as determined by angiography at 30 minutes) of *de novo* lesions in native coronary arteries.

   Exclusion Criteria: Lesions >20 mm in length and in vessels <2.5 mm diameter, diffuse disease, or severe tortuosity.

   Treatment: Balloon angioplasty (PTCA) alone or PTCA followed by elective coronary stenting.

   Results: 13.5% of patients crossed over to stenting. Angiographic restenosis and TVR rates were similar [19.2% (stent) vs. 16. 4% (PTCA); 17.5% vs. 13.5%]. Immediate and follow-up angiography showed that acute gain was significantly higher in the stent than in the PTCA group (1.95 vs. 1.50 mm; $p < 0.03$), but this was offset by a higher late loss (0.63 vs. 0.26 mm; $p = 0.01$). Overall costs (hospital and follow-up) were lower in the PTCA group ($398,480 vs. $591,740; $p < 0.02$).

32. Optimal PTCA and Provisional Stent versus Primary Stent Trial (**OPUS**). Preliminary results presented at the 48th ACC Scientific Session in New Orleans, LA, March 1999.

   This prospective, randomized trial was composed of 479 patients 21–81 years of age with stable or unstable angina or MI >24 hours earlier and 70% coronary artery stenosis (≤2 mm length, vessel diameter ≥3 mm). Palmaz-Schatz stenting was recommended, and intravascular ultrasonography was used at the physician's discretion. Abciximab was used in <15% of patients. Provisional stenting was undertaken if residual stenosis post-PTCA was >20%, if there was impending abrupt closure, stenosis was ≥2 mm, or flow-limiting dissection was a factor. At 6 months, the primary stenting group had a significantly lower incidence in the primary composite end points of death, MI, and TVR (6.1% vs. 14.9%; $p = 0.003$). The majority of this benefit was due to a lower TVR rate (4% vs. 10%; $p = 0.007$). The optimal PTCA and provisional stent groups had lower initial costs ($8,434 vs. $9,234, $p <$ 0.01), but by 6 months, the overall costs were lower in the primary stent group due to a lower readmission rate ($10,206 vs. $10,490, $p < 0.01$).

Atherectomy Studies

33. **Topol EJ**, et al., Coronary Angioplasty versus Excisional Atherectomy Trial (**CAVEAT**). A comparison of directional atherectomy with coronary angioplasty in patients with coronary artery disease. *N Engl J Med* 1993;329:221–227.
    Design: Prospective, randomized, controlled, multicenter study. Primary end point was angiographic restenosis at 6 months.
    Purpose: To compare outcomes in patients undergoing balloon angioplasty (PTCA) with those having DCA.
    Population: 1,012 patients with symptomatic CAD and no prior intracoronary interventions.
    Exclusion Criteria: Lesions 12 mm in length and MI in prior 5 days.
    Treatment: PTCA or DCA.
    Results: Atherectomy group had a higher initial success rate (≤50% stenosis; 89% vs. 80%), but was associated with a higher rate of early complications (11% vs. 5%) and higher hospital costs. At 6-month angiography, the atherectomy group showed a trend toward lower restenosis (50% vs. 57%; $p = 0.06$) and a higher probability of death or MI (8.6% vs. 4.6%; $p = 0$).

34. **Adelman AG**, et al. Canadian Coronary Atherectomy Trial (**CCAT**). A comparison of directional atherectomy with balloon angioplasty for lesions of the left anterior descending coronary artery. *N Engl J Med* 1993;329:228–233.
    Design: Prospective, randomized, open label, multicenter study. Primary end point was restenosis at follow-up angiography (median 5.9 months).
    Purpose: To compare restenosis rates for balloon angioplasty and directional atherectomy in lesions of the proximal LAD artery.
    Population: 274 patients with *de novo* 60% stenosis of the LAD artery.
    Exclusion Criteria: MI in prior 7 days, severe left ventricular dysfunction.
    Treatment: Balloon angioplasty or directional atherectomy.
    Results: Atherectomy group had a nonsignificantly higher success rate (94% vs. 88%; $p = 0.06$); no difference in complication rates was observed (5% vs. 6%). At follow-up angiography, restenosis rates and minimal luminal diameters were similar [43% (angioplasty) vs. 46% (atherectomy); 1.61 vs. 1.55 mm).

35. **CAVEAT-II.** Holmes DR Jr, et al. A multicenter, randomized trial of coronary angioplasty vs directional atherectomy for patients with saphenous vein bypass graft lesions. *Circulation* 1995; 91:1966–1974.

Design: Prospective, randomized, open label, multicenter study.
Purpose: To compare outcomes after directional atherectomy versus balloon angioplasty in patients with *de novo* venous bypass graft stenosis.
Population: 305 patients with *de novo*, nonocclusive saphenous vein graft stenoses (≥60%) who were suitable candidates for atherectomy or angioplasty.
Exclusion Criteria: MI in prior 5 days.
Treatment: Balloon angioplasty or directional atherectomy.
Results: Higher initial angiographic success was observed with atherectomy (89.2% vs. 79.0%, $p = 0.019$). No significant differences in either angiographic restenosis [45.6% (atherectomy) vs. 50.5% (angioplasty)] or target vessel reintervention [18.6% (atherectomy) vs. 26.2% (PTCA), $p = 0.09$] were observed. No difference in death or Q-wave MI rates were observed. However, the atherectomy group did have more frequent distal embolization (13.4% vs. 5.1%; $p = 0.012$) and a trend toward increased incidence of non–Q-wave MI (16.1% vs. 9.6%; $p = 0.09$).

36. **Simonton CA**, et al. Optimal directional atherectomy. Final results of the Optimal Atherectomy Restenosis Study (**OARS**). *Circulation* 1998; 97:332–339.
    Design: Prospective, multicenter registry study. Primary end point was angiographic restenosis at 6 months.
    Purpose: To determine if use of an optimal atherectomy technique would translate into a lower rate of late clinical and angiographic restenosis.
    Population: 199 patients 18–80 years of age with angina or a positive functional study and following angiographic criteria: (a) target vessel reference diameter 3.0–4.5 mm; (b) culprit lesion(s) with 60% stenosis; and (c) mild to moderate tortuosity and mild or no target lesion calcification. DCA and adjunctive angioplasty were performed if necessary to achieve <15% residual stenosis; 213 lesions met the criteria.
    Exclusion Criteria: Adjacent nontreated lesions with >40% stenosis, MI in prior 5 days, stroke in prior year, and bleeding diathesis.
    Treatment: DCA (7F device).
    Results: Frequent (87%) postatherectomy angioplasty was performed. The short-term procedural success rate was 97.5%. The mean rate of residual stenosis was only 7%. The major complication rate was 2.5% (death, emergency bypass surgery, Q-wave MI). Non–Q-wave MI (CK-MB more than three times normal) occurred in 14%. At 1-year follow-up, the target lesion revascularization rate was 17.8%. The 6-month restenosis rate was 28.9% (major predictor: smaller postprocedural lumen diameter).
    Comments: A lower restenosis rate was observed than in prior directional atherectomy trials.

37. **Baim DS**, et al. for the Balloon vs Optimal Atherectomy Trial (**BOAT**) Investigators. Final results of the Balloon vs Optimal Atherectomy Trial (BOAT). *Circulation* 1998;97:322–331 (editorial pp. 309–311).
    Design: Prospective, randomized, double-blind, multicenter study. Primary end point was restenosis rate at follow-up angiography (median 6.9 months).

Purpose: To compare the optimal DCA technique with conventional balloon angioplasty on restenosis.

Population: 1,000 patients with single *de novo,* native vessel lesions in vessels >3 mm in diameter.

Exclusion Criteria: Bifurcated lesion and stroke in prior 3 months.

Treatment: DCA (large device used) with aggressive tissue removal and use of adjunctive PTCA if indicated, or PTCA alone.

Results: DCA group had a higher procedural success rate (99% vs. 97%; $p = 0.02$) and a lower rate of residual stenosis (15% vs. 28%; $p < 0.0001$). Similar rates of major complication were observed (2.8% vs. 3.3%). However, DCA was associated with more frequent CK-MB elevations (more than 3 times normal; 16% vs. 6%; $p < 0.0001$). At follow-up angiography, the DCA group had a lower restenosis rate (primary end point): 31.4% vs. 39.8% ($p = 0.016$). At 1-year follow-up, the DCA group had nonsignificant reductions in mortality (0.6% vs. 1.6%; $p = 0.14$), target-vessel revascularization (17.1% vs. 19.7%; $p = 0.33$), target-site revascularization (15.3% vs. 18.3%; $p = 0.23$), and target vessel failure (death, Q-wave MI, or TVR) (21.1% vs. 24.8%; $p = 0.17$).

Comments: The results show that DCA can provide a relatively safe and enduring alternative to conventional angioplasty; comparisons of DCA to stenting require future study.

38. Study to Determine Rotablator and Transluminal Angioplasty Strategy (**STRATAS**). Preliminary results.

   This prospective, multicenter trial randomized 500 patients to aggressive rotablator therapy (70%–90% burr-to-artery ratio) or standard rotablator (50%–70% burr-to-artery ratio). At 6 months, there were no significant differences between the two groups in mean luminal diameter, restenosis, or clinical events.

Excimer Laser

39. **Litvack F**, et al. Percutaneous excimer laser coronary angioplasty: results in the first consecutive 3,000 patients. *J Am Coll Cardiol* 1994;23:323–329.

   This registry study showed a 90% procedural success rate (final stenosis <50% and no in-hospital Q-wave MI, bypass surgery, or death). Complications included coronary artery perforation [1.2% (0.4% in last 1,000 patients)], angiographic dissection (13%), sustained occlusion (3.1%), in-hospital bypass surgery (3.8%), Q-wave MI (2.1%), and death (0.5%). Most treated lesions were complex (B2 or C type, no difference in outcomes between two groups).

40. **Deckelbaum LI**, et al. Percutaneous Excimer Laser Coronary Angioplasty (**PELCA**) Trial. Effect of intracoronary saline infusion on dissection during excimer coronary angioplasty: a randomized trial. *J Am Coll Cardiol* 1995;26:1264–1269.

   This small randomized study was composed of 63 patients who received 1–2 mL/s of normal saline or a blood medium during excimer laser angioplasty. Saline-treated patients had a lower mean dissection grade [0. 43 vs. 0.91 (scale 0–5)] and 71% fewer significant dissections (grade 2: 7% vs. 24%; $p < 0.05$). The proposed mechanism of benefit was minimization of blood irradiation leading to less arterial wall damage.

41. **Appelman YEA**, et al., Amsterdam-Rotterdam (**AMRO**) Trial. Randomised trial of excimer angioplasty vs balloon angioplasty

for treatment of obstructive coronary artery disease. *Lancet* 1996;347:79–84.

Design: Prospective, randomized, double-blind, multicenter study. Primary clinical end point was cardiac death, MI, bypass surgery, and repeat angioplasty. Primary angiographic end point was minimal lumen diameter at 6 months.

Purpose: To evaluate initial and long-term clinical and angiographic outcome of excimer laser angioplasty in patients with long coronary lesions.

Population: 308 patients with stable angina and coronary lesions >10 mm in length.

Exclusion Criteria: Unstable angina and MI in prior 2 weeks.

Treatment: Excimer laser or balloon angioplasty.

Results: Similar angiographic success rates (80% vs. 79%) were observed. No significant differences in lumen gain [0.4 mm (laser) vs. 0.48 mm (angioplasty); $p = 0.34$] or restenosis rate (51.6% vs. 41.2%; $p = 0.13$) were observed. The clinical event rates were similar (MI, 4.6% vs. 5.7%; bypass surgery, 10.6% vs. 10.8%; repeat angioplasty, 21.2% vs. 18.5%).

42. **Reifart N**, et al. Excimer Laser, Rotational Atherectomy and Balloon Angioplasty Comparison Study (**ERBAC**). Randomized comparison of angioplasty of complex lesions at a single center. *Circulation* 1997;96:91–98.

Design: Prospective, randomized, single center study. Primary end point was procedural success rate (defined as <50% stenosis without in-hospital death, MI, or coronary bypass surgery).

Purpose: To compare three percutaneous interventional techniques in patients with complex coronary lesions.

Population: 685 patients with type B or C lesions.

Exclusion Criteria: MI or balloon angioplasty in prior 4 months, saphenous vein graft disease, and total occlusion not traversable by guidewire.

Treatment: Balloon angioplasty (PTCA), laser, or rotational atherectomy.

Results: Rotational atherectomy group had best procedural success rate (defined as residual stenosis <50% and no death, MI, or bypass surgery): 89% vs. 80% [PTCA] and 77% [laser] ($p = 0.0019$). No difference in incidence of in-hospital complications was observed. At 6-month follow-up, the PTCA group had undergone less revascularization of target lesions [31.9% vs. 42.4% (atherectomy) and 46% (laser); $p = 0.013$] and had a lower restenosis rate [47% vs. 57% ($p = NS$) and 59% ($p < 0.05$)].

43. **Stone GW**, et al., for the Laser Angioplasty vs Angioplasty (**LAVA**) Trial Investigators. Prospective, randomized, multicenter comparison of laser-facilitated balloon angioplasty vs standalone balloon angioplasty in patients with obstructive coronary artery disease. *J Am Coll Cardiol* 1997;30:1714–1721.

Design: Prospective, randomized, multicenter study. Primary composite end point was freedom from death, MI, or need for CABG surgery or repeat balloon angioplasty.

Purpose: To evaluate the acute and late outcomes of laser-facilitated angioplasty compared with standard balloon angioplasty.

Population: 215 patients with 244 lesions in vessels ≥2 mm in diameter that were successfully crossed with a guidewire.

Treatment: Holmium laser–facilitated balloon angioplasty or balloon angioplasty.

Results: Similar in-hospital clinical success rates were observed [89.7% (laser) vs. 93.9% (angioplasty alone); $p = 0.27$]. No difference was observed in postprocedural diameter stenosis (18.3% vs. 19.5%). However, the laser group had significantly more major and minor procedural complications (18.0% vs. 3.1%; $p = 0.0004$), MIs (4.3% vs. 0%; $p = 0.04$), and total in-hospital major adverse events (10.3% vs. 4.1%; $p = 0.08$). At mean follow-up of 11 months, no significant differences in late or event-free survival between the two groups was observed.

Adjunctive Pharmacologic Therapy

Aspirin (see reference 112).

Heparin

44. **Friedman HZ**, et al. Randomized prospective evaluation of prolonged vs abbreviated intravenous heparin treatment after PTCA. *J Am Coll Cardiol* 1994;24:1214–1219.

    Design: Prospective, randomized, open, single-center study.

    Purpose: To compare continuous prolonged heparin therapy with abbreviated heparin therapy with early sheath removal after uncomplicated coronary angioplasty.

    Population: 238 patients who underwent successful elective coronary angioplasty (46 were excluded because of unfavorable procedural results).

    Exclusion Criteria: Recent MI, unstable angina, and uncompensated left ventricular dysfunction.

    Treatment: All patients received an initial bolus of 10,000–15,000 U of heparin then an infusion at 10 U/kg/h (titrated to ACT 160–190 seconds) for 24 hours or no additional heparin with sheath removal 3–4 hours later.

    Results: Abbreviated heparin group had fewer bleeding complications [zero vs. eight patients (one blood transfusion, seven inguinal hematomas), $p < 0.001$]. Abbreviated infusion patients also were discharged earlier (after 23 vs. 42 hours; $p < 0.001$), resulting in a cost savings of $1,370/patient.

45. **Garachemani AR**, et al. Prolonged heparin after uncomplicated coronary interventions: a prospective, randomized trial. *Am Heart J* 1998;136:352–356 (editorial pp. 183–185).

    This prospective randomized trial was composed of 191 consecutive patients who underwent successful coronary angioplasty. Patients received prolonged intravenous heparin (12–20 hours) or no postprocedural heparin. Stents were used in 33% and 36% of patients. MIs occurred in 3% and 4%, whereas vascular complications were seen in 3% and 1%. Accompanying editorial contains results from a meta-analysis of six studies comprising 2,186 patients. Post-procedural heparin was associated with a nonsignificant odds ratio of 0.91 (0.45– 1.84) for ischemic complications and an odds ratio of 2.54 (1.44–4.47) for bleeding complications (~27 additional episodes/1,000 patients treated).

46. **Popma JJ**, et al. Heparin dosing in patients undergoing coronary intervention. *Am J Cardiol* 1998;82(suppl 8B):19P–24P.

    This review describes current pretreatment, procedural, and postprocedural heparin dosing regimens. Prolonged infusions after uncomplicated procedures are not recommended because increased bleeding complications arise without any decrease in ischemic complications. The lower heparin dosing requirements in conjunction with glycoprotein IIb/IIIa inhibitors are discussed. Other sections review complication rates and activated partial thromboplastin time monitoring.

47. **Lincoff AM**, et al. Precursor to EPILOG (**PROLOG**) Investigators. Standard versus low-dose, weight-adjusted heparin in patients treated with the platelet glycoprotein IIb/IIIa receptor antibody fragment abciximab (c7E3 Fab) during percutaneous coronary revascularization. *Am J Cardiol* 1997;79:286–291.

This randomized 2x2 factorial pilot study was composed of a total of 103 patients undergoing PCI with concomitant abciximab (0.25 mg/kg intravenous bolus, then 10 µg/min for 12 hours) were randomized to standard or high-dose heparin (100 U/kg bolus prior to PCI then hourly boluses to keep ACT 300–350 seconds, or continuous infusion at 10 U/kg/h without further ACT measurements) or low-dose heparin (70 U/kg then 30 U/kg boluses during the procedure or continuous infusion at 7 U/kg/h without further ACT measurements). There was a separate randomization to early or late sheath removal. The early sheath removal group had heparin discontinued immediately after PCI and sheaths removed at 6 hours, whereas the late group had heparin continued for 12 hours and sheaths removed 4–6 hours later. There was no difference between the groups in the incidence of ischemic events at 7 days. The early sheath removal group had a smaller decrease in mean hemoglobin from baseline ($p = 0.03$), and there were nonsignificant trends toward less minor non-CABG bleeding with low-dose heparin and early sheath removal.

48. **Rabah MM**, et al. Enoxaparin in PTCA. *J Am Coll Cardiol* 1999;31:14A.

Sixty patients were randomized to enoxaparin 1 mg/kg intravenously or heparin with a target ACT of >300 seconds prior to PTCA. Sheaths were taken out 8 hours after enoxaparin was given or when ACT was <140 seconds. The two groups had similar incidences of ischemic complications, procedural success, and bleeding. Of note, enoxaparin patients had a higher Xa to IIa ratio than unfractionated heparin patients (2.79 vs. 1.27).

Antithrombotic Regimens to Prevent Stent Thrombosis

49. **Schomig A**, et al. Intracoronary Stenting and Antithrombotic Regimen (**ISAR**). A randomized comparison of antiplatelet and anticoagulant therapy after the placement of coronary artery stents. *N Engl J Med* 1996;334:1084–1089 (editorial pp. 1126–1128).
Design: Prospective, randomized, open, multicenter study. Primary cardiac end points were cardiovascular death, MI, bypass surgery, and repeat target vessel intervention. Additional noncardiac end point was death from noncardiac causes, cerebrovascular accidents, severe hemorrhage, and peripheral vascular events.
Purpose: To compare the early outcome of patients given a combined antiplatelet regimen or conventional anticoagulation after coronary stent placement.
Population: 517 patients who underwent successful stenting.

Exclusion Criteria: Cardiogenic shock and stenting intended as a bridge to CABG surgery.

Treatment: Intravenous heparin for 12 hours, ticlopidine 250 mg twice daily, and aspirin; or intravenous heparin for 5–10 days, phenprocoumon, and aspirin.

Results: At 30 days, the antiplatelet group had 75% fewer cardiac end points (1.6% vs. 6.2%), including a significant reduction in MI (0.8% vs. 4.2%; $p = 0.02$). The antiplatelet group had a 90% reduction in the primary noncardiac end point (1.2% vs. 12.3%; $p < 0.001$), including an 87% reduction in peripheral vascular events (0.8% vs. 6.2%; $p = 0.001$) and no bleeding complications (vs 6.5%; $p < 0.001$). Antiplatelet therapy also was associated with 86% fewer stent reocclusions (0.8% vs. 5.4%; $p = 0.004$).

50. **Karrillon GJ**, et al. **French Multicenter Registry**. Intracoronary stent implantation without ultrasound guidance and with replacement of conventional anticoagulation by antiplatelet therapy. *Circulation* 1996;94:1519–1527.

The results of this large registry study of 2,900 patients confirm that the benefits of antiplatelet regimen can be achieved without ultrasonographic guidance. Patients were treated with aspirin 100 mg/day and ticlopidine 250 mg/day for 1 month. Low-molecular-weight heparin use was reduced in four stages (1 month to none). At 1 month, the subacute closure rate was 1.8% (peak incidence at 5–8 days; 12 of 51 died) and the acute MI rate was 0.6%; coronary artery bypass surgery was performed in 0.3%. A higher stent thrombosis rate was seen with balloons <3 mm (≤2.5 mm, 10%; 3 mm, 2.3%; 3.5 mm, 1%), in bail-out situations (6.7% vs. 1.4%), and in patients with unstable angina or acute MI (2.2% vs. 1.1%; $p = 0.02$).

51. **Bertrand ME**, et al. Full Anticoagulation versus Aspirin and Ticlopidine (**FANTASTIC**). Randomized multicenter comparison of conventional anticoagulation versus antiplatelet therapy in unplanned and elective coronary stenting. *Circulation* 1998;98:1597–1603.

Design: Prospective, randomized, multicenter study. Primary end point was bleeding and peripheral vascular complications. Secondary end points were death, MI, and stent occlusion.

Purpose: To compare the effects of aggressive antiplatelet treatment with anticoagulation after implantation of a Wiktor stent on bleeding rates and stent thrombosis rates.

Population: 485 patients undergoing elective (58%) or unplanned (42%) coronary stenting.

Exclusion Criteria: Platelet count <150,000, bleeding disorders, recent (<6 months) gastrointestinal bleeding, recent stroke, angiographic evidence of thrombus at target site, and allergy to aspirin or ticlopidine.

Treatment: Antiplatelet therapy with aspirin 100–325 mg/day and ticlopidine 250 mg twice daily for 6 weeks [first dose (500 mg) given in catheterization laboratory], or anticoagulation with heparin (target activated partial thromboplastin time 2.0–2.5 times control), then warfarin for 6 weeks (target international normalized ratio 2.5–3.0). The anticoagulation group also received aspirin. All patients received heparin 10,000-U bolus prior to procedure.

Results: Successful stent implantation was achieved in 99%. The antiplatelet group had fewer bleeding and peripheral vascular complications (13.5% vs. 21%, odds ratio 0.6; $p = 0.03$). Major cardiac events in electively stented patients were less common in the antiplatelet group (2.4% vs. 9.9%, odds ratio 0.23; $p = 0.01$). Antiplatelet patients had a shorter average hospital stay (4.3 vs. 6.4 days; $p = 0.0001$).

52. **Urban P**, et al. for the Multicenter Aspirin and Ticlopidine Trial after Intracoronary Stenting (**MATTIS**) investigators. Randomized evaluation of anticoagulation versus antiplatelet therapy after coronary stent implantation in high-risk patients. *Circulation* 1998;98:2126–2132.

    Design: Prospective, randomized, multicenter study. Primary composite end point was cardiovascular death, MI, and repeat revascularization at 30 days.

    Purpose: To compare antiplatelet therapy with anticoagulation in high-risk patients undergoing coronary stent implantation.

    Population: 350 patients randomized within 6 hours of stent implantation who met the eligibility criteria: (a) stent(s) was placed to treat abrupt closure after balloon angioplasty; (b) suboptimal angiographic result was achieved; (c) the stented segment measured >45 mm (or was composed of three stents); (d) the vessel in question was small (i.e., largest balloon used was ≤2.5 mm). Eight different stent types were used by investigators.

    Exclusion Criteria: Recent MI, persistent ischemia, administration of glycoprotein IIb/IIIa inhibitors before or during procedure, and intervention planned within 30-day follow-up period.

    Treatment: Aspirin 250 mg once daily and ticlopidine 250 mg twice daily for 30 days or aspirin 250 mg once daily and oral anticoagulation (target international normalized ratio 2.5–3.0).

    Results: Antiplatelet group demonstrated a trend toward fewer cardiac end points (5.6% vs. 11%; $p = 0.07$) and significant reduction in major vascular and bleeding complications (1.7% vs. 6.9%; $p = 0.02$). The incidence of subacute stent thrombosis was not precisely known (no angiographic end point). Three patients (1.7%) treated with ticlopidine developed asymptomatic agranulocytopenia.

53. **Leon MB**, et al. for the Stent Anticoagulation Restenosis Study (**STARS**) investigators. A clinical trial comparing three antithrombotic-drug regimens after coronary-artery stenting. *N Engl J Med* 1998;339:1665–1671.

    Design: Prospective, randomized, open, multicenter study (50). 30-day primary composite end point was death, MI, revascularization of target lesion, and angiographically evident thrombosis.

    Purpose: To compare clinical outcomes for three antithrombotic regimens after elective coronary stenting.

    Population: 1,653 patients who underwent successful stenting of a >60% stenosis in a native coronary artery with a diameter of 3–4 mm.

    Exclusion Criteria: MI in prior 7 days, abciximab administration, and planned revascularization within 30 days.

    Treatment: Aspirin 325 mg daily, aspirin 325 mg daily and intravenous heparin followed by warfarin (target international normalized ratio 2.0–2.5), or aspirin 325 mg daily and ticlopidine 250 mg twice daily.

    Results: Aspirin plus ticlopidine group had a significant reduction in the incidence of primary composite end points for aspirin and warfarin (0.5% vs. 2.7%) and for aspirin alone (3.6%; $p <$

0.001 for comparison of all three groups). Hemorrhagic and vascular surgical complications occurred less frequently with aspirin alone: 1.8% vs. 5.5% (aspirin plus ticlopidine), and 6.2% (aspirin and warfarin) and 0.4% vs. 2.0% and 2.0%. No significant differences were observed in the incidences of neutropenia or thrombocytopenia (overall incidence 0.3%).

54. Clopidogrel Aspirin Stent International Cooperative Study (**CLASSICS**). Preliminary results presented at ACC 48th Scientific Session in New Orleans, LA, March 1999.

   The results of this prospective, randomized trial of 1,020 stented patients demonstrate that clopidogrel has an efficacy similar to and better tolerability than ticlopidine. Patients were randomized to ticlopidine 250 mg twice daily for 4 weeks, clopidogrel 75 mg once daily for 4 weeks, or clopidogrel 300 mg loading dose followed by 75 mg once daily (days 2–28). All patients received aspirin 325 mg once daily. The clopidogrel groups had a significantly lower incidence of the primary composite end points, which consisted of major bleeding, neutropenia, thrombocytopenia, and early discontinuation of therapy: 2.9% (loading dose group) and 6.3% (clopidogrel .75 mg/day [all clopidogrel patients:4.6%] vs 9.1% for ticlopidine ($p = 0.005$)). This difference was due to lower discontinuation rates in the clopidogrel groups (2% and 5.1% vs. 8.2%). Major cardiac events occurred in 1.3% of clopidogrel patients vs 0.9% of ticlopidine patients ($p =$ NS; see Fig. 2–1).

55. **Hall P**, et al. A randomized comparison of combined ticlopidine and aspirin therapy versus aspirin therapy alone after successful intravascular ultrasound-guided stent implantation. *Circulation* 1996;93:215–222.

   A total of 226 patients were randomized to aspirin 325 mg/day or ticlopidine 250 mg twice daily for 1 month and aspirin for 5 days. One-month stent thrombosis rates were 2.9% vs. 0.8% ($p = 0.2$). The rates were 2.9% vs. 0% for death and 3.9% vs. 0.8% for major clinical events ($p = 0.1$). Thus, there was a trend toward benefit with the combined aspirin and ticlopidine regimen. Severe neutropenia occurred in one ticlopidine patient.

56. **Goods CM**, et al. Utilization of the coronary balloon-expandable stent without anticoagulation or intravascular ultrasound. *Circulation* 1996;93:1803–1808.

   This retrospective analysis of 216 patients demonstrated that the benefits of antiplatelet regimen can be achieved without the routine use of intravascular ultrasonography. Patients were treated with aspirin and ticlopidine for 1 month. Patients were excluded if stenting provided inadequate dissection coverage, filling defects were present, or flow was less than TIMI grade 3. At 30-day follow-up, stent thrombosis had occurred in only two patients. One patient died, two patients had coronary artery bypass surgery, and four required blood transfusions.

57. **Goods CM**, et al. Comparison of aspirin alone versus aspirin and ticlopidine after coronary artery angioplasty stenting. *Am J Cardiol* 1996;78: 1042–1044.

   The results of this prospective, nonrandomized study show that aspirin alone is not an adequate antithrombotic regimen after stenting. Aspirin and ticlopidine were used in 338 patients and aspirin alone in only 46 patients. Inclusion criteria included adequate coverage of intimal dissections, absence of residual filling defects, and normal flow in the stented vessel at the end of the procedure. The aspirin and ticlopidine group had a significantly lower stent thrombosis rate (0.9% vs. 6.5%; $p = 0.02$), fewer deaths (0.3% vs. 4.4%; $p = 0.04$), and fewer Q-wave MIs (0% vs. 6.5%; $p = 0.002$).

58. **Gregorini L**, et al. Ticlopidine and aspirin pre-treatment reduces coagulation and platelet activation during coronary dilation procedures. *J Am Coll Cardiol* 1997;29:13–20.

This small study was composed of 85 patients, all on aspirin 250 mg/day and 70 on ticlopidine 250 mg twice daily (≤1 day, n = 28; ≥3 days, n = 42). This group of patients had 35 stents, 30 PTCAs (15 on ticlopidine, all 72 hours), and 20 rotational atherectomies. Ticlopidine patients had less thrombin generation before and after treatment. The group on ticlopidine for 72 hours had decreased platelet activation and lower plasma serotonin.

59. **Albiero M**, et al. Results of a consecutive series of patients receiving only antiplatelet therapy after optimized stent implantation. Comparison of aspirin alone vs combined ticlopidine and aspirin therapy. *Circulation* 1997;95:1145–1156 (editorial pp. 1098–1100).

This analysis focused on 801 patients treated with antiplatelet therapy only (aspirin, n = 264; aspirin plus ticlopidine, n = 537). The first 575 patients were not randomized. At 1 month, no difference in subacute stent thrombosis (1.9% vs. 1.3%; $p = 0.5$) or major clinical events (1.9%, 2.0%) was observed. The combination therapy group had a higher discontinuation rate [1.9% (0.6% with neutropenia) vs. 0%; $p = 0.04$]. The accompanying editorial points out some weaknesses of this primarily observational study: six different stent types were used, the aspirin arm was smaller, and the use of antiplatelets for abrupt closure, acute MI, or with suboptimal results was not addressed.

60. **Steinbuhl SR**, et al. The duration of pretreatment with ticlopidine prior to stenting is associated with the risk of procedure-related non–Q-wave MIs. *J Am Coll Cardiol* 1998;32:1366–1380.

This retrospective study showed the benefits of beginning ticlopidine several days prior to stenting. Outcomes were analyzed in 175 consecutive patients treated with ticlopidine prior to stenting. Non–Q-wave MI was defined as CK greater than the upper limit of normal and the CK-MB fraction ≥4%. Longer duration of ticlopidine pretreatment was strongly associated with a lower incidence of procedure-related non–Q-wave MI: <1 day, 29%; 1–2 days, 14%; ≥3 days, 5% (chi square for trend 9.6; $p = 0.002$).

61. **Berger PB**, et al. Safety and efficacy of ticlopidine for only 2 weeks after successful intracoronary stent placement. *Circulation* 1999; 99:248–253.

This analysis of 827 patients undergoing successful stent implantation showed 2 weeks of ticlopidine to be associated with no cases of neutropenia as well as no cases of stent thrombosis after ticlopidine was stopped. Of note, patients requiring chronic warfarin were excluded and 11% of patients at increased risk of stent thrombosis were treated with enoxaparin for 10–14 days.

62. **Berger PB**, et al. Clopidogrel versus ticlopidine for coronary stents. *J Am Coll Cardiol* 1999;31(suppl A):34A.

This analysis focused on 1,327 stented patients; ticlopidine was used in 827 and clopidogrel in 500 (beginning in March 1998).

Clopidogrel was dosed as follows: (a) for unscheduled interventions, 300 mg prior to procedure then 75 mg once daily for 2 weeks; (b) for interventions scheduled <72 hours in advance, 300 mg once, then 75 mg once daily; and (c) for interventions planned >72 hours in advance, 75 mg once daily. Despite the clopidogrel group having more baseline adverse characteristics, there were no significant differences in major event rates, consisting of death, MI, stent thrombosis, and repeat PCI/CABG, at 30 days. Platelet inhibition studies, using 5 μmol ADP, showed that the clopidogrel group receiving a loading dose achieved >60% platelet inhibition in ~24 hours versus 4–5 days with no loading dose and 5–6 days with ticlopidine (250 mg twice daily).

63. **Moussa I**, et al. Effectiveness of clopidogrel and aspirin versus ticlopidine and aspirin in preventing stent thrombosis after coronary stent implantation. *Circulation* 1999;99:2364–2366.

This observational study was composed of 1,689 patients undergoing coronary stent implantation; 1,406 received ticlopidine (500 mg loading dose then 250 mg twice daily) and aspirin (325 mg once daily), and 283 received clopidogrel (300 mg loading dose then 75 mg once daily) and aspirin. Exclusion criteria included requirement for oral anticoagulation, abciximab administration, and procedural failure. At one month follow-up, the two groups had a similar incidence of stent thrombosis [1.5% (ticlopidine plus aspirin) vs. 1.4%] and major adverse cardiac events (3.1% vs. 2.4%). The clopidogrel plus aspirin group had a significantly lower incidence of side effects, consisting of neutropenia, diarrhea, or rash (5.3% vs. 10.6%, RR 0.53; *p* = 0.006).

Glycoprotein IIb/IIIa Inhibitors

64. Evaluation of 7E3 for the Prevention of Ischemic Complications (**EPIC**). Use of a monoclonal antibody directed vs platelet glycoprotein IIb/IIIa receptor in high-risk percutaneous transluminal coronary angioplasty. *N Engl J Med* 1994;330:956–961.

Design: Prospective, randomized, double-blind, multicenter study. 30-day primary composite end point was death, MI, CABG surgery, repeat percutaneous intervention for acute ischemia, and stenting due to procedural failure, or placement of an intraaortic balloon pump.

Purpose: To determine whether the monoclonal antibody c7E3 Fab provides clinical benefit in patients undergoing coronary angioplasty or atherectomy.

Population: 2,099 high-risk patients, defined as having experienced acute MI with onset of symptoms within previous 12 hours, two episodes of postinfarct angina within previous 24 hours with ECG changes, or high-risk clinical or angiographic features, who underwent percutaneous intervention (PTCA, 90%; directional atherectomy, 5%; both, 5%).

Exclusion Criteria: Age 80 years, bleeding diathesis, major surgery in prior 6 weeks, and stroke in prior 2 years.

Treatment: Abciximab 0.25 mg/kg intravenous bolus (started 10 minutes before procedure) then 10 μg/min infusion for 12 hours, abciximab or placebo. All patients received heparin (10,000- to 12,000-U bolus; target ACT 300–350 seconds).

Results: Abciximab bolus plus infusion group had 35% fewer end points (death, MI, unplanned surgical revascularization, repeat percutaneous procedure, need for intraortic balloon pump): 12.8% vs. 11.4% (bolus only; $p = 0.43$) and 8.3% (placebo; $p = 0.008$). A significant reduction was observed in the MI rate only: 5.2% vs. 8.6% for placebo ($p = 0.013$). Abciximab was associated with more bleeding episodes: 14% vs. 7% ($p = 0.001$). Follow-up studies have shown abciximab to be associated with persistent significant reductions at 6 months (27% vs. 35.1%, $p = 0.001$; see Lancet 1994;343:881) and 3 years [41.1% vs. 47.4% (bolus only) and 47.2% (placebo), $p = 0.009$; see JAMA 1997; 278:479]. Three-year follow-up also showed that the subgroup of patients with an evolving MI or refractory unstable angina (28% of patients) had a significant 60% reduction in mortality rate (5.1% vs. 12.7%; $p = 0.01$). *Comments:* Significant bleeding likely was due to high heparin dosing. A subsequent cost analysis showed abciximab use to be associated with $1,407 higher in-hospital costs per patient that were nearly offset by subsequent savings of $1,270/patient (due to 23% fewer hospitalizations, 22% less repeat revascularization).

65. Integrelin to Minimise Platelet Aggregation and Coronary Thrombosis II (**IMPACT II**). Randomised placebo-controlled trial of effect of eptifibatide on complications of percutaneous coronary intervention: IMPACT-II. *Lancet* 1997;349:1422–1428 (editorial pp. 1409–1410).
   Design: Prospective, randomized, double-blind, multicenter study. 30-day primary composite end point was death, MI, unplanned surgical or repeat percutaneous revascularization, or stenting for abrupt closure.
   Purpose: To determine the effectiveness of eptifibatide in reducing ischemic complications in patients undergoing nonsurgical coronary revascularization.
   Population: 4,010 patients who underwent elective, urgent, or emergent percutaneous intervention (PTCA, 91%–93%).
   Exclusion Criteria: Bleeding diathesis, major surgery in prior 6 weeks, and any history of stroke.
   Treatment: Eptifibatide 135 µg/kg intravenous bolus (10–60 minutes before procedure), then 0.5 or 0.75 µg/kg/min for 20–24 hours; or placebo.
   Results: At 30 days, a nonsignificant reduction in the primary composite end point was observed: 9.2% (135/0.5 group) and 9.9% (135/0.75 group) vs. 11.4% (placebo) ($p = 0.063, 0.22$). On-treatment analysis showed that the 135/0.5 group had a significant 22% reduction in composite primary end point (9.1% vs. 11.6%; $p = 0.035$). No significant differences in bleeding or transfusion rates were observed.

66. c7E3 Fab Antiplatelet Therapy in Unstable Refractory Refractory Angina (**CAPTURE**). Randomized, placebo-controlled trial of abciximab before and during coronary intervention in refractory unstable angina: the CAPTURE study. *Lancet* 1997;349: 1429–1435 (editorial pp. 1409–1410).
   Design: Prospective, randomized, placebo-controlled, multicenter study. 30-day primary end point was death, MI, or urgent intervention for recurrent ischemia.
   Purpose: To assess whether abciximab given before and until briefly after percutaneous intervention improves outcome in patients with refractory unstable angina.
   Population: 1,265 patients with chest pain at rest with ST-segment depression or elevation or abnormal T waves, with one

or more episodes (rest pain and/or ECG changes) occurring >2 hours after the start of intravenous heparin and nitrate therapy. *Exclusion Criteria:* Recent MI, persisting ischemia that required immediate intervention, and left main stenosis as shown by angiography.

Treatment: After angiography, patients were randomized to abciximab (0.25 mg/kg bolus then 10 μg/min) or placebo for 18–24 hours before and 1 hour after percutaneous intervention (balloon angioplasty with stenting only if necessary to maintain vessel patency). Goal ACT was 300 seconds.

Results: Trial was stopped early due to significant treatment effect (1,400 patients planned). The abciximab group had a 29% reduction in 30-day primary end points of death, MI, and ischemia requiring intervention (11.3% vs. 15.9%; $p = 0.012$). Most of this difference was due to fewer MIs (defined as CK or CK-MB three times the upper limit of normal in two samples): 4.1% vs. 8.2% ($p = 0.002$). MIs occurred less frequently before and after PTCA in abciximab patients (0.6% vs. 2.1%, $p = 0.029$; 2.6% vs. 5.5%, $p = 0.043$). Importantly, no difference in event rates was seen at 6 months (31% vs. 30.8%). A twofold higher major bleeding rate was observed in the abciximab group (3.8% vs. 1.9%; $p = 0.043$). An ECG ischemia substudy (332 patients monitored from start of treatment to 6 hours after intervention) showed that the abciximab group had a lower incidence of two episodes of significant (≥1 mm) ST segment deviation (5% vs. 14%; $p < 0.01$) (*see Circulation* 1998;98:1358).

Comments: In contrast to other studies, patients given abciximab for a substantial period prior to intervention and only briefly afterward had a reduction in events during the 18- to 24-hour interval prior to intervention. Lack of long-term benefits are likely due to lack of 12-hour postintervention infusion.

67. Evaluation in PTCA to Improve Long-term Outcome with Abciximab Glycoprotein IIb/IIIa Blockade (**EPILOG**) investigators. Platelet glycoprotein IIb/IIIa receptor blockade and low-dose heparin during percutaneous coronary revascularization. *N Engl J Med* 1997;336:1689–1696 (editorial pp. 1748–1749).

Design: Prospective, randomized, double-blind, multicenter study. Thirty-day composite primary end point was death, MI, ischemia requiring urgent coronary bypass surgery, or repeat percutaneous coronary revascularization.

Purpose: To determine whether the clinical benefits of abciximab extend to all patients undergoing coronary intervention and to evaluate if hemorrhagic complications are reduced by adjusting heparin dosing.

Population: 2,792 patients undergoing urgent or elective revascularization.

Exclusion Criteria: Acute MI or unstable angina with ECG changes in preceding 24 hours, planned stenting or atherectomy, PCI in prior 3 months, anticoagulant therapy, and major surgery or bleeding in prior 6 weeks.

Treatment: Abciximab [0.25 mg/kg intravenous bolus (10–60 minutes preprocedure) then 0.125 μg/kg/min for 12 hours] plus heparin (100 U/kg bolus), abciximab plus heparin 70 U/kg, or placebo plus heparin 100 U/kg.

Results: Abciximab groups had lower 30 day incidences of death, MI, and urgent revascularization: 5.4% and 5.2% vs.

11.7% (odds ratio 0.45, 0.43; both $p < 0.001$). Fewer large non–Q-wave MIs also were observed (CK five times normal): 2.5% and 2% vs. 5.6% ($p < 0.001$). Similar major bleeding rates were observed, but abciximab plus standard heparin was associated with more minor bleeds [7.4% vs. 4% (low heparin); $p < 0.001$). At 6 months, similar rates of repeat revascularization and a smaller reduction in composite end points were observed (death, MI, and any revascularization): 22.3% and 22.8% vs. 25.8% ($p = 0.04$). One-year follow-up showed persistent benefit in abciximab groups (incidences of primary end points were 9.6% and 9.5% in abciximab plus low-dose heparin and abciximab plus standard heparin groups, respectively, vs. 16.1% in placebo group; *see Circulation* 1999;99:1951).

Comments: In an effort to reduce bleeding rates, sheaths were removed as soon as possible, and no routine postprocedural heparin was administered.

68. Randomized Efficacy Study of Tirofiban for Outcomes and Restenosis (**RESTORE**) Investigators. Effects of platelet GPIIb/IIIa blockade with tirofiban on adverse cardiac events in patients with unstable angina or acute MI undergoing coronary angioplasty. *Circulation* 1997;96:1445–1453.

Design: Prospective, randomized, double-blind, placebo-controlled, multicenter study. Primary composite end point was death, MI, CABG due to failed PTCA or recurrent ischemia, repeat PTCA of target vessel due to ischemia or stenting for actual or threatened abrupt closure.

Purpose: To evaluate the effectiveness of tirofiban in patients undergoing high-risk coronary interventions.

Population: 2,139 patients presenting within 72 hours of onset of symptoms with a 60% stenosis.

Exclusion Criteria: Thrombolytic therapy in prior 24 hours, bleeding disorder, history of stroke, and scheduled stenting or adjunctive rotablation.

Treatment: Tirofiban (10 µg/kg intravenous bolus over 3 minutes then 0.15 µg/kg/min for 36 hours) or placebo. All patients were on aspirin and heparin.

Results: For the initial procedure, PTCA was performed in 92%–93%, atherectomy in 7%–8% of patients. At 30 days, a similar incidence of primary composite end points was observed (10.3% vs. 12.2%; $p = 0.16$). If only urgent/emergent CABG and PTCA are included, the rates are 8% vs. 10.5% ($p = 0.052$). However, the tirofiban group had significantly fewer events at 2 days and 7 days (RR 0.62, $p \leq 0.005$; RR 0.73, $p = 0.022$), mostly due to less reinfarction and repeat PTCA [at 2 days, 2.7% vs. 4.4% ($p = 0.039$) and 1.1% vs. 3.2% ($p = 0.001$); at 7 days, 3.6% vs. 5.3% ($p = 0.055$) and 2.7% vs. 4.4% ($p = 0.034$)]. Similar rates of major bleeding and thrombocytopenia were observed [5.3% vs. 3.7% ($p = 0.096$) and 1.1% vs. 0.9%).

69. Evaluation of Platelet IIb/IIIa Inhibitor for Stenting (**EPIS-TENT**) Investigators. Randomized placebo-controlled and balloon-angioplasty-controlled trial to assess safety of coronary stenting with use of platelet glycoprotein IIb/IIIa blockade. *Lancet* 1998; 352:87–92.

Design: Prospective, randomized, double-blind, placebo-controlled multicenter study. Primary composite end point was death, MI, and urgent revascularization at 30 days.

Purpose: To evaluate the effects of platelet glycoprotein IIb/IIIa blockade with abciximab in conjunction with elective coronary stenting in patients with 60% coronary lesions.

Population: 2,399 patients with ischemic heart disease and suitable coronary artery lesions (e.g., stenosis ≥60%).

Exclusion Criteria: Unprotected left main stenosis, stroke within prior 2 years, PCI in past 3 months, SBP >180 mm Hg, and DBP >100 mm Hg.

Treatment: Stent plus placebo, stent plus abciximab [0.25 mg/kg bolus up to 60 minutes prior to intervention, then 0.125 µg/kg/min (maximum 10 µg/min) for 12 hours], or balloon angioplasty plus abciximab. All patients were given aspirin and heparin (70 U/kg and 100 U/kg boluses in abciximab and placebo groups, respectively). Ticlopidine administration prior to enrollment was encouraged.

Results: Stent plus abciximab group had >50% reduction in 30-day composite end points compared with the stent plus placebo group (5.3% vs. 10.8%; $p < 0.01$), whereas the balloon angioplasty plus abciximab group had a 36% reduction (6.9%; $p = 0.007$). Death and large MIs (defined as CK greater than five times normal) occurred less frequently in the abciximab groups [3.0% and 4.7% vs. 7.8% (placebo)]. However, the rates of Q-wave MI were similar (0.9%–1.5%). No significant differences were seen in major bleeding complications (1.4%–2.2%).

70. **Lincoff AM**, et al. Complementary clinical benefits of coronary-artery stenting and blockade of platelet glycoprotein IIb/IIa receptors. *N Engl J Med* 1999;341:319–327.

This report of the 6 month EPISTENT results demonstrates persistent benefits of stenting in combination with abciximab. The incidence of composite endpoints was 6.4% in the stent plus abciximab group, 9.2% in the angioplasty plus abciximab group, and 12.1% in the stent alone group. The mortality rate with stent plus abciximab was also significantly lower than angioplasty plus abciximab (0.5% vs 1.8%, $p = 0.02$ [stent alone: 1.2%, $p = 0.12$]). This mortality benefit persists at 1 year (71st AHA Scientific Session in Dallas, Texas, November 1998; see Fig. 2–3).

71. Evaluation of Oral Xemilofiban in Controlling Thrombotic Events (**EXCITE**). Preliminary results presented at the 48th ACC Scientific Session in New Orleans, LA, March 1999

This prospective, randomized, multicenter trial was composed of 7,232 patients with stable or unstable angina or MI >24 hours earlier who had undergone successful percutaneous translumi-nal coronary revascularization. Patients received xemilofiban 20 mg 20–90 minutes prior to percutaneous transluminal coronary revascularization (stents placed in ~70%), then 10 or 20 mg three times daily for 6 months or placebo. Of note, CK values were measured routinely in all patients; MI was defined as CK-MB greater than three times the upper limit of normal in the first 24 hours (or twice the upper limit of normal subsequently) or as new Q waves in at least two leads. At 6-month follow-up, the treatment groups had a similar incidence of the primary com-posite end points, consisting of death, MI, and urgent revascu-larization: 9.1% for placebo, 9.3% for xemilofiban 10 mg, and 8.2% for xemilofiban 20 mg [$p = 0.238$ (placebo vs. xemilofiban 20 mg)]. Interestingly, there were significantly fewer events in the xemilofiban 20 mg group at 2 days due to fewer MIs, but this difference disappeared after several days.

Thrombin Inhibitors

72. **Bittl A**, et al. Hirulog Angioplasty Study (**HAS**). Treatment with bivalirudin (hirulog) as compared with heparin during coronary angioplasty for unstable or postinfarction angina. *N Engl J Med* 1995;333:764–769
Design: Prospective, randomized, double-blind, multicenter study. Primary composite end point was death in hospital, MI, abrupt vessel closure, or rapid clinical deterioration of cardiac origin. Follow-up period was 6 months.
Purpose: To evaluate whether bivalirudin is more effective than heparin in reducing mortality and ischemic events in unstable or postinfarction angina patients undergoing angioplasty.
Population: 4,098 patients undergoing coronary angioplasty (PTCA) for unstable angina or postinfarct angina.
Exclusion Criteria: Thrombolysis in prior 24 hours, scheduled percutaneous coronary intervention, and creatinine >3.0 mg/dL.
Treatment: Bivalirudin 1.0 mg/kg bolus, then 2.5 mg/kg/h for 4 hours and 1.0 mg/kg/h for 14–20 hours, or heparin 175 U/kg bolus, then 15 U/kg/h for 18–24 hours. Agents were started immediately before angioplasty and doses adjusted according to activated clotting times. All patients received aspirin (300–325 mg daily).
Results: Overall, the incidence of composite end points was similar in both groups (11.4% vs. 12.2%). Among postinfarction angina patients, bivalirudin was associated with a significant reduction in composite end points (9.1% vs. 14.2%; $p = 0.04$), although at 6 months cumulative rates of death, MI, and repeat revascularization were similar (20.5% vs. 25.1%; $p = 0.1$). Bivalirudin was associated with decreased bleeding (3.8% vs. 9.8%; $p < 0.001$).

Special Situations

Chronic Total Occlusions

Review Article

73. **Puma JA**, et al. Percutaneous revascularization of chronic coronary occlusions: an overview. *J Am Coll Cardiol* 1995;26:1–11.
This review begins by providing definitions and histologic and pathophysiologic findings associated with chronic occlusions. Predictors of success are then discussed in detail. The final two sections cover pharmacologic therapies and use of new devices, including atherectomy and excimer laser angioplasty.

Angioplasty

74. **Stone G**, et al. Procedural outcome of angioplasty for total coronary artery occlusion: an analysis of 971 lesions in 905 patients. *J Am Coll Cardiol* 990;15:849–856.
This retrospective analysis focused on 905 patients with 971 occlusions. Complication rates were 0.8% for death, 0.6% for MI, and 0.8% for urgent bypass surgery. Regarding nonoccluded (690 patients) vs. occluded lesions, the lower angioplasty success rates were 72% vs. 96% ($p = 0.001$) and more complications rates were 3.5% vs. 1.9% ($p = 0.01$).

75. **Ivanhoe RJ**, et al. Percutaneous transluminal coronary angioplasty of chronic total occlusions. *Circulation* 1992;85:106–115.

This retrospective analysis focused on 480 patients treated from 1980 to 1988. Initial success (66%) was associated with fewer MIs and cardiac deaths (7% vs. 11%; $p = 0.0044$) and lower 4-year coronary artery grafting surgery rate (13% vs. 36%; $p < 0.0001$). Predictors of failure included diseased vessels ($p < 0.001$), vessel location (right coronary artery and left circumflex; $p = 0.016$), and absence of distal antegrade filling ($p = 0.00$).

76. **Violaris AG**, et al. Long-term luminal renarrowing after successful elective coronary angioplasty of total occlusion. *Circulation* 1995;91:2140–2150 (editorial pp. 2113–2114).

This analysis focused on 2,930 patients from four prospective restenosis trials, 7% with chronic occlusions. The occluded group had a higher restenosis rate (44.7% vs. 34.0%, RR 1.58; $p < 0.001$), mostly due to more reocclusions (19.2% vs. 5.0%). The occluded group also had more absolute mean luminal diameter loss (0.43 vs. 0.31 mm; $p < 0.001$). The accompanying editorial points out that the occluded group had more prior MIs. Subsequent decreased distal bed flow could lead to slower flow, especially after angioplasty, causing increased reocclusion.

Stenting

77. **Sirnes PA**, et al. Stenting in Chronic Coronary Occlusion (**SICCO**): a randomized, controlled trial of adding stent implantation after successful angioplasty. *J Am Coll Cardiol* 1996;28:1444–1451.

Design: Prospective, randomized, multicenter study. Primary end point was restenosis rate at 6 months.

Purpose: To assess the potential benefit of additional stent implantation after successful angioplasty of a chronic coronary occlusion.

Population: 119 patients undergoing balloon angioplasty of an occluded native coronary artery.

Exclusion Criteria: Indications for stenting (e.g., major dissection), occlusions <2 weeks old, vessel diameter <2.5 mm, and visible thrombus.

Treatment: Stenting (or not) after successful balloon angioplasty.

Results: Stent group had less restenosis at 6 months (32% vs. 74%; $p < 0.001$). At long-term follow-up (33 ± 6 months), the stent group had fewer cardiac events (cardiovascular death, lesion-related acute MI, repeat lesion-related revascularization, or angiographic documentation of reocclusion): 24.1% vs. 59.3%, odds ratio 0.22 ($p = 0.002$; *see J Am Coll Cardiol* 1998;22:305).

78. **Rubatelli P**, et al. Gruppo Italiano di Studio sullo Stent nelle Occlusioni Coronariche (**GISSOC**). Stent implantation vs balloon angioplasty in chronic coronary occlusions: results from the GISSOC trial. *J Am Coll Cardiol* 1998;32:90–96.

This randomized study was composed of 110 patients who underwent successful PTCA of a chronically occluded vessel 3 mm in diameter. Patients were randomized to Palmaz-Schatz stenting and warfarin for 1 month, or to no other therapy. Repeat angiography (at mean 9 months) revealed that the stent group had a larger mean luminal diameter (1.74 vs. 0.85mm; $p < 0.001$), lower restenosis rate (32% vs. 68%; $p < 0.001$), and less reocclusion (8% vs. 34%; $p = 0.003$). The stent group also had less recurrent ischemia (14% vs. 46%; $p = 0.002$) and target lesion revascularization (5.3% vs. 22%; $p = 0.038$), although hospitalization was prolonged.

79. **Buller CE**, et al. Total Occlusion Study of Canada (**TOSCA**) Investigators. Primary stenting versus balloon angioplasty in occluded coronary arteries. *Circulation* 1999;100:236–242.

    This prospective, multicenter, randomized trial of primary stenting (with heparin-coated Palmaz-Schatz stent) vs. balloon angioplasty was composed of 410 patients with symptomatic nonacute total occlusion (TIMI grade 0/1 flow) of native coronary arteries. Randomization occurred after successful placement of a guidewire across the occlusion and was stratified by duration of occlusion (≤6 weeks vs. >6 weeks/unknown). The crossover rate to the stent arm was 10%. The overall incidence of the primary end point, failure of sustained TIMI grade 3 flow at 6 months (confirmed by angiography), was significantly lower in the stent group (10.9% vs. 19.5%; $p = 0.024$). The stent group also had a lower restenosis rate (<50% diameter stenosis; 55% vs. 70%, $p < 0.01$) and less TVR at 6 months (8.4% vs 15.4%, $p = 0.03$).

Saphenous Vein Graft Lesions

Angioplasty

80. **Feyter PJ**, et al. Balloon angioplasty for the treatment of lesions in saphenous vein grafts. *J Am Coll Cardiol* 1993;21:1539–1549.

    This review estimates an initial success rate of 90% and restenosis rate of 42%. The poorest outcomes were seen in patients with chronic total occlusions, diffuse saphenous vein graft disease, and presence of chronic graft thrombus.

Stenting

81. **Piana RN**, et al. Palmaz-Schatz stenting for treatment of focal vein graft stenosis: immediate results and long-term outcome. *J Am Coll Cardiol* 1994;23:1296–1304.

    This retrospective analysis focused on 200 consecutive saphenous vein graft lesions treated with either coronary (n = 146) or biliary (n = 46) stents; a 98.5% procedural success rate was achieved. Complications included one hospital death, one acute thrombosis, and vascular repair in 8.5%. At follow-up angiography (3–6 months), a 17% rate of restenosis was observed. The 2-year revascularization rate (49%) also reflects progressive disease at other sites (stent failure in only 22%).

82. **Wong SC**, et al. Immediate results and late outcomes after stent implantation in saphenous vein graft lesions: the multicenter U.S. Palmaz-Schatz stent experience. *J Am Coll Cardiol* 1995; 26:704–712.

    This analysis focused on 589 stented patients; a 97% procedural success rate was achieved. The anticoagulant regimen used consisted of aspirin 325 mg four times daily and dipyridamole 75 mg three times daily started 24–48 hours prior to the procedure, dextran and heparin during the procedure, then warfarin (target prothrombin [PT] time 16–18 seconds) and dipyridamole for 1 month, and aspirin indefinitely. Stent thrombosis occurred in 1.4% and major vascular or bleeding complications in 14%. The 6-month restenosis rate was 29.7%. Independent predictors included (a) restenotic lesions (46% vs. 18%); (b) small reference size (<3 mm; 47% vs. 26%); (c) history of diabetes; and (d) higher post-stent residual stenosis. Of note, these results compare favorably with those observed in similar patients with PTCA. In CAVEAT II, a 51% restenosis rate was seen with PTCA.

83. **Savage MP**, et al. Saphenous Vein *de novo* (**SAVED**). Stent placement compared with balloon angioplasty for obstructed coronary bypass grafts. *N Engl J Med* 1997;338;740–747.

    Design: Prospective, randomized, multicenter study. Primary end point was restenosis.

    Purpose: To compare stent implantation with balloon angioplasty for the treatment of obstructive disease of venous bypass grafts.

    Population: 220 patients with obstructed coronary bypass grafts.

    Exclusion Criteria: MI in prior 7 days, ejection fraction <25%, diffuse disease that would require more than stents, and presence of thrombus.

    Treatment: Palmaz-Schatz stent or balloon angioplasty.

    Results: Stent group had higher procedural efficacy, defined as residual stenosis <50% without cardiac complications (92% vs. 69%; $p < 0.001$). However, the stent group had more hemorrhagic complications (17% vs. 5%; $p < 0.01$). Restenosis rates were not significantly different [37% (stent group) vs. 46%; $p = 0.24$], but the stent group did have a lower incidence in the composite end points of freedom from death, MI, repeat bypass surgery, and target lesion revascularization (73% vs. 58%; $p = 0.03$).

Other

84. **Braden GA**, et al. Transluminal extraction catheter atherectomy followed by immediate stenting in treatment of saphenous vein grafts. *J Am Coll Cardiol* 1997;30:657–663.

    This observational study evaluated transluminal extraction catheter atherectomy followed by Palmaz-Schatz stenting in 49 consecutive patients with 53 vein grafts >9 years old. The procedural success rate was 98%, with minimal lumen diameter increasing from 1.3 mm at baseline to 3.9 mm after the transluminal extraction catheter–stent procedure. The event-free survival rate to hospital discharge was 90%. At follow-up (mean 13 months), only 26% had experienced one adverse outcome (revascularization rate was 11%, nonfatal MI rate 9%, death rate 11%).

Small Vessels

85. **Elezi S**, et al. Vessel size and long-term outcome after coronary stent placement. *Circulation* 1998;98:1875–1880.

    This retrospective analysis of 2,602 patients who underwent successful stenting showed that small vessel size predisposes to restenosis. Patients were divided into three groups: <2.8 mm, 2.8–3.2 mm, and >3.2 mm vessels. the <2.8 mm group had the lowest 1-year event-free survival (69.5% vs. 77.5% and 81%; $p < 0.001$). Late lumen loss was similar between the three groups, but the <2.8 mm group had a higher angiographic restenosis rate (38.6% vs. 28.4% and 20.4%). The highest restenosis rate (53.5%) was seen in the <2.8 mm patients with diabetes and complex lesions.

86. **Akiyama T**, et al. Angiographic and clinical outcome following coronary stenting of small vessels. *J Am Coll Cardiol* 1998; 32:1610–1618.

    This analysis showed that stenting of small vessels is associated with poorer outcomes. A total of 1,298 consecutive patients with 1,673 lesions were identified; angiographic follow-up was done in 75%. Patients with <3 mm vessels vs. 3 mm showed no difference in procedural success or subacute stent thrombosis rates (95.9% vs. 95.4%; 1.4% vs. 1.5%) but had a higher restenosis rate (32.6% vs. 19.9%; $p < 0.0001$) and a lower rate of event-free survival (63% vs. 71.3%; $p = 0.007$).

Diabetes

87. **Kip KE**, et al. Coronary angioplasty in diabetic patients: the NHLBI PTCA Registry. *Circulation* 1996;94:1818–1825 (editorial pp. 1804–1806).

    In this analysis of the 1985–1986 NHLBI Registry, 281 diabetic and 1,833 nondiabetic patients were studied. The diabetic group was older and had more three-vessel coronary disease, atherosclerotic lesions, and comorbidities. At 9-year follow-up, diabetic patients had a twofold higher mortality rate (35.9% vs. 17.9%) and increased incidences of nonfatal MI (29% vs. 18.5%), CABG surgery (36.7% vs. 27.4%), and repeat PTCA (43.7% vs. 36.5%).

88. **Elezi S**, et al. Diabetes mellitus and the clinical and angiographic outcomes after coronary stent placement. *J Am Coll Cardiol* 1998;32:1866–1873.

    This analysis of 715 patients with diabetes and 2,839 patients without diabetes showed less favorable outcomes in the diabetic group. At 6 months, the incidence of angiographic restenosis and stent vessel occlusion was higher among diabetics (37.5% vs. 28.3%; $p < 0.001$; 5.3% vs. 3.4%; $p = 0.037$). At 1 year, the diabetic group had lower rates of event-free survival and survival free of MI (73.1% vs. 78.5%, $p < 0.001$; 89.9% vs. 94.4%, $p < 0.001$). Multivariate analyses found that diabetes was an independent predictor of adverse clinical events and restenosis.

Complications
Review Article

89. **O'Meara JJ**, Dehmer GJ. Care of the patient and management of complications after percutaneous coronary artery interventions. *Ann Intern Med* 1998;127:458–471.

    This review focused on common postintervention complications, including acute closure and thrombosis, vascular access problems, chest pain, elevated CK levels, contrast-induced nephropathy, and radiation-induced skin injury. The middle section covers management considerations after 48 hours, such as restenosis and functional studies. The concluding section covers issues specific to atherectomy, excimer laser angioplasty, and stents.

Postintervention CK/CK-MB Studies

90. **Klein LW**, et al. Incidence and clinical significance of transient CK elevations and the diagnosis of non—Q wave MI associated with coronary angioplasty. *J Am Coll Cardiol* 1991;17:621–626.

    This prospective analysis of 272 patients undergoing coronary angioplasty (33 excluded because of acute or recent MI) showed that abnormal cardiac enzyme release after successful angioplasty is relatively common. The procedural success rate was 92%. Fifteen patients had a CK level of 200 IU/L and CK-MB 5%, four patients had an elevated CK only, and 19 had only a high CK-MB. The first group had more events than the other groups

(87% vs. 48%; $p < 0.01$) and more events associated with persistent ECG changes ($p = 0.05$) and chest pain ($p < 0.05$).

91. **Abdelmeguid AE**, et al. Defining the appropriate threshold of CK elevation after percutaneous coronary interventions. *Am Heart J* 1996;131:1097–1105.

This analysis focused on 4,664 consecutive patients who underwent successful PTCA or directional atherectomy. CK level was no greater than that of the controls in 4,480 patients, 361–900 IU/L in 123 patients, and >900 IU/L (and CK-MB >4%) in 61 patients. At follow-up (average 3 years), enzyme elevations correlated with increased cardiac death; risk ratio was 2.19 (Kaplan-Meier survival analysis adjusted with Cox proportional hazard regression). No differences were observed in cardiac death and cardiac-related hospitalization between groups 2 and 3.

92. **Abdelmeguid AE**, et al. Significance of mild transient release of CK-MB fraction after percutaneous coronary interventions. *Circulation* 1996;94:1528–1536.

This retrospective analysis focused on 4,484 patients post-PTCA or directional atherectomy. No elevations were detected in 3,776 patients, the CK level was 100–180 IU/L and MB >4% in 450 patients, and CK 181–360 IU/L and MB >4% in 258 patients. CK-MB elevation predictors included atherectomy (odds ratio 4.1) and catheterization laboratory complications (odds ratio 2.6). At 3 years, the group with elevated CK and CK-MB had more MIs (RR 1.3), cardiac deaths (RR 1.3), and ischemic complications (death, MI, revascularization; 48.9% vs. 43.3% vs. 37.3%).

93. **Kong TQ Jr**, et al. Prognostic implication of CK elevation following elective coronary artery interventions. *JAMA* 1997;277: 461–466 (editorial pp. 495–497).

This retrospective cohort study was composed of 253 consecutive patients with CK and CK-MB elevations and 120 patients without CK elevations. The CK elevation group had increased cardiac mortality ($p = 0.02$), highest if more than three times normal (RR 1.05 per 100 U/L CK increase). The effect was independent of procedure type and outcome. Top mortality predictors were peak CK and ejection fraction (both $p < 0.001$).

94. **Tardiff BE**, et al. Clinical outcomes after detection of elevated cardiac enzymes in patients undergoing percutaneous intervention. *J Am Coll Cardiol* 1999;33:88–96.

This analysis of the IMPACT-II database showed that even small elevations in cardiac enzymes are associated with an increased short-term risk of adverse outcomes. No CK-MB elevation was seen in 1,779 patients (76%), whereas levels were elevated to one to three times the upper limit of normal in 323 patients (13.8%), three to five times the upper limit of normal in 3.6%, five to ten times normal in 3.7%, and more than 10 times normal in 2.9%. For all devices, including stents, CK-MB elevations of any magnitude were associated with an increased incidence of the composite end point at 30 days and 6 months (at 6 months normal CK-MB level was 20.2%–27.3%, CK-MB one to three times the upper limit of normal was 29.6%–40.0%). The degree of risk correlated with the rise in enzymes, even for patients who had undergone successful procedures without abrupt closure. As seen in other studies, atherectomy performed in conjunction with angioplasty was associated with a greater incidence of postprocedural CK-MB elevations than was angioplasty alone ($p < 0.0001$).

Stent Thrombosis

95. **Mak KH**, et al. Subacute stent thrombosis: evolving issues and current concepts. *J Am Coll Cardiol* 1996;27:494–503.

This excellent review discusses the advances in stenting technique and antithrombotic regimens that have led to a significant reduction in incidence of subacute stent thrombosis. The importance of antiplatelet therapy is emphasized.

96. **Hasdai D**, et al. Coronary angioplasty and intracoronary thrombolysis are of limited efficacy in resolving early intracoronary stent thrombosis. *J Am Coll Cardiol* 1996;28:361–367 (editorial pp. 368–370).

This retrospective analysis focused on 29 of 1,761 consecutive patients with early (≤30 days) stent thrombosis occurring in 44 stents. Acute MI occurred in 90% of patients, and five patients died (17%). Fourteen patients were treated with balloon angioplasty (PTCA), seven with PTCA and urokinase, and two with urokinase only. Among these treated patients, flow was restored in 48% (6 of 14, 4 of 7, and 1 of 2). The accompanying editorial points out that risk factors for stent thrombosis include emergency use and preexisting thrombus (*see Circulation* 1994; 89:1126).

97. **Moussa I**, et al. Subacute stent thrombosis in the era of intravascular ultrasound-guided coronary stenting without anticoagulation: frequency, predictors and outcome. *J Am Coll Cardiol* 1997; 29:6–12.

This retrospective analysis focused on 1,001 patients with 1,334 lesions. Subacute stent thrombosis occurred in 1.9%. Predictors of subacute stent thrombosis included low ejection fraction ($p = 0.019$), combination of different stents ($p = 0.013$) and postprocedural dissection ($p = 0.014$), and slow flow ($p = 0.0001$).

Other

98. **de Feyter PJ**, et al. Acute coronary artery occlusion during and after percutaneous transluminal coronary angioplasty. *Circulation* 1991;83:927–936.

This retrospective analysis focused on 1,423 consecutive patients who underwent elective coronary angioplasty. Multivariate analysis found three independent predictors of acute coronary occlusion: unstable angina, multivessel disease, and complex lesions. Occlusion was associated with a high incidence of major complications, including MI in 36%.

99. **Lincoff AM**, et al. Abrupt vessel closure complicating coronary angioplasty: clinical, angiographic, and therapeutic profile. *J Am Coll Cardiol* 1992;19:926–935.

This analysis focused on 109 patients (8.3%) who had abrupt vessel closure during 1,319 consecutive angioplasty procedures. Abrupt vessel closure occurred at a median of 27 minutes from the first balloon inflation. Thrombus was visualized in 20% of cases, and dissection was identified in 28%. The incidence of death, emergency coronary bypass surgery, and Q-wave and non—Q-wave MI was 8%, 20%, 9%, and 11%, respectively. Successful reversal of closure (TIMI grade 3 flow and no Q-wave MI, emergent bypass surgery, or death) was achieved in 43% of patients. Multivariate analysis demonstrated prolonged balloon inflation time (odds ratio 5.11; $p = 0.001$) and stenting (odds ratio 4.37; $p = 0.049$) as independent correlates of successful outcome.

100. **Baumbach A**, et al. Acute complications of excimer laser coronary angioplasty: a detailed analysis of multicenter results. *J Am Coll Cardiol* 1994;23:1305–1313.

   In this retrospective analysis of 1,469 patients, 7% had major complications (death, emergent or urgent bypass surgery). ACTs were obtained before, after 10,000-U bolus of heparin, and at the end of the procedure. The group with complications had lower ACTs during and after the procedure: <250 seconds in 61% vs. 27%. Complications were seen in all patients with a final ACT <250 seconds, but only in 0.3% with ACT >300 seconds.

101. **Narins CR**, et al. Relation between activated clotting time during angioplasty and abrupt closure. *Circulation* 1996;93:667–671.

   This study correlated low ACTs with adverse outcomes. The analysis focused on 62 of 1,290 consecutive nonemergent angioplasty patients with in- or out-of-catheterization laboratory closure and 124 matched controls. Abrupt closure patients had a lower initial and minimum ACT (350 vs. 380 seconds; 345 vs. 370 seconds). High ACTs were not associated with more major bleeding complications.

102. **Schaub F**, et al. Management of 219 consecutive cases of postcatheterization pseudoaneurysm. *J Am Coll Cardiol* 1997;30: 670–675.

   This analysis focused on 219 patients with postcatheterization pseudoaneurysm. A compression bandage was reapplied in 132 patients with 32% success [more likely if small (610 mm; 71% vs. 95%) and not anticoagulated (72% vs. 93%)]. Ultrasound-guided compression repair was undertaken in 124 patients (primary treatment modality in 49). The success rate was 84%, higher if preceded by reapplied bandage (89% vs. 76%; $p = 0.04$). Overall, surgical repair was necessary in only 7% of patients.

103. **Piana RN**, et al. Effect of transient abrupt vessel closure during otherwise successful angioplasty for unstable angina on clinical outcome at six months. *J Am Coll Cardiol* 1999;33:73–78 (editorial pp. 79–81).

   This analysis of 4,098 patients undergoing angioplasty in the Hirulog Angioplasty Study (HAS) showed that uncomplicated abrupt vessel closure is a powerful predictor of adverse clinical outcomes following successful angioplasty. Ninety-five percent of patients had a successful procedure without in-hospital death, emergent bypass surgery, or clinical evidence of MI. Multivariate analysis found abrupt vessel closure to be the strongest independent predictor of major adverse cardiac events at 6 months [odds ratio 3.6, 95% confidence interval (CI) 2.5–5.1; $p < 0.001$]. Other predictors included multivessel angioplasty, target lesion in the LAD artery, and diabetes (all $p \leq 0.02$).

Restenosis

Review Articles and Miscellaneous

104. **Dangas G**, Fuster V. Management of restenosis after coronary intervention. *Am Heart J* 1996;132:428–436.

   This review begins with an extensive description of the pathogenesis of restenosis. The largest section describes medical therapies targeted at preventing this process, including potential new molecular therapies.

105. **Frishman WH**, et al. Medical therapies for the prevention of restenosis after coronary interventions. *Curr Probl Cardiol* 1998;23:538–635.

This extensive review covers the definition and pathophysiologic characteristics of restenosis. The largest section discusses the pharmacologic approaches to restenosis, including antiplatelet and antithrombotic agents, anti-inflammatory drugs, lipid-lowering agents, and radiotherapy.

106. **Violaris AG**, et al. Role of angiographically identifiable thrombus on long-term renarrowing after PTCA. *Circulation* 1996;93: 889–897.

This analysis focused on 2,950 patients with 3,583 lesions, 160 with thrombus. Thrombotic lesions were associated with a 45% higher restenosis rate (at 6 months, 43% vs. 34%; $p = 0.01$), mostly due to increased total occlusion rate (13.8% vs. 5.7%; $p < 0.001$).

Balloon Angioplasty

107. **Tardif JC**, et al. for the Multivitamins and Probucol (**MVP**) Study Group. Probucol and multivitamins in the prevention of restenosis after coronary angioplasty. *N Engl J Med* 1997;337:365–372 (editorial pp. 418–419).

Design: Prospective, randomized, double-blind, placebo-controlled, multicenter study. Primary end point was reduction in minimal luminal diameter (MLD).

Purpose: To evaluate whether the antioxidant probucol, multivitamins (vitamins E and C and beta carotene), or the combination reduce restenosis after angioplasty.

Population: 317 patients undergoing elective angioplasty of *de novo* lesion(s) in native coronary vessels.

Exclusion Criteria: MI in prior 7 days and angioplasty in prior 6 months.

Treatment: Probucol 500 mg, multivitamins (vitamin C 500 mg, vitamin E 700 IU, beta carotene 30,000 IU), or both twice daily, started 1 month prior to angioplasty and continued for 6 months after. Twelve hours prior to angioplasty, an extra 1 g of probucol, 2,000 IU of vitamin E, both, or placebo are administered.

Results: Probucol therapy resulted in a significantly smaller mean reduction in luminal diameter: 0.12 vs. 0.22 mm (combined treatment), 0.33 mm (multivitamins), and 0.38 mm (placebo) ($p = 0.006$ for those receiving vs. those not receiving probucol). The probucol group had less restenosis per segment: 20.7% vs. 28.9%, 40.3%, and 38.9% ($p = 0.003$ for probucol vs. no probucol). Probucol also was associated with less repeat angioplasty (11.2% vs. 16.2%, 24.4%, and 26.6%; $p = 0.009$). Of note, high-density lipoproteins decreased by >40% in the probucol group.

Comments: Subsequent retrospective analysis showed that the probucol group had significantly less lumen loss in vessels <3 mm diameter (see *Circulation* 1998;97:429–436; editorial pp. 416–420). It is unclear if 1 month of pretreatment is necessary to achieve benefits and if discontinuation of probucol at 6 months will lead to catch-up phenomenon.

108. **Watanabe K**, et al. Preventive effects of probucol on restenosis after percutaneous transluminal coronary angioplasty. *Am Heart J* 1996;132:23–29.

    In this small trial, 118 patients were randomized to probucol 0.5 mg/day (>7 days before to 3 months after angioplasty) or nothing. The probucol group had a 51% lower restenosis rate (19.7% vs. 39.7%).

109. **Yokoi H**, et al. Probucol Angioplasty Restenosis Trial (**PART**). Effectiveness of an antioxidant in preventing restenosis after percutaneous transluminal coronary angioplasty: the Probucol Angioplasty Restenosis Trial. *J Am Coll Cardiol* 1997;30:855–862.

    This prospective, randomized study of 101 patients showed that probucol started well before elective angioplasty appears to reduce restenosis rates. Patients received probucol 1,000 mg/day or control (no lipid-lowering) therapy starting 4 weeks before angioplasty, and continued until follow-up angiography at 24 weeks. The angiographic restenosis rate was ~60% lower in the probucol group: 23% vs. 58% ($p = 0.001$).

110. **Kosuga K**, et al. Effectiveness of tranilast on restenosis after directional coronary atherectomy. *Am Heart J* 1997;134:712–718.

    This nonrandomized study was composed of 192 patients who underwent successful DCA. After the procedure, 40 patients were given oral tranilast for 3 months and 152 were not. Angiographic follow-up at 3 and 6 months showed that the tranilast patients had a significantly lower minimal luminal diameter (2.08 vs. 1.75 mm, $p = 0.004$; 2.04 vs. 1.70 mm, $p = 0.003$). The restenosis rate at 3 months was >50% lower in the tranilast group (11% vs. 26%; $p = 0.03$). At 1 year, the tranilast group had also experienced fewer clinical events ($p = 0.013$).

111. **Ohsawa H**, et al. Preventive effects of an antiallergic drug, pemirolast potassium, on restenosis after percutaneous transluminal coronary angioplasty. *Am Heart J* 1998;136:1081–1087.

    This prospective, randomized trial was composed of 205 patients with restenosis in native vessels. Patients received pemirolast 20 mg/day starting 1 week before PTCA until 4-month follow-up angiography. Of note, pemirolast has been shown to markedly inhibit migration and proliferation of vascular smooth muscle cells and intimal hyperplasia in animal models. The pemirolast group had a significantly lower restenosis rate (24.0% vs. 46.5% of patients, 18.6% vs. 35.3% of lesions; both $p < 0.01$). At 8-month follow-up, the pemirolast group also had lower incidences of death, MI, bypass surgery, and repeat PTCA (18.3% vs. 36.6%; $p = 0.013$).

Negative Trials

112. **Schwartz L**, et al. Aspirin and dipyridamole in the prevention of restenosis after PTCA. *N Engl J Med* 1988;318:1714–1719.

    Design: Prospective, randomized, double-blind, placebo-controlled, multicenter study.

    Purpose: To determine whether an aspirin–dipyridamole combination reduces the rate of restenosis after successful coronary angioplasty.

    Population: 376 patients undergoing coronary angioplasty.

    Treatment: Aspirin 330 mg/day and dipyridamole 75 mg three times daily (started 24 hours prior to angioplasty), or placebo.

Dipyridamole was given by continuous intravenous infusion (10 mg/h) from 16 hours prior to procedure until 8 hours after. *Results:* Among 249 patients who underwent follow-up angiography, similar restenosis rates [37.7% vs. 38.6% (placebo)] were observed. The drug therapy group did have 77% fewer periprocedural Q-wave MIs (1.6% vs. 6.9%; $p = 0.01$).

113. **Serruys PW**, et al. Coronary Artery Restenosis Prevention on Repeated Thromboxane Antagonism (**CARPORT**). Prevention of restenosis after percutaneous transluminal coronary angioplasty with thromboxane A_2-receptor blockade. *Circulation* 1991;84:1568–1580.
    Design: Prospective, randomized, double-blind, placebo-controlled, parallel-group study. Follow-up period was 6 months.
    Purpose: To evaluate the effectiveness of thromboxane A_2 blockade on restenosis after successful balloon angioplasty.
    Population: 697 patients with successful balloon angioplasty of *de novo* native coronary artery lesion. Follow-up angiography was available in 575 patients.
    Exclusion Criteria: MI in prior 2 weeks, use of platelet-inhibiting or nonsteroidal antiinflammatory agents in prior 7 days, and oral anticoagulation.
    Treatment: Thromboxane A2-receptor antagonist (GR32191B) 80 mg before angioplasty and 40 mg/day for 6 months, or aspirin 250 mg intravenously before angioplasty and placebo for 6 months.
    Results: No significant differences were observed in mean coronary artery diameter (postangioplasty to follow-up angioplasty, –0.31 mm in both groups) or in severity of clinical events between the treatment and placebo groups.

114. **Faxon DP**, et al. Enoxaparin Restenosis after Angioplasty (**ERA**). Low molecular weight heparin in prevention of restenosis after angioplasty. Results of enoxaparin restenosis (ERA) trial. *Circulation* 1994;90:908–914.
    Design: Prospective, randomized, double-blind, placebo-controlled, multicenter study. Primary end point was angiographic or clinical evidence of restenosis.
    Purpose: To evaluate whether treatment with enoxaparin after angioplasty would reduce the restenosis rate.
    Population: 458 patients who underwent successful angioplasty.
    Exclusion Criteria: Abrupt closure after angioplasty, MI in prior 5 days, bleeding diathesis, and history of heparin-associated thrombocytopenia.
    Treatment: Enoxaparin 40 mg subcutaneously once daily for 1 month, or placebo.
    Results: Similar restenosis rates were observed between the two groups [51% (placebo) vs. 52%; $p = 0.63$]. Clinical event rates also were similar, except for minor bleeding, which was more frequent in the enoxaparin group.

115. **Weintraub WS**, et al. Lack of effect of lovastatin on restenosis after coronary angioplasty. *N Engl J Med* 1994;331:1331–1337.
    Design: Prospective, randomized, double-blind, placebo-controlled, multicenter study. Primary end point was degree of stenosis at 6-month angiography.
    Purpose: To determine the effect of aggressive lipid-lowering therapy with lovastatin on restenosis.
    Population: 404 patients undergoing successful elective coronary angioplasty of native coronary vessels.

Exclusion Criteria: Prior coronary angioplasty, recent MI, and total cholesterol <160 or >300 mg/dL.

Treatment: Lovastatin 40 mg twice daily started 7–10 days before angioplasty, or placebo.

Results: A 92% procedural success rate was observed. At 6-month angiography (321 patients), no significant reduction was seen in luminal diameter (preangioplasty, 64% vs. 63%; at 6 months, 44% vs. 46%; $p = 0.50$).

116. **Maresta A**, et al. Studio Trapidil versus Aspirin nella Restenosi Coronarica (**STARC**). Trapidil (triazolopyrimidine), a platelet-derived growth factor antagonist, reduces restenosis after PTCA. *Circulation* 1994;90:2710–2715.

Design: Prospective, randomized, double-blind, comparative study. Primary end point was restenosis at follow-up angiography.

Purpose: To evaluate the effects of trapidil on restenosis after balloon angioplasty.

Population: 254 evaluable patients <75 years of age undergoing coronary angioplasty of *de novo* lesions.

Exclusion Criteria: MI or thrombolytic therapy in prior 2 weeks and total occlusions.

Treatment: Trapidil 300 mg orally every 8 hours or acetylsalicylic acid 100 mg three times daily for 6 months.

Results: Trapidil group had a significantly lower restenosis rate (24.2% vs. 39.7%; $p < 0.01$). Clinical events were similar in the two groups, except that recurrent angina occurred less frequently in the trapidil group (25.8% vs. 43.7%).

117. Multicenter American Research with Cilazapril after Angioplasty to Prevent Transluminal Obstruction and Restenosis (**MARCATOR**). Effect of high-dose ACE inhibition on restenosis: final results of MARCATOR study, a multicenter, double-blind, placebo-controlled trial of cilazapril. *J Am Coll Cardiol* 1995;25: 362–369.

Design: Prospective, randomized, double-blind, multicenter study. Primary end point was change in minimal lumen diameter by quantitative angiography.

Purpose: To evaluate the effect of low- and high-dose inhibition with cilazapril on restenosis after coronary angioplasty.

Population: 1,436 patients 25–80 years of age undergoing coronary angioplasty.

Exclusion Criteria: MI in prior 5 days and prior coronary revascularization.

Treatment: Cilazapril 1.0 or 2.5 mg after angioplasty then 1, 5, or 10 mg twice daily for 6 months, or placebo. All patients received aspirin.

Results: No significant difference was observed between any groups regarding post-PTCA vs. follow-up angiography minimal lumen diameter changes (range −0.35 to −0.45 mm). Predictors of lumen loss included angina <6 months, history of MI, diameter pre- and post-PTCA, and proximal lesion location (traditional atherosclerosis risk factors did not correlate).

Comments: A similar study of 693 patients enrolled at European sites (MERCATOR) showed no significant differences in minimal luminal diameter and major events at 6 months between cilazapril and placebo groups (*see Circulation* 1992;86:100).

118. **Serruys PW**, et al. The **HELVETICA** Investigators. A comparison of hirudin with heparin in the prevention of restenosis after coronary angioplasty. *N Engl J Med* 1995;333:757–763.
Design: Prospective, randomized, double-blind, multicenter study. Primary end point was event-free survival at 30 weeks. Secondary end point was minimal luminal diameter at 6-month angiography.
Purpose: To evaluate whether hirudin compared with heparin reduced the frequency of restenosis in patients undergoing coronary angioplasty.
Population: 1,141 unstable angina patients.
Exclusion Criteria: Stable angina, planned multistage coronary intervention, and MI in prior 2 weeks.
Treatment: Group 1. Heparin 10,000-U bolus, continuous infusion for 24 hours, then subcutaneous placebo twice daily for 3 days. Group 2. Hirudin 40 mg, intravenous infusion for 24 hours, then subcutaneous placebo twice daily for 3 days. Group 3. Same as group 2, except hirudin 40 mg subcutaneously twice daily for 3 days.
Results: Hirudin-treated patients had decreased early (96-hour) cardiac events (7.9% and 5.6% vs. 11%), but no significant differences were seen in event-free survival at 7 months (67.3%, 63.5%, 68%).

119. Subcutaneous Heparin and Angioplasty Restenosis Prevention Trial (**SHARP**). The SHARP trial: results of a multicenter randomized trial investigating the effects of high dose unfractionated heparin on angiographic restenosis and clinical outcome. *J Am Coll Cardiol* 1995;26:947–954.
Design: Prospective, randomized, parallel-group, open-label, multicenter study. Primary end point was change in minimal lumen diameter at follow-up angiography.
Purpose: To determine whether high-dose subcutaneous heparin after balloon angioplasty reduces restenosis and clinical events/
Population: 339 patients who had undergone successful coronary angioplasty of *de novo* lesions.
Exclusion Criteria: Chronic occlusion.
Treatment: Heparin 12,500 U subcutaneously twice daily for 4 months, or no treatment. All patients received aspirin.
Results: No significant differences were observed between treatment groups in change in mean lumen diameter as assessed by immediate postangioplasty and follow-up (mean 4.2 months) angiography. Incidence of clinical events and angina at 4 months were also similar.

120. **Savage MP**, et al. for the Multi-Hospital Eastern Atlantic Restenosis Trial (**M-HEART II**) Study Group. Effect of thromboxane A_2 blockade on clinical outcome and restenosis after coronary angioplasty. *Circulation* 1995;92:3194–3200.
Design: Prospective, randomized, double-blind, placebo-controlled, multicenter study. 6-month primary composite end points were death, MI, and restenosis associated with recurrent angina or need for revascularization.
Purpose: To determine whether aspirin or sulotroban improves clinical outcomes and reduces restenosis after coronary angioplasty.

Population: 752 patients undergoing elective angioplasty of 60% restenosis

Exclusion Criteria: Q-wave MI or thrombolytic therapy within 3 days of angioplasty and increased bleeding risk.

Treatment: Aspirin 325 mg once daily, sulotroban 800 mg four times daily, or placebo, started 1–6 hours before PTCA and continued for 6 months.

Results: Aspirin group had significant reduction in composite end points [30.2% vs. 44.0% (sulotroban), $p = 0.006$; 30.2% vs. 40.6% (placebo), $p = 0.046$]. The aspirin group had fewer MIs than the placebo group (1.2% vs. 5.7%; $p = 0.03$). The aspirin group also had less angiographic restenosis (by lesion) than did the sulotroban group (39% vs. 53%; $p = 0.006$).

121. **Cairns JA**, et al. Enoxaparin MaxEPA Prevention of Angioplasty Restenosis (**EMPAR**). Fish oils and low-molecular-weight heparin for the reduction of restenosis after percutaneous transluminal coronary angioplasty. *Circulation* 1996;94:1553–1560.

Design: Prospective, randomized, partially open, 2×2 factorial, multicenter study. Primary end point was restenosis at follow-up angiography (18 ± 2 weeks).

Purpose: To evaluate the effects of both enoxaparin and omega-3 polyunsaturated fatty acid (maxEPA) on restenosis after balloon angioplasty.

Population: 814 patients undergoing elective angioplasty of *de novo* lesions in native coronary vessels.

Exclusion Criteria: MI in prior 4 weeks, unstable angina necessitating angioplasty in <48 hours, and increased bleeding risk.

Treatment: maxEPA 18 capsules/day (5.4 g n-3 fatty acids) or placebo started a median 6 days before angioplasty and continued for 18 weeks. After sheath removal, 653 patients had one successfully dilated lesion randomized to enoxaparin 30 mg subcutaneously twice daily or control (no treatment) for 6 months.

Results: No significant differences were observed in restenosis rates per patient and per lesion (fish oils, 46.5% vs. 39.7%; placebo, 44.7% vs. 38.7%; enoxaparin, 45.8% vs. 38.0%; control, 45.4% vs. 40.4%). Incidence of ischemic events was similar in all four groups.

122. **Karsch KR**, et al. Reduction of Restenosis after PTCA, Early Administration of Reviparin in a Double-blind, Unfractionated Heparin and Placebo-controlled Evaluation (**REDUCE**). Low-molecular weight heparin (reviparin) in percutaneous transluminal coronary angioplasty. *J Am Coll Cardiol* 1996;28: 1437–1443.

Design: Prospective, randomized, double-blind, multicenter study. Primary end point was death, MI, reintervention, and coronary artery bypass surgery.

Purpose: To evaluate whether reviparin is more effective than unfractionated heparin or placebo in reducing the incidence of restenosis after angioplasty.

Population: 625 stable or unstable angina patients with single lesions suitable for elective coronary angioplasty.

Exclusion Criteria: MI in prior 2 weeks, history of heparin-associated thrombocytopenia, and bleeding disorders.

Treatment: Reviparin 7,000 U before angioplasty, followed by 10,500 U over 24 hours, then 3,500 U twice daily for 28 days, or heparin 10,000 U over 24 hours then placebo subcutaneously.

Results: At 30 weeks, the treatment groups had similar incidences of composite end points [33.3% (reviparin) vs. 32%], loss of lumen diameter, or bleeding. The reviparin group had fewer acute events (3.9% vs. 8.2%; $p < 0.03$).

123. **Lablanche J-M**, et al. Angioplastie Coronaire Corvasal Diltiazem (**ACCORD**). Effect of the direct nitric oxide donors linsidomine and molsidomine on angiographic restenosis after coronary balloon angioplasty. *Circulation* 1997;95:83–89.

This prospective, randomized, multicenter trial was composed of 700 patients. Patients were randomized 12–24 hours prior to angioplasty to linsidomine infusion followed by oral molsidomine or oral diltiazem 60 mg three times daily for 6 months. The nitric oxide donor group had a better mean luminal diameter (initial, 1.94 vs. 1.81 mm, $p = 0.001$; 3 months, 1.54 vs. 1.38, $p = 0.007$) and lower restenosis rate (38% vs. 46.5%; $p = 0.026$). However, no significant differences in major clinical events were observed (32.2% vs. 32.4%).

124. **Bertrand ME**, et al. Prevention of Restenosis by Elisor after Transluminal Coronary Angioplasty Trial (**PREDICT**). Effect of pravastatin on angiographic restenosis after coronary balloon angioplasty. *J Am Coll Cardiol* 1997;30:863–869.

Design: Prospective, randomized, double-blind, placebo-controlled, multicenter study. Primary end point was minimal lumen diameter at follow-up angiography.

Purpose: To determine whether treatment with pravastatin could reduce restenosis after balloon angioplasty.

Population: 695 patients 25–75 years of age with total cholesterol 200–310 mg/dL undergoing elective angioplasty.

Exclusion Criteria: MI in past 15 days and prior angioplasty or coronary bypass graft surgery of target vessel.

Treatment: Pravastatin 40 mg/day or placebo for 6 months.

Results: No significant difference was observed in mean lumen diameter between the two groups [1.54 mm (pravastatin) vs. 1.54 mm; $p = 0.21$). Late loss and net gain did not differ significantly between groups. Restenosis rates (defined as >50% restenosis) were also similar [39.2% (pravastatin) vs. 43.8%; $p = 0.26$].

125. **Lablanche J-M**, et al. Fraxiparine Angioplastie Coronaire Transluminale (**FACT**). Effect of nadroparin, a low-molecular-weight heparin, on clinical and angiographic restenosis after coronary balloon angioplasty. *Circulation* 1997;96:3396–3402.

Design: Prospective, randomized, double-blind, placebo-controlled, multicenter study. Primary end point was restenosis at 3-month angiography.

Purpose: To evaluate the effect of nadroparin, a low-molecular-weight heparin, on angiographic restenosis after balloon angioplasty.

Population: 354 patients ≤ 75 years of age undergoing elective angioplasty of *de novo* lesions.

Exclusion Criteria: Chronic total occlusion, MI in prior 3 weeks, and increased bleeding risk.

Treatment: Daily subcutaneous nadroparin (0.6 mL of 10,250 anti-Xa IU/mL) or placebo injections started 3 days before angioplasty and continued for 3 months.

Results: No significant differences in mean lumen diameter and mean residual stenosis (1.37 vs. 1.48 mm; 51.9% vs. 48.8%) or in incidence of major cardiac events were observed between the nadroparin and placebo groups.

126. Coronary Angioplasty Restenosis Trial (**CART**). n-3 fatty acids do not prevent restenosis after coronary angioplasty: results from the CART study. *J Am Coll Cardiol* 1999;33:1619–1626.
Design: Prospective, randomized, double-blind, placebo-controlled study.
Purpose: To evaluate the effect of dietary supplementation of n-3 fatty acids on restenosis after coronary angioplasty.
Population: 500 patients undergoing elective coronary angioplasty.
Exclusion Criteria (Angiographic): Diffuse lesions (>2 cm long), excessive tortuosity of proximal segment, and chronic (>3 months) total occlusions.
Treatment: n-3 fatty acids 5.1 g/day or corn oil (placebo) starting at least 2 weeks prior to and continued for 6 months after angioplasty.
Results: Similar restenosis rates were observed in the two groups (restenosis defined as minimal luminal diameter <40% of the reference diameter): 40.6% in the n-3 fatty acid group and 35.4% in the placebo group ($p = 0.21$).

127. **Gimple LW**, et al. Usefulness of subcutaneous low molecular weight heparin (ardeparin) for reduction of restenosis after percutaneous transluminal coronary angioplasty. *Am J Cardiol* 1999;83:1524–1529.
Design: Prospective, randomized, double-blind, placebo-controlled, multicenter study. Primary end point was angiographic restenosis at 3–5 months.
Purpose: To evaluate whether low-molecular-weight heparin reduces angiographic restenosis after successful balloon angioplasty (PTCA).
Population: 565 patients >25 years of age who had undergone successful PTCA of one or two *de novo* lesions.
Treatment: Ardeparin subcutaneously twice daily (50 or 100 antiXa µ/kg) or placebo for 3 months.
Results: Ardeparin had no effect on the incidence of angiographic restenosis (41.5% vs 42.1%).

128. Nisoldipine in Coronary Disease in Leuven (**NICOLE**). Preliminary results presented at the 20th Congress of the European Society of Cardiology in Vienna, Austria, August 1998.
This single-center, placebo-controlled trial of the calcium-channel blocker nisoldipine was composed of 826 patients who underwent successful intervention in native coronary arteries. Patients were randomized to nisoldipine (20 mg/day for 2 weeks then 40 mg/day for 3 years), or placebo. At 6 months, there was no significant difference between groups in minimum lumen diameter, initial gain, late loss, or diameter stenosis.

Stenting and Atherectomy

129. **Moussa I**, et al. Coronary stenting after rotational atherectomy in calcified and complex lesions. *Circulation* 1997;96:128–136.
This study of 75 consecutive patients with 106 lesions showed that stenting after rotablation in calcified and complex lesions can be performed with high success rates and minimal procedural complications and can result in a low restenosis rate. Intravascular ultrasound-guided stent placement was used, and

the procedural success rate was 93.4%. Acute stent thrombosis occurred in two patients (1.9%), and subacute stent thrombosis occurred in one patient (0.9%). Angiographic follow-up at 4.6 ± 1.9 months showed a restenosis rate of 27.5%. Clinical follow-up at 6.4 ± 3 months found that 18% had undergone target lesion revascularization.

130. **Kastrati A**, et al. Restenosis after coronary stent placement and randomized to a 4-week combined antiplatelet or anticoagulant therapy. *Circulation* 1997;96:462–467 (editorial pp. 383–385).

This analysis of 432 ISAR patients who underwent 6-month angiography showed no favorable effects on restenosis in patients receiving an antiplatelet regimen. Antiplatelet versus anticoagulant therapy showed no significant differences in restenosis rate (26.8% vs. 28.9%), mean luminal diameter (1.95 vs. 1.90 mm), late lumen loss (1.10 vs. 1.15 mm), or TVR (14.6% vs. 15.6%). The accompanying editorial points out that this analysis was poorly powered to detect a restenosis difference. This trial also did not address the potential impact on restenosis of long-term anti-platelet therapy (>1 month).

131. **Erbel R**, et al. Coronary-artery stenting compared with balloon angioplasty for restenosis after initial balloon angioplasty. *N Engl J Med* 1998;339:1672–1678.

Design: Prospective, randomized, multicenter study. Primary end point was angiographic evidence of restenosis at 6 months.

Purpose: To determine whether coronary stenting, as compared with balloon angioplasty, reduces restenosis after prior successful balloon angioplasty.

Population: 383 patients with clinical and angiographic evidence of restenosis after successful balloon angioplasty.

Treatment: Standard balloon angioplasty or Palmaz-Schatz stent implantation; crossover to stenting was allowed if symptomatic dissection occurred that could not be managed by repeated balloon inflations.

Results: Stent group had a significantly lower restenosis rate (18% vs. 32%; $p = 0.03$) and less TVR (10% vs. 27%; $p = 0.001$). The difference resulted from smaller mean luminal diameter in angioplasty (1.85 vs. 2.04 mm; $p = 0.01$). The stent group had better event-free survival at 250 days (84% vs. 72%; $p = 0.04$), but there was a nonsignificant increase in death and MI (at 6 months, 5.6% vs. 2.3%). Subacute thrombosis occurred more frequently in the stent group (3.9% vs. 0.6%).

Comments: These results are consistent with prior studies (26–29) that have shown a reduction in TVR but an excess of the hard end points of death and MI.

132. **Mahdi NA**, et al. Directional coronary atherectomy for the treatment of Palmaz-Schatz in-stent restenosis. *Am J Cardiol* 1998;82:1345–1351.

This single-center experience in 45 patients with 46 lesions found that DCA resulted in a large postprocedural lumen diameter (2.7 ± 0.7 mm, 17% residual stenosis), low rate of TVR (28.3% at 10 ± 4.6 months), and few major clinical events (non–Q-wave MI in 9%; no Q-wave MIs or emergent bypass surgery).

133. **LeMay MR**, et al. Predictors of long-term outcome after stent implantation in a saphenous vein graft. *Am J Cardiol* 1999; 83:681–686.

This analysis was performed on 18 month follow-up data from 106 patients who had 128 stents placed in saphenous vein grafts. A high initial procedural success rate was observed (98.1%), but event-free survival, defined as freedom from death, MI, repeat bypass surgery, and repeat PCI, was seen in only 44%. A Cox proportional hazards model found predictors of survival were the absence of a high-profile lesion in any nonstented patent graft ($p = 0.004$) and the use of lipid-lowering agents at follow-up ($p = 0.01$).

134. Evaluation of Reopro and Stenting to Eliminate Restenosis (**ERASER**) Investigators. Acute platelet inhibition with abciximab does not reduce in-stent restenosis. *Circulation* 1999;100: 799–806.

     This prospective, multicenter, double-blind, placebo-controlled trial randomized 225 patients undergoing primary stent implantation to abciximab (12- or 24-hour infusion) or placebo. Target lesions were *de novo* 60% stenoses in native coronary arteries with a diameter of 3.0–3.5 mm. At 6-month follow-up, there were no significant differences between groups in in-stent volume obstruction (primary end point).

Radiation

135. **Teirstein PS**, et al. Scripps Coronary Radiation to Inhibit Proliferation Post-Stenting (**SCRIPPS**). Catheter-based radiotherapy to inhibit restenosis after coronary stenting. *N Engl J Med* 1997;336:1697–1703 (editorial pp. 1748–1749).

     This small study showed promising results with a gamma radiation source. Fifty-five patients with restenosis (in-stent, 62%) were randomized to ^{192}Ir (20- to 45-minute exposure, dose of 800–3,000 cGy) or placebo. Of note, the iridium group had less diabetes mellitus. Angiographic follow-up in 53 patients at 6.7 ± 2.2 months showed that the iridium group had a larger mean luminal diameter (2.43 vs. 1.85 mm; $p = 0.02$) and an impressive 69% lower restenosis rate (17% vs. 54%; $p = 0.01$). No apparent complications were seen with iridium use, although long-term follow-up is necessary. At 2-year follow-up (*see Circulation* 1999;99:243), the incidence of death, MI, or target lesion revascularization was 55% lower in the radiation group (23.1% vs. 51.7%; $p = 0.03$). Most of this benefit was due to a 75% lower target lesion revascularization rate (15.4% vs. 44.8%; $p < 0.001$).

136. **King SB III**, et al. Beta Energy Restenosis Trial (**BERT**). Endovascular beta-radiation to reduce restenosis after coronary balloon angioplasty. *Circulation* 1998;97:2025–2030.

     This small study (23 patients) demonstrated the safety and feasibility of beta-radiation after angioplasty. A ^{90}Sr/Y source was used to deliver 12, 14, or 16 Gy at 2 mm. Source delivery was successful in 21 of 23 patients (91%). No in-hospital morbidity or mortality occurred, and follow-up angiography in 20 patients showed a late lumen loss of only 0.5 mm and restenosis in 15%. A larger, randomized, double-blind study is ongoing. Subsequent 6-month follow-up data on 64 patients showed an overall restenosis rate of 14% (20% in the 12-Gy group and 11% in the 14- and 16-Gy groups).

137. Washington Radiation for In-Stent Restenosis Trial (**WRIST**). Preliminary results presented at 71st AHA Scientific Session in Dallas, TX, November 1998.

A total of 130 patients with in-stent restenosis in native coronary arteries (n = 100) and saphenous vein grafts (n = 30) were randomized to catheter-delivered gamma-radiation (^{192}Ir source, mean dwell time 22 minutes) or placebo. At 6 months, the radiation therapy group had a significant reduction in the primary composite end points of death, MI, and TVR, including a marked 41.5% absolute reduction in TVR (26.2% vs. 57.7%). Angiographic restenosis was significantly reduced in the radiation group (16% vs. 48%), especially among diabetic patients (13.8% vs. 63.1%).

138. Beta Washington Radiation for In-Stent Restenosis Trial (**BETA-WRIST**). Preliminary results.

This open-label registry study was composed of 49 consecutive patients with in-stent restenosis in native vessels 2.5–4.0 mm in diameter and lesion length <47 mm. Exclusion criteria included MI within the preceding 72 hours and ejection fraction <20%. An yttrium source was used; delivery device dwell time was 182 seconds. After controlling for lesion length, patients who received radiation had a significantly lower restenosis rate: 32.7% vs. 67.8% ($p = 0.001$).

139. **GAMMA-1.** Preliminary results presented at the 48th ACC Scientific Session in New Orleans, LA, March 1999.

This prospective, randomized, double-blind, multicenter trial was composed of 252 patients with 60% restenosis of stented native vessels 2.75–4 mm in diameter and lesion length ≤45 mm. Exclusion criteria included MI in prior 72 hours, visible thrombus, ejection fraction <40%, and anticipated abciximab administration (actual use <10%). Most treated lesions (>70%) were complex (type B2 or C). An ^{192}Ir radiation source was used (6, 10, or 14 seeds). Lesions were irradiated with 800–3,000 cGy; delivery device dwell time was ~20 minutes. The radiation group had a 58% lower stent restenosis rate ($p < 0.001$). Treatment of long lesions with this radiation source is being examined in the GAMMA-2 and Long-WRIST trials.

Other

140. **Belle EV**, et al. Restenosis rates in diabetic patients. *Circulation* 1997;96:1454–1460 (editorial pp. 1374–1377).

This retrospective analysis showed an increased risk of restenosis among diabetic patients undergoing balloon angioplasty but not stenting. A total of 300 stented patients (single native vessel procedure, no high-pressure balloon inflation; 19% diabetics) and 300 balloon angioplasty (PTCA) patients were analyzed. The PTCA group had a nearly twofold higher restenosis rate (63% vs. 36%; $p = 0.0002$), whereas among stented patients, diabetics and nondiabetics had a similar rate of restenosis (25% vs. 27%) as well as similar late loss and occlusion rates. The accompanying editorial points out that these findings suggest that vascular remodeling (vs. neointimal proliferation) drives the excess in post-PTCA restenosis in diabetics. However, these findings contradict those of other studies that have shown no special benefit with stenting in diabetics: [*see* Carrozza JP, et al. *Ann Intern Med* 1993;118:344, restenosis in 55% (diabetics) vs. 20%; *see* Elezi S, et al. *JACC* 1997;29:188A, 40% vs. 24%; *see* Yokoi H, et al. *JACC* 1997;29:455A, 29% vs. 23%]. One possible explanation for the differences in results between this and other studies is that the lack of high-pressure balloon inflation in this stented population led to less vessel damage and subsequently less intimal proliferation (the latter may be especially important in the restenotic process in diabetics).

CABG Surgery

Review Articles, Meta-Analyses

141. **Kirklin JW**, et al. ACC/AHA Guidelines. Guidelines and indications for coronary artery bypass graft surgery; a report of the ACC/AHA Task Force on Assessment of Diagnostic and Therapeutic Cardiovascular Procedures (Subcommittee on CABG Surgery). *J Am Coll Cardiol* 1991;17:543–589.

142. **Yusuf S**, et al. Effect of coronary artery bypass graft surgery on survival: overview of 10-year results from randomised trials by the CABG Trialists Collaboration. *Lancet* 1994;344:563–570.
    This review of data focuses on 1,324 patients assigned to CABG surgery and 1,325 patients who received medical management. The CABG group had a significantly lower mortality rate at 5 years (10.2% vs. 15.8%, odds ratio 0.61; $p = 0.0001$), 7 years (15.8% vs. 21.7%, odds ratio 0.68; $p < 0.001$), and 10 years (26.4% vs. 30.5%, odds ratio 0.83; $p = 0.03$). The risk reduction was most marked in patients with left main CAD and three-vessel disease or one- or two-vessel disease [odds ratios 0.32, 0.58 vs. 0.77 (two- and one-vessel disease)]. High-risk patients (defined as those with two of following: severe angina, history of hypertension, prior MI, and ST segment depression at rest) had a 29% mortality reduction at 10 years compared with a 10% reduction in patients at moderate risk and a nonsignificant trend toward higher mortality in low-risk patients [no risk factors (except ST depression allowed)].

143. **Nwasokwa ON**. Coronary artery bypass graft disease. *Ann Intern Med* 1995;123:528–545.
    This thorough review of the literature showed only an ~50% patency of saphenous vein grafts at 10 years after bypass surgery versus >90% patency achieved with IMA grafts. The use of IMA grafts leads to less frequent symptoms, better left ventricular function, decreased need for reoperation, and improved survival. The role of antiplatelet agents in decreasing graft occlusion rates is also reviewed.

144. **Pocock SJ**, et al. Meta-analysis of randomised trials comparing coronary angioplasty with bypass surgery. *Lancet* 1996; 346:1184–1189.
    This analysis of data was derived from 3,771 patients in eight trials (CABRI, RITA, EAST, GABI, MASS, ERACI, Toulouse, Lausanne). The average follow-up period was 2.7 years. No differences were demonstrated in overall cardiac mortality between PTCA and CABG. However, CABG patients had 90% fewer first year reinterventions (3.3% vs. 33.7%) and less angina. A CABG was performed in 18% of PTCA patients within 1 year. Importantly, the impact of longer follow-up is unknown (e.g., increased saphenous venous graft disease).

145. **Roach G**, et al. Adverse cerebral outcomes after coronary bypass surgery. *N Engl J Med* 1996;335:1857–1863.
    This prospective study was composed of 2,108 patients, 6.1% with cerebral events: type I 3.1% (focal injury, or stupor or coma

at hospital discharge (D/C); 55 of 66 had nonfatal strokes) or type II 3% (deterioration in intellectual function, memory deficit, or seizures). Events were associated with increased in-hospital mortality [21% (type I) and 10% vs. 2%], longer hospital stay (25 days, 21 days, 10 days), and more patients discharged to intermediate or long-term care (47%, 30%, 8%). Type I predictors included proximal aortic atherosclerosis, history of neurologic disease, and age; type II predictors included age, hypertension, pulmonary disease, and alcohol consumption.

Studies

CABG vs Medical Therapy

146. European Coronary Surgery Study (**ECSS**) Group. Long-term results of prospective randomised study of coronary artery bypass surgery in stable angina pectoris. *Lancet* 1982;320:1173–1180.
     Design: Prospective, randomized, open study. Primary end point was all-cause mortality. Follow-up period was 5–8 years.
     Purpose: To compare coronary bypass surgery with initial medical management in patients with angina and multivessel CAD.
     Population: 768 men ≤65 years of age with mild to moderate angina, ≥50% stenosis in two major vessels, and good left ventricular function.
     Treatment: CABG surgery or medical therapy.
     Results: Surgery was beneficial in the total population (88.6% survival vs. 79.9% at 8 years), although most of the benefit was seen in patients with proximal LAD artery stenoses (10-year survival, 76% vs. 66%). No benefit was present if left main disease was present. Independent predictors of surgical benefit were abnormal rest ECG, ST-depression 1.5 mm with exercise, peripheral vascular disease, and increased age.

147. Coronary Artery Surgery Study (**CASS**) Principal Investigators and their associates. Myocardial infarction and mortality in the CASS randomized trial. *N Engl J Med* 1984;310:750–758.
     Design: Prospective, randomized, open, parallel-group study. Primary end point was all-cause mortality. Mean follow-up period was 6 years.
     Purpose: To determine whether coronary bypass surgery reduces mortality and MI rates in patients with mild angina and angiographically documented CAD.
     Population: 780 patients ≤65 years of age with coronary artery stenosis ≥70%.
     Treatment: CABG surgery or medical therapy.
     Results: Lower mortality trend was observed with CABG (1.1%/yr vs. 1.6%/yr), strongest in patients with ejection fraction ≤50% ($p = 0.085$) and three-vessel disease and ejection fraction ≤50% ($p = 0.063$). Among patients with three-vessel disease and ejection fraction of 35%–49%, there was a significant mortality difference at subsequent follow-up [12% (CABG) vs. 35% mortality, $p = 0.009$; *see N Engl J Med* 1985;312:1665). At 10-year follow-up (*see Circulation* 1990;82:1629), CABG had been performed in 40% of medical patients, and there was still no overall survival difference (medical group 79%, surgical group 82%). However, the results of CABG were significantly better than medical therapy in patients with an ejection fraction <50% (79% vs. 61%; $p = 0.01$).
     Comments: Long-term follow-up in 912 patients with left main equivalent disease (e.g., severe proximal left anterior descending

and left circumflex disease) showed that surgery prolongs life (13.1 vs. 6.2 years), but not if normal left ventricular function is present (15 year survival, 63% vs. 54%; p = NS), even with right coronary artery stenosis ≥70% (see *Circulation* 1995;91:2335).

148. **VA** Coronary Artery Bypass Surgery Cooperative Study Group. Eleven year survival in Veterans Affairs randomized trial of coronary bypass surgery for stable angina. *N Engl J Med* 1984; 311:1333–1339.

Design: Prospective, randomized, multicenter, open study. Primary end point was all-cause mortality. Average follow-up was 11.2 years.

Purpose: To compare bypass surgery (CABG) with medical therapy in patients with stable angina.

Population: 686 patients with stable angina pectoris of >6 months' duration.

Exclusion Criteria: MI in prior 6 months, unstable angina, DBP >100 mm Hg, uncompensated congestive heart failure.

Treatment: CABG surgery or medical therapy.

Results: Overall, a significant mortality difference was observed between groups at 7 years (77% survival in CABG group vs. 70%; p = 0.043) but not at 11 years (57% vs. 58%). Surgery was beneficial in the following subgroups: (a) three-vessel disease plus left ventricular dysfunction (per angiography), 50% vs. 38% survival at 11 years (p = 0.026); (b) clinically high-risk patients (at least two of the following: resting ST depression, history of MI, history of hypertension), 49% vs. 36% survival (p = 0.015); and (c) combined angiographic and clinically high risk, 54% vs. 24% (p = 0.005). Patients with left ventricular dysfunction (ejection fraction <45%, end-diastolic pressure >14 mm Hg, or any contraction abnormality) benefited from surgery at 7 years (survival 74% vs. 63%; p = 0.049) but not at 11 years (53% vs. 49%).

Comments: Subsequent 18-year follow-up report showed no benefit of surgery, even in the high-risk subgroups. Overall, the benefits of surgery began to diminish after 5 years, a time course that parallels the development of graft disease.

149. **Luchi RJ**, et al., **VA Cooperative Study 28**. Comparison of medical and surgical therapy for unstable angina pectoris. *N Engl J Med* 1987;316:977–984.

Design: Prospective, randomized, multicenter study.

Purpose: To compare CABG with medical therapy in patients with unstable angina.

Population: 468 men <70 years of age with unstable angina (MI excluded by serial ECG and serum CK measurements).

Treatment: CABG plus medical therapy or medical therapy alone.

Exclusion Criteria: MI in prior 3 months, no unstable angina in 10 days prior to admission, and prior operation for angina.

Results: Surgical group had 4.1% operative mortality (defined as death occurring within 30 days after surgery) and 75% 1-year graft patency. There was no difference in all-cause mortality rates between the CABG and medical therapy groups; however, mortality at 2 years was lower with CABG among patients with an ejection fraction of 30% to 59% (p = 0.01). Similar nonfatal MI rates were observed [11.7% (most perioperative) vs. 12.2%].

CABG Surgery vs PTCA

150. Coronary angioplasty vs coronary artery bypass surgery: the Randomised Intervention Treatment of Angina (**RITA**) trial. *Lancet* 1993;341:573–580.

Design: Prospective, randomized, multicenter study. Primary end point was death and MI. Mean follow-up period was 2.5 years.

Purpose: To compare bypass surgery with coronary angioplasty in patients in whom equivalent myocardial revascularization could be achieved by either treatment method.

Population: 1,011 patients with multivessel coronary disease (55% with at least two diseases of the coronary arteries).

Exclusion Criteria: Left main disease, prior coronary angioplasty or bypass surgery, and significant valve disease.

Treatment: CABG surgery or PTCA.

Results: No difference was observed in the primary composite end point of death or MI at 5 years (8.6% vs. 9.8%, RR 0.88, 95% CI 0.59–1.29). CABG patients had a longer recovery but fewer additional measures. At 2 years, repeat angiography was performed in 7% vs. 31% ($p < 0.001$) and revascularization or a primary event occurred in 11% vs. 38% ($p < 0.001$). CABG patients also had less angina (22% vs. 31% at 2 years). A subsequent report showed that the PTCA group had a higher out-of-work rate at 2 years (26% vs. 22%) (*see Circulation* 1996;94:135).

151. **Hamm CW**, et al. German Angioplasty Bypass Surgery Investigation (**GABI**). A randomized study of coronary angioplasty compared with bypass surgery in patients with symptomatic multivessel coronary disease. *N Engl J Med* 1994;331:1037–1043.

Design: Prospective, randomized, multicenter study. Primary end point was freedom from angina at 1 year.

Purpose: To compare the clinical efficacy of bypass surgery with balloon angioplasty in patients with symptomatic multivessel CAD.

Population: 8,981 patients <75 years of age were screened, and 359 were enrolled (total revascularization of at least two major vessels needed and feasible technically).

Exclusion Criteria: Totally occluded vessels, left main stenosis >30%, MI in prior 4 weeks, and prior bypass or angioplasty.

Treatment: CABG surgery or PTCA.

Results: CABG group had longer hospitalization (19 vs. 5 days) and more MIs (8.1% vs. 2.3%; $p = 0.022$) due to procedures. However, CABG patients had similar in-hospital mortality rates (2.5% vs. 1.1%), fewer interventions (6% vs. 44%; $p < 0.001$), and less angina at hospital discharge (7% vs. 18%; no difference at 1 year), and fewer patients were on antianginal medications (12% vs. 22%; $p = 0.041$).

152. **King SB**, et al. Emory Angioplasty vs Surgery Trial (**EAST**). A randomized trial comparing coronary angioplasty with coronary bypass surgery. *N Engl J Med* 1994;331:1044–50 (editorial pp. 1086–1087).

Design: Prospective, randomized, multicenter study. Composite primary end point was death, Q-wave MI, and large defect on thallium scan at 3 years.

Purpose: To compare outcomes of bypass surgery with angioplasty in patients with multivessel disease.

Population: 392 patients with two- or three-vessel CAD (5,118 patients screened; 842 eligible).

Exclusion Criteria: Prior bypass surgery or coronary angioplasty, old (>8 weeks) chronic occlusions, left main stenosis >30%, and ejection fraction <25%.

Treatment: CABG surgery or PTCA.

Results: No significant difference was observed between groups in 3-year mortality (7.1% vs. 6.3%) or primary composite end points (28.8% vs. 27.3%). However, CABG patients required less repeat coronary artery bypass surgery (1% vs. 22%; *p* < 0.001) and fewer angioplasties (13% vs. 41%; *p* < 0.001), and reported less angina (12% vs. 20%).

153. CABRI Trial Participants. First year results of **CABRI** (Coronary Angioplasty vs Bypass Revascularization Investigation). *Lancet* 1995;346:1179–1184.

Design: Prospective, randomized, multicenter, open study. Primary outcomes were 1-year mortality and symptom status (based on angina class) at 1 year.

Purpose: To compare bypass surgery with angioplasty in patients with multivessel coronary disease requiring intervention.

Population: 1,054 patients ≤75 years of age with multivessel disease and typical angina or unstable angina, 62% with class III angina.

Treatment: CABG surgery or PTCA.

Exclusion Criteria: MI in prior 10 days, ejection fraction <35%, and prior PTCA or CABG.

Results: At 1-year follow-up, mortality rates were similar between groups (2.7% for CABG, 3.9% for PTCA). The CABG group did have 81% fewer reinterventions (6.5% vs. 33.6%; *p* < 0.001) and 35% less angina, and patients were on fewer medications. The 1-year mortality rate was highest in patients with grade IV angina or unstable angina (5% vs. 2.7%).

Comments: Complete revascularization was not required, and patients with total occlusions were not excluded.

154. **Frye RL**, et al. Bypass Angioplasty Revascularization Investigation (**BARI**). Comparison of coronary bypass surgery with angioplasty in patients with multivessel disease. *N Engl J Med* 1996;335:217–225 (editorial pp. 275–276).

Design: Prospective, randomized, multicenter study. Primary end point was all-cause mortality. Follow-up period was 5.4 years.

Purpose: To compare outcomes of bypass surgery with angioplasty in patients with multivessel disease and severe angina or ischemia.

Population: 1,829 patients; 41% had three-vessel CAD.

Treatment: CABG surgery or PTCA.

Results: CABG and PTCA groups had similar in-hospital mortality rates [1.3% (CABG) vs. 1.1%] and 5-year survival rates (89% vs. 86%; *p* = 0.19). The CABG group had more in-hospital Q-wave MIs (4.6% vs. 2.1%; *p* < 0.01), but had an 85% lower 5-year revascularization rate (8% vs. 54%) and 44% better 5-year survival in patients with diabetes (19% of enrolled patients; 81% vs. 66%; *p* = 0.003). The PTCA group had a 31% 5-year CABG rate.

Comments: Accompanying editorial reports that combining data from the BARI, EAST, and CABRI trials, CABG is associated with nonsignificant 14% mortality reduction (95% CI + 16% to −37%). A subsequent cost and quality of life analysis of 934 patients showed that the initial costs were 35% lower in the

PTCA group but only 5% lower at 5 years ($56,000 vs. $58,900; $p = 0.047$). Also, the cost of surgery was –$26,000/yr of life added, and surgical patients returned to work 5 weeks later but had better functional status at 3 years (*see N Engl J Med* 1997; 336:92). Another analysis showed that more lesions were favorable for revascularization by CABG (92% vs. 78%; $p < 0.001$), especially 99%–100% lesions (78% vs. 22%) (*see Am J Cardiol* 1996;77:805).

155. Arterial Revascularization Therapy Study (**ARTS**). Preliminary results presented at the 71st AHA Scientific Session in Dallas, TX, November 1998.

   In this prospective, randomized, multicenter trial, 1,200 patients with multivessel CAD were randomized to CABG or stenting. Primary outcome was the 1-year incidence of death, MI, stroke, or need for revascularization. At 30 days, primary events occurred in 6.8% of CABG patients and 8.7% of stent patients (p = NS). CABG patients underwent repeat revascularization significantly less frequently (0.8% vs. 3.7%).

156. **Rodriguez A**, et al. Estudio Randomizado Argentino de Angioplastia versus Cirugia (**ERACI**). Argentine randomized trial of PTCA vs coronary artery bypass surgery in multivessel disease: in-hospital results and one year follow-up. *J Am Coll Cardiol* 1993;22:1060–1067.

   In this prospective, single center study, 127 patients were randomized to angioplasty or bypass surgery. No differences were seen in in-hospital deaths, periprocedural MIs, emergency revascularization, or 1-year mortality rate. However, coronary artery bypass patients did have less angina and fewer reinterventions and combined cardiac events (83.5% vs. 63.7%; $p < 0.005$).

157. **Goy JJ**, et al. Coronary angioplasty vs left internal mammary artery grafting for isolated proximal left anterior descending artery stenosis. *Lancet* 1994;343:1449–1453.

   This prospective, randomized study was composed of 134 patients. The follow-up period was 2.5 years. No differences between the two groups were seen in in-hospital complications, cardiac deaths, or MIs, but the angioplasty group was on more antianginal drugs and had more adverse events [57% (mostly restenosis requiring repeat percutaneous intervention or CABG) vs. 14%].

158. **Bourassa MG**, et al. Asymptomatic Cardiac Ischemia Pilot (**ACIP**) study. ACIP study: effects of coronary angioplasty and CABG surgery on recurrent angina and ischemia. *J Am Coll Cardiol* 1995;26:606–614.

   This analysis focused on 78 CABG and 92 PTCA patients enrolled in the ACIP trial. Of note, the study was nonrandomized with the decision about CABG or PTCA made by clinical staff. At baseline, the CABG patients had more multivessel disease (86% vs. 62%) and ischemic episodes. However, at 8 weeks, CABG patients had significantly less ambulatory ischemia (30% vs. 54% of PTCA patients; $p = 0.002$), less ST depression (54% vs. 77%), less angina (10% vs. 32%), and increased treadmill time (+2.4 vs. +1.4 minutes; $p = 0.02$).

159. **Hueb WA**, et al. Medicine, Angioplasty or Surgery Study (**MASS**): a prospective, randomized trial of medical therapy, bal-

loon angioplasty or bypass surgery for single proximal left anterior descending stenoses. *J Am Coll Cardiol* 1995;26:1600–1605.

This prospective, randomized, multicenter study was composed of 214 patients with stable angina, normal left ventricular function, and >80% proximal LAD stenosis. Patients were randomized to CABG, PTCA, or medical therapy alone. At an average follow-up of 3 years, no CABG patients needed revascularization (vs. 8 and 7 patients; $p = 0.019$) and only 3% [vs. 24% (PTCA), $p = 0. 0002$; and vs. 17%, $p = 0.006$] had experienced a primary end point (death, Q wave MI, or large ischemic defect on thallium scan at 3 years). However, there was no significant difference in mortality or infarction rates. CABG and PTCA groups did have greater symptom relief and decreased ischemia on treadmill.

Graft and Patency Studies

160. **Loop FD**, et al. Influence of the internal mammary graft on 10 year survival and other cardiac events. *N Engl J Med* 1986; 314:1–6.

This retrospective analysis focused on 5,931 patients who underwent CABG from 1971 to 1979; 3625 patients had saphenous vein grafts only. IMA patients had better survival. Ten-year rates were 93.4% vs. 88% ($p = 0.05$) for one-vessel disease; 90% vs. 79.5% ($p < 0.0001$) for two-vessel disease; and 82.6% vs. 71% ($p < 0.001$) for three-vessel disease. A Cox multivariate analysis was performed, and for the saphenous vein graft group, the RR of death was 1.61, late MI RR 1.14, hospitalization for cardiac events RR 1.25, and cardiac reoperation RR 2.0.

161. **Cameron A**, et al. Coronary bypass surgery with internal thoracic artery grafts—effects on survival over a 15-year period. *N Engl J Med* 1996;334:216–219 (editorial pp. 263–265).

This analysis focused on 5,637 CASS registry patients, including 749 patients who received arterial grafts. In multivariate analysis, internal thoracic artery patients had a 27% lower mortality rate at 15-year follow-up. Benefit was seen in all major subgroups, with the mortality difference widening over time. The accompanying editorial refers to specific situations where internal thoracic artery grafting is contraindicated: radiation damage, extensive brachiocephalic atherosclerosis, and subclavian steal.

162. **Fitzgibbon GM**, et al. Coronary bypass graft fate and patient outcome: angiographic follow-up of 5065 grafts related to survival and reoperation in 1388 patients during 25 years. *J Am Coll Cardiol* 1996;28:616–626.

This retrospective analysis focused on 1,388 patients (mostly male veterans) who underwent surgery between 1969 and 1994; 91% of grafts were venous. Saphenous vein graft patency was 88% at early angiography, 81% at 1 year, 75% at 5 years, and 50% at 15 years. At 15 years, 44% had >50% stenoses. Arterial patency rates were significantly better: early, 95%; late (5 years), 80%. Reoperative mortality (6.6% vs. 1.4% for isolated first CABG) and morbidity were mostly due to vein graft atheroembolism.

163. **Goldman S**, et al. Predictors of graft patency 3 years after coronary artery bypass graft surgery. *J Am Coll Cardiol* 1997; 29:1563–1568.

This retrospective analysis focused on 266 male VA patients with 656 grafts patent at 7–10 days. Multivariate analysis predictors of 3-year patency (related to operative technique vs. antiplatelet therapy) included total cholesterol ≤225 mg/dL (p = 0.024), no more than two proximal anastomoses (p = 0.032), vein preservation solution temperature ≤5°C (p = 0.004), and recipient artery diameter >1.5 mm (p = 0.034).

Transmyocardial Revascularization

164. **Schofiel PM**, et al. Transmyocardial laser revascularization in patients with refractory angina: a randomised controlled trial. *Lancet* 1999;353:519–524.

   In this prospective trial, 188 patients were randomized to surgical TMR plus normal medication(s) or medical management alone. The perioperative mortality rate in TMR patients was 5%. One-year survival was 89% in the TMR group and 96% in the medical management group (p = 0.14). Most of the excess mortality in the TMR group was due to perioperative deaths. At 1 year, the TMR group did not have a significantly longer mean exercise treadmill time (+40 seconds; p = 0.152) or greater mean 12-minute walk distance (+33 meters; p = 0.108). The TMR group did have a significant improvement in Canadian Cardiovascular Society angina score: 25% of patients had a two-class improvement (at 1 year) versus only 4% of medical management patients (p < 0.001). Of note, necropsy reports of three patients showed dense fibrous scarring and no open channels.

165. **Kantor B**, et al. Transmyocardial revascularization and percutaneous myocardial revascularization: current and future role in the treatment of coronary artery disease. *Mayo Clin Proc* 1999; 74:585–592.

   This review discusses the available trial data on both the surgical and catheter-based procedures, the possible pathophysiologic mechanisms by which benefits are achieved, and current controversies and future directions.

166. **Burkhoff D**, et al. The Angina Treatments–Lasers and Normal Therapies in Comparison (**ATLANTIC**) Investigators. Transmyocardial laser revascularisation compared with continued medical therapy for treatment of refractory angina pectoris: a prospective randomized trial. *Lancet* 1999;354:885–890.

   This prospective, randomized, multicenter study was composed of 182 patients with Canadian Cardiovascular Society Angina (CCSA) score of III or IV, reversible ischemia, and incomplete response to other therapies. Patients were assigned to transmyocardial laser revascularisation (TMR) and continued medication, or continued medication alone. At 1 year, the TMR group had improved exercise tolerance (+65 seconds vs −46 seconds, p < 0.0001) and better CCSA scores (II or lower in 47.8% vs 14.3%, p < 0.001).

167. Potential Angina Class Improvement from Intramyocardial Channels (**PACIFIC**). Preliminary results presented at the 48th ACC Scientific Session in New Orleans, LA, March 1999.

   This prospective, randomized, multicenter trial was composed of 220 patients with stable class III or IV angina symptoms refractory to medical therapy who were not PTCA or CABG candidates and had an ejection fraction <30%. Percutaneous transmyocardial revascularization (PTMR) was achieved with pulsed laser energy that achieved an average 6-mm channel depth. PTMR patients had significant angina improvement at 3 months (average −1.3 Canadian Cardiovascular Society classes) and 6 months [−1.4 vs. −0.25 (medical therapy)]. PTMR patients also had significantly better exercise tolerance at 6 months (+30%; p = 0.0002). The PTMR complication rate was low: tamponade, 1%;, heart block requiring permanent pacemaker, 1%; death, MI, and stroke, 0%.

168. **Oesterle SN**, et al. Preliminary results presented at the ACCIS Session in New Orleans, LA, March 1999.

In this prospective study, 335 patients with wall thickness ≥9mm were randomized to PTMR or maximal medical management. Success without major complications was achieved in 95.8%. Complications included death (one patient), tamponade (five patients; 3.0%), non–Q-wave MI (six patients; 3.6%), ventricular tachycardia (one patient), and stroke (one patient). At 3-month follow-up, PTMR patients had an improvement of two Canadian Heart Association classes in 50% (vs. 17%; p < 0.0001) and a longer average exercise time (529 vs. 415 seconds; p = 0.0002). The PTMR group had a lower 3-month incidence of PCI (0.8% vs. 5.6%), whereas the non–Q-wave MI rate was higher (7.6% vs. 1.6%). Similar rates of death (3% vs. 1.6%), CABG (0% vs. 0.8%), and rehospitalization (33% vs. 36%) were observed.

3

Unstable Angina/Non-ST Elevation MI

EPIDEMIOLOGY

Each year in the United States, there are approximately 750,000 hospital admissions for unstable angina and approximately 350,000 for non-ST elevation myocardial infarction (non-STEMI). Unstable angina precedes MI in approximately half of cases.

PATHOPHYSIOLOGY (see page 146)

Unstable angina and non-STEMI are typically the result of nonocclusive coronary artery thrombus due to ruptured plaque(s). Other causes include vasoconstriction (e.g., Prinzmetal's angina, microcirculatory angina); progressive mechanical obstruction; and secondary causes (e.g., tachycardia, fever, thyrotoxicosis, anemia, and hypotension). Data also support the role of inflammation (e.g., activated neutrophils) (5).

CLASSIFICATION (see page 145)

1. Unstable angina: Canadian Cardiovascular Society (CCS) and Braunwald systems are the most commonly used today (1).
2. Non-STEMI: One third to one half of patients in unstable angina trials actually had a non-STEMI.

CLINICAL AND LABORATORY FINDINGS

History and Symptoms

Chest discomfort typically occurs at rest or with increasing frequency and lasts 5 to 20 minutes but can last several hours. Temporary/incomplete relief is provided by sublingual nitroglycerin. Most chest pain episodes respond to sublingual nitroglycerin.

Electrocardiogram

In unstable angina, ST-segment depression is seen in approximately 30% of cases, T-wave inversion in approximately 20%, and ST-segment elevation in 2% to 5%; these changes are predictive of adverse outcomes.

Cardiac Enzymes

Creatine Kinase and CK-MB

The current gold standard for the diagnosis of myocardial necrosis, creatine kinase (CK) and CK-MB levels typically rise approximately 6 hours after onset of ischemic symptoms.

Troponin T and I (see page 166)

More sensitive than CK and CK-MB, in a meta-analysis of 21 published studies, the two types of troponins were found to be equally sensitive and specific (see Am J Cardiol 1998;81:1405). Approximately one in three patients previously diagnosed with unstable angina are now known to have suffered a small non–ST elevation MI (microinfarctions). In one study of patients with rest pain, troponin T was detected in 39%, whereas CK-MB was elevated in less than 10% (54). Troponin levels also remain elevated for several days and, thus, are a reliable marker for diagnosing MI within the preceding 2 to 5 days.

Treatment

Aspirin (see page 147)

Aspirin (160 to 325 mg initially then 81 to 325 mg daily) has been shown to reduce the risk of fatal or nonfatal MI by approximately 70% during acute phase in patients with unstable angina or non-STEMI and by approximately 50% to 60% at 3 months to 3 years (9,10,12,13).

For patients with clear contraindications to aspirin (allergy, history of major gastrointestinal bleed), alternatives include ticlopidine and clopidogrel, although both have a delayed onset of action (maximal antiplatelet effect achieved after a few days).

Ticlopidine (250 mg twice daily) reduced cardiovascular mortality and reinfarction rates by nearly 50% in one study (11); however, long-term ticlopidine use is associated with a significant risk of neutropenia.

Clopidogrel (75 mg once daily) has been approved by the U.S. Food and Drug Administration (FDA) for long-term secondary prevention based on the results of the Clopidogrel versus Aspirin in Patients at Risk of Ischaemic Events (CAPRIE) trial (see Chapter 1). No increased neutropenic risk has been observed, but clopidogrel has not yet been studied in patients with unstable angina.

Heparin (see pages 145–150)

Heparin [60–70 U/kg bolus then 12–15 U/kg/h; goal activated partial thromboplastin time (aPTT) 1.5–2.0 times control], in a meta-analysis of six trials, showed a strong trend toward reducing rates of reinfarction and recurrent ischemia [odds ratio 0.67, 95% confidence interval (CI) 0.44–1.02] when used with aspirin; results showed the combination to be more effective than aspirin alone (4). After discontinuation of heparin infusion, there is a rebound phenomenon, with patients at increased risk of reactivation of unstable angina and MI (16).

Low-Molecular-Weight Heparins (see pages 150–152)

The Efficacy and Safety of Subcutaneous Enoxaparin in Non–Q-wave Coronary Events (ESSENCE) and Thrombolysis. In myocardial infarction (TIMI-11B) trials showed enoxaparin (1 mg/kg subcutaneously twice daily) to be superior to unfractionated heparin, resulting in 15% to 20% fewer major events (death, MI, and urgent revascularization) at 6 weeks (20,22).

In the Fragmin during Instability in CAD (FRISC) trial (18), dalteparin (120 IU/kg subcutaneously twice daily for 6 days, then 7,500 IU/day for 35–45 days) showed a significant reduction in death and MI at 6 days compared with placebo, whereas the Fragmin in Unstable Coronary Artery Disease (FRIC) trial showed equivalence between dalteparin and intravenous unfractionated heparin (19). In FRISC II (21), extended use of dalteparin (120 IU/kg twice daily for 3 months) was associated with a significant reduction in death or MI at 30 days, but the reduction did not remain significant at 3 months.

In the Fraxiparine in Ischemic Syndrome (FRAXIS) trial (22), fraxiparine showed no benefit compared with unfractionated heparin; of note, this study enrolled many low-risk patients.

Note: Enoxaparin has a higher ratio of anti–Factor Xa to anti-thrombin activity (3.8:1.0) than does dalteparin or fraxiparine.

β-Blockers

Metoprolol (5 mg intravenously every 5 minutes for three doses, then 25–50 mg orally every 6 hours), propranolol (0.5–1.0 mg intravenously, then 40–80 mg orally every 6–8 hours), and atenolol (5 mg intravenously, then 50–100 mg orally daily), used alone or in combination with nitrates or calcium-channel blockers, have been shown to reduce the incidence of MI and recurrent ischemia, including silent or asymptomatic episodes.

Nitrates

Nitrates are useful for treating episodes of recurrent ischemia [reducing both left ventricular end-diastolic pressure and systolic blood pressure (SBP)]. If no relief is gained from three sublingual nitroglycerin tablets, intravenous nitroglycerin (10–200 μg/min) should be started.

Calcium-Channel Blockers (see page 153)

Calcium-channel blockers are as effective in relieving symptoms, but an overview of randomized trials showed no reduction in mortality or MI rates (*see Br Med J* 1989;299:1887.)

Diltiazem confers a possible benefit in non–Q-wave MI patients (majority with non-ST elevation MI). In the Diltiazem Reinfarction Study, diltiazem use (90 mg four times daily) was associated with a significant reduction in in-hospital mortality (24). However, no overall benefit was observed by the Multicenter Diltiazem Postinfarction Trial Research Group (60 mg four times daily), although a post hoc analysis showed benefit in patients without evidence of left ventricular dysfunction.

Glycoprotein IIb/IIIa Inhibitors (see pages 154–168)

In the Platelet Receptor Inhibition in Ischemic Syndrome Management in Patients Limited by Unstable Signs and Symptoms (PRISM-PLUS) trial, tirofiban (0.4 μg/kg/min for 30 minutes, then 0.10 μg/kg/min for 48–72 hours), heparin, and aspirin resulted in decreased death, MI, and refractory ischemia at 7 days compared with heparin alone (28), and death and MI were decreased by approximately 30% at 30 days.

In the large Platelet Glycoprotein IIb/IIIa in Unstable Angina Receptor Suppression Using Integrelin Therapy (PURSUIT) trial, eptifibatide (180 μg/kg bolus, then 2.0 μg/kg/min) showed an approximately 10% reduction in death and MI at 30 days (31).

Abciximab (0.25 μg/kg bolus, then 0.10 μg/min for 12 hours) also has been shown to confer some benefit. The Evaluation of 7E3 for the Prevention of Ischemic Complications (EPIC), Evaluation in PTCA to Improve Long-term Outcome with Abciximab Glycoprotein IIb/IIIa Blockade (EPILOG), and c7E3 Fab Antiplatelet Therapy in Unstable Refractory Refractory Angina (CAPTURE) trials were interventional studies that enrolled some unstable angina patients, and all showed substantial reductions (30%–60%) at 30 days in the rates of death, MI, and ischemia-provoked intervention or revascularization (*see* Chapter 2). The 6-month results of the Evaluation of Platelet IIb/IIIa Inhibitor for Stenting (EPISTENT) trial, an interventional study comparing stenting alone versus stenting plus abciximab versus balloon angioplasty plus abciximab, showed an impressive 10% absolute reduction in death and MI in the subgroup of patients with unstable angina. CAPTURE analysis found that the benefits of abciximab in the unstable angina cohort undergoing percutaneous coronary intervention (PCI) were restricted to patients with elevated troponin T levels (59).

A small Canadian study (365 patients) showed a 69% reduction in death and MI at 30 days in two high-dose lamifiban groups compared with placebo, whereas the larger Platelet IIb/IIIa Antagonism for the Reduction of Acute Coronary Syndrome Events in a Global Organization Network (PARAGON) A trial (2,282 patients) showed no difference (30). The PARAGON B trial is ongoing.

Oral Agents (see pages 157, 158)

The phase II TIMI-12 study showed that sibrafiban induced longer term (4 weeks) platelet inhibition, but at the expense of increased minor bleeding (33). The interventional ORBIT study showed that xemilofiban was well tolerated over a 4-week treatment period and, although underpowered, demonstrated a trend toward fewer cardiovascular events at 3 months. In the Evaluation of Oral Xemilofiban in Controlling Thrombotic Events (EXCITE) study, a larger inventional trial, xemilofiban showed no significant clinical benefit (*see* Chapter 2). Orbofiban showed no significant clinical benefit in the large Orbofiban in Patients with Unstable Coronary Syndromes (OPUS)/TIMI-16 trial (32). Trials with second generation agents are ongoing.

Direct Thrombin Inhibitors (see page 158)

In the Global Utilization of Strategies to Open Occluded Arteries (GUSTO) IIb trial, hirudin in patients with acute coronary syndromes [chest pain with electrocardiographic (ECG) changes] resulted in a nonsignificant 11% reduction in death and MI at 30 days compared with heparin (34). In the Organization to Assess Strategies for Ischemic Syndromes (OASIS-2) trial, medium-dose hirudin (0.4 mg/kg bolus then 0.15 mg/kg/h) resulted in a nonsignificant (16%) reduction in cardiovascular death and MI at 7 days (35).

Thrombolytic Therapy (see pages 160, 161)

Thrombolytic therapy was not found to be beneficial in the Unstable Angina Study Using Eminase (UNASEM) and TIMI III (39,40). Use was associated with increased bleeding and MI rates, and no benefit of adjunctive intracoronary thrombolytic therapy was observed during percutaneous transluminal coronary angioplasty (PTCA) in the Thrombolysis and Angioplasty in Unstable Angina (TAUSA) trial (41).

Invasive Strategy (see pages 161–164)

Coronary Angiography

Using coronary angiography, three-vessel disease was found in approximately 40%, two-vessel disease in approximately 20%, left main disease in approximately 20%, single-vessel disease in approximately 10%, and no critical obstruction in approximately 10% of patients screened. The routine use of angiography is debated. TIMI IIIB showed that early angiography followed by revascularization (if indicated) did not reduce major cardiac events but did result in fewer hospital readmissions (42), whereas the Veteran Affairs Non–Q-wave Infarction Strategies in Hospital (VANQWISH) study, which enrolled medium- to high-risk patients, showed no benefit of an invasive strategy and a trend toward higher mortality (43). Of note, the invasive group in the VAN-QWISH study had a high coronary artery bypass graft (CABG) operative mortality rate (12%). The FRISC II trial reported a significantly lower incidence of death or MI with an invasive strategy compared with a noninvasive strategy (at 6 months: 9.4% vs 12.1%, $p = 0.031$) (45); subgroup analysis showed that this benefit was restricted to men.

A more conservative strategy may be most appropriate in low-risk patients [e.g., patients with new-onset angina (<2 weeks) or no ECG changes during pain who do not have a positive stress test), whereas higher risk patients may be more likely to benefit from an invasive strategy.

Percutaneous Coronary Intervention

The success rate of PCI is 90%–95%. Ischemic complications are reduced by concomitant administration of intravenous glycoprotein IIb/IIIa inhibitor. (Routine use is recommended, but cost is an issue.)

Coronary Artery Bypass Surgery (see page 165)

The operative mortality rate with coronary artery bypass surgery is approximately 4% in patients with refractory unstable angina (vs. ~2% for patients with chronic stable angina). Improved survival has been demonstrated in patients with left main disease and three-vessel disease with significant left ventricular dysfunction (*see* Chapter 2). An intraaortic balloon pump may be needed for stabilization prior to surgery.

One observational study showed that patients treated by cardiologists (vs. internists) tended to have lower mortality rates ($p = 0.06$). Cardiologists prescribed more appropriate medications and ordered more invasive testing (48).

Noninvasive Evaluation

Exercise Treadmill Test (ETT)

Treadmill testing should not be performed in the acute phase. Once the patient is stable, it can be performed 48 to 72 hours later. If the patient is high risk (e.g., ≥2 mm ST segment depression), catheterization should be considered.

ETT with Nuclear Imaging

ETT is helpful if the ECG results are nondiagnostic. The size of perfusion defect(s) is predictive of mortality and major cardiac events.

Echocardiography

In patients with chest pain but no ECG changes or an obscured ECG picture (left bundle branch block, paced rhythm), echocardiography can be used to evaluate whether a wall motion abnormality is present.

Prognosis

Unstable Angina (see page 171)

The hospital mortality rate is 1% to 2%, 1-year mortality rate 7% to 10% and 1-month reinfarction rate approximately 5%. Twenty percent to 25% of patients are rehospitalized within 1 year. Recurrent ischemia is associated with a near tripling of mortality (72).

Non-ST Evaluation Myocardial Infarction

The in-hospital mortality rate is 3% to 4%, reinfarction rate 8% to 10%, and 1-year mortality rate 10% to 15%. (The latter is similar to that of ST-elevation patients.)

Prior Aspirin Use (Aspirin Failures) (see page 166)

Prior aspirin use is associated with an increased risk of death or MI at 30 days (54).

Electrocardiography (see page 171)

TIMI III Registry analysis showed an increased risk of death and MI at 1 year with left bundle branch block on admission ECG [relative risk (RR) 2.8] and 0.5 mm of ST deviation (RR 2.5). Of note, T-wave inversion was not associated with increased risk (72).

Echocardiography (see page 170)

Routine use of echocardiography may not be necessary in all non-STEMI patients. Studies have shown that 97% of patients with non-anterior MIs, no Q waves, total CK less than 1000 IU, and no evidence of congestive heart failure have normal left ventricular function (68).

Troponin Levels (see page 167)

Troponin levels have been shown to provide substantial prognostic information. TIMI IIIB and FRISC analyses showed a strong correlation between troponin T levels and adverse outcomes (57,58). In the FRISC trial, the benefit of low-molecular-weight heparin over aspirin was limited to patients with elevated troponin T levels (56). Similarly, in the CAPTURE trial, the benefit of abciximab was seen only in patients with elevated troponin T levels (58). Whether troponins will be helpful in improving outcomes based on triaging to an invasive or conservative strategy is being tested in ongoing prospective trials.

C-Reactive Protein (see page 169)

Elevated levels of C-reactive protein (CRP) are found in patients who die. A TIMI 11-A analysis showed patients at highest risk of subsequent adverse events if both CRP and troponin are elevated (63).

Von Willebrand Factor (see page 169)

Analysis of a small group of ESSENCE patients (63) showed lower levels among enoxaparin-treated patients; further studies are needed.

Fibrinogen (see page 168)

High fibrinogen levels were associated with increased mortality in a FRISC analysis (62) and higher incidence of death, MI, and spontaneous ischemia in a TIMI III B analysis (62).

REFERENCES

Review Articles and Meta-Analysis

1. **Braunwald E.** Unstable angina: a classification. *Circulation* 1989; 80:410–414.
   This article provides the original description of one of the two most commonly used unstable angina classification systems (the other one being the CCS). The reader is referred to Calvin et al. (53) for prospective validation of this system.

   Severity:

   Class I. New-onset (<2 months), severe, or accelerated; no rest pain in preceding 2 months.
   Class II. Subacute (angina at rest >48 hours to 1 month previously).
   Class III. Acute (at least one episode in preceding 48 hours).

   Clinical:

   Class A. Secondary unstable angina (e.g., triggered by anemia, infection thyrotoxicosis).
   Class B. Primary unstable angina.
   Class C. Postinfarction unstable angina (<2 weeks after documented MI).

   Intensity of therapy:

   1. Absence of or minimal therapy.
   2. Occurring in the presence of standard therapy for chronic stable angina (e.g., oral β-blockers, nitrates, calcium antagonists).
   3. Occurring despite maximal therapy (oral therapy and intravenous nitroglycerin).

2. **Theroux P**, Lidon RM. Unstable angina: pathogenesis, diagnosis and treatment. *Curr Probl Cardiol* 1993;18:163–231.
   This extensive review covers the classification, risk stratification, diagnosis, and treatment of unstable angina.

3. **Braunwald E**, et al. Diagnosing and managing unstable angina. *Circulation* 1994;90:613–622.
   The Unstable Angina Guidelines provide supporting evidence for all aspects of the diagnosis and management of unstable angina and both the inpatient and outpatient settings.

4. **Oler A**, et al. Adding heparin to aspirin reduces the incidence of MI and death in patients with unstable angina: a meta-analysis. *JAMA* 1996;276:811–815.
   This meta-analysis was derived from six randomized trials enrolling 1,353 patients. Aspirin and heparin tended to be preferable to aspirin alone (RR of death and MI 0.67; 95% CI 0.44–1.02). Combination therapy also was associated with nonsignificant reduction in recurrent ischemia (RR 0.82; 95% CI 0.40–1.17). No difference in revascularization rates was observed (RR 1.03; 95% CI 0.74–1.43), whereas aspirin and heparin were associated with a nonsignificant increase in major bleeding (RR 1.99; 95% CI 0.52–7.65).

5. **Azar RR**, Waters DD. The inflammatory etiology of unstable angina. *Am Heart J* 1996;132:1101–1106.
   This review discusses the role of inflammation in coronary plaque disruption, especially the evidence for activation of circulating leukocytes.
6. **Ribeiro PA**, Shah PM. Unstable angina: new insights into pathophysiology, characteristics, prognosis, and management strategies. *Curr Probl Cardiol* 1996; 21:675–731.
   This extensive review includes sections on the pathophysiology, diagnosis, assessment, and treatment of unstable angina. The latter section discusses the use of aspirin, heparin, nitrates, β-blockers, calcium-channel blockers, thrombin inhibitors, glycoprotein IIb/IIIa inhibitors, thrombolysis, balloon angioplasty, and surgical revascularization.
7. **Theroux P**, Fuster V. Acute coronary syndromes: unstable angina and non–Q-wave MI. *Circulation* 1998;97:1195–1206.
   This review provides a detailed discussion of the pathophysiology and pathogenesis of unstable angina, as well as its evaluation and management.
8. **Braunwald E**. Unstable angina: an etiologic approach to management. *Circulation* 1998;98:2219–2222.
   This editorial describes five different, though not mutually exclusive, causes of unstable angina: (a) nonocclusive thrombus on pre-existing plaques (most common); (b) dynamic obstruction (e.g., Prinzmetal's variant angina, microcirculatory angina); (c) progressive mechanical obstruction; (d) inflammation and/or infection; and (e) secondary causes (e.g., fever, thyrotoxicosis, hypotension).

Drugs and Studies

Aspirin and Ticlopidine

9. **Lewis HD Jr**, et al., **VA Cooperative Study**. Protective effects of aspirin against acute MI and death in men with unstable angina. *N Engl J Med* 1983;309:396–403.
   Design: Prospective, randomized, double-blind, placebo-controlled, multicenter study. 12-week primary end point was death or MI.
   Purpose: To determine whether aspirin can decrease the incidence of death and acute MI in patients with unstable angina.
   Population: 1,266 men with pain at rest beginning within previous month and present within last week and evidence of coronary artery disease (CAD), defined as one or more of the following: history of MI, ST depression ≥1 mm, angiogram showing 75% stenosis of at least one vessel, exercise test with ≥1 mm ST depression, and exertional angina relieved by nitroglycerin within 5 minutes.
   Exclusion Criteria: Included new Q waves or ST elevation on ECG, elevated screening enzymes (more than twice the normal level), severe heart failure (New York Heart Association Class IV), ventricular arrhythmia, oral anticoagulation, bleeding diasthesis, allergy or intolerance to aspirin, recent aspirin ingestion (on >3 days of the previous 7), MI within previous 6 weeks, bypass surgery in previous 12 weeks, and cardiac catheterization in prior week.
   Treatment: Buffered aspirin 324 mg daily or placebo for 12 weeks.

Results: At 12 weeks, the aspirin group had a 51% lower incidence of death and MI (5% vs. 10%; $p < 0.0005$), with both death and nonfatal MI being reduced by 51% (3.4% vs. 6.9%, $p = 0.005$; 1.6% vs. 3.3%, $p = 0.054$). No difference was observed in gastrointestinal symptoms or evidence of blood loss between the two treatment and placebo groups.

10. **Cairns JA**, et al. Aspirin, sulfinpyrazone, or both in unstable angina: results of a Canadian multicenter trial. *N Engl J Med* 1985;313:1369–75.

    Design: Prospective, randomized, double-blind, placebo-controlled, multicenter study. Primary end point was cardiac death and nonfatal MI. Mean follow-up period was 18 months.

    Purpose: To evaluate the efficacy of aspirin, sulfinpyrazone, or both in the acute management of unstable angina.

    Population: 555 patients 70 years of age with evidence of myocardial ischemia (exertional angina, transient ST- or T-wave changes with pain, or relief with sublingual nitroglycerin in <10 minutes on at least three occasions in hospital) and unstable pain pattern (crescendo pain or pain 15 minutes in duration).

    Exclusion Criteria: Included MI in preceding 12 weeks, contraindications to study medications, new Q waves on ECG, severe chest pain lasting ≥30 minutes, and elevated (more than twice the upper limit of normal) enzymes (at least two of following: serum aspartate aminotransferase, lactic dehydrogenase, CK), with positive CK-MB fraction or MB >5%.

    Treatment: Aspirin 325 mg four times daily, sulfinpyrazone 200 mg four times daily, both, or neither.

    Results: Aspirin groups had 51% less cardiac death and MI versus nonaspirin groups (8.6% vs. 17%; $p = 0.008$). The aspirin groups also had 71% lower all-cause mortality rates (3.0% vs. 11.7%; $p = 0.004$). Intention-to-treat analysis showed aspirin groups to have 30% lower rates of cardiac death and nonfatal MI ($p = 0.072$), 56% fewer cardiac deaths ($p = 0.009$), and 43% lower all-cause mortality rate ($p = 0.035$). Sulfinpyrazone showed no benefit for any outcome event.

11. **Balsano F**, et al. Antiplatelet therapy with ticlopidine in unstable angina: controlled, multicenter clinical trial. *Circulation* 1990; 82:17–26 (editorial pp. 296–298).

    In this randomized trial, 652 patients received conventional therapy (without aspirin) or ticlopidine 250 mg twice daily. At 6 months, the ticlopidine group had 46% fewer primary end points, consisting of vascular death or nonfatal MI (7.3% vs. 13.6%; $p = 0.009$). There was a 53% reduction in risk of fatal or nonfatal MI (5.1% vs. 10.9%, $p = 0.006$).

Unfractionated Heparin and Warfarin

12. **Theroux P**, et al. **Montreal Heart Study**. Aspirin, heparin, or both to treat acute unstable angina. *N Engl J Med* 1988;319: 1105–1111.

    Design: Prospective, randomized, double-blind, placebo-controlled, dual-center study. Major end points were death, MI, and refractory angina.

    Purpose: To evaluate the usefulness of aspirin, intravenous heparin, and their combination in the early management of unstable angina.

Population: 479 patients ≤75 years of age with accelerating pattern of chest pain occurring at rest or with minimal exercise, or pain lasting 20 minutes with last episode in previous 24 hours. Their ECG changes had to be consistent with ischemia; if absent, diagnosis had to be confirmed by two cardiologists. CK levels had to be less than twice the upper limit of normal.

Exclusion Criteria: Included regular use of aspirin, contraindications to heparin or aspirin, coronary angioplasty within previous 6 months, and bypass surgery within previous 12 months (or scheduled).

Treatment: Aspirin 325 mg twice daily or intravenous heparin 1,000 U/h (given for average 6 days).

Results: Incidence of MI was significantly reduced in groups receiving aspirin [3% vs. 12% (placebo); $p = 0.01$], heparin (0.8%; $p < 0.001$), and aspirin plus heparin (1.6%; $p = 0.003$). No deaths occurred in these three treatment groups. Heparin was associated with a trend toward refractory angina compared with aspirin (RR 0.47; 95% CI 0.21–1.05; $p = 0.06$). Combination therapy was associated with more serious bleeding [3.3% vs. 1.7% (heparin alone)].

Comments: An additional 245 patients were randomized to either aspirin or heparin to allow for an adequately powered comparison (*see Circulation* 1993;88:2045). A total of 484 patients were randomized to these two treatments, and the heparin group demonstrated a 78% lower MI rate at 5.7 ± 3.3 days (0.8% vs. 3.7%; $p = 0.035$). Only one death occurred (aspirin patient).

13. **Wallentin LW**, et al. Research on Instability in CAD (**RISC**). Risk of MI and death during treatment with low dose aspirin and intravenous heparin in men with unstable coronary artery disease. *Lancet* 1990;336:827–830.

Design: Prospective, randomized, double-blind, placebo-controlled, 2×2 factorial, multicenter study. Primary end point was death and MI.

Purpose: To evaluate the efficacy of aspirin and/or heparin in acute treatment of unstable and non–Q-wave MI and to assess the long-term effects of aspirin compared with placebo in these patients.

Population: 796 men <70 years of age with non–Q-wave MI or increasing angina within previous 4 weeks, with last episode of pain within 72 hours and ischemia on resting ECG or predischarge exercise test.

Exclusion Criteria: Included Q-wave MI, myocardial dysfunction due to prior MI, previous coronary bypass surgery, left bundle branch block or pacemaker, concurrent anticoagulant or aspirin therapy, and increased bleeding risk.

Treatment: Aspirin 75 mg daily for 1 year, or placebo and intravenous heparin boluses (10,000 U every 6 hours for four doses, then 7,500 U every 6 hours for 4 days), or placebo alone.

Results: Trial was stopped early due to publication of ISIS-2 results (minimum follow-up reduced to 3 months vs. 12 months). Aspirin patients had a markedly reduced risk of MI and death at 5 days (odds ratio 0.43; $p = 0.033$), 1 month (odds ratio 0.31; $p < 0.0001$), and 3 months (odds ratios 0.36; $p < 0.0001$). No benefits were seen with heparin alone. The aspirin and heparin group had fewer events in the first 5 days [1.4% vs. 3.7% (aspirin alone), $p = $ NS; 5.5% (heparin alone), $p = 0.045$; 6.0% (both placebos), $p = 0.027$]. Gastrointestinal symptoms with aspirin became more frequent after 3 months.

14. **Cohen M**, et al. Antithrombotic Therapy in Acute Coronary Syndromes **(ATACS)**. Prospective comparison of unstable angina vs non-Q wave MI during antithrombotic therapy. *J Am Coll Cardiol* 1993;22:1338–1343.

    Design: Prospective, randomized, open, parallel-group, multicenter study. Primary end point was death, MI, and recurrent ischemia at 12 weeks.

    Purpose: To evaluate whether the combination of aspirin and anticoagulant therapy is superior to either agent alone in reducing ischemic events in patients with unstable angina or non–Q-wave MI.

    Population: 358 patients >21 years of age with ischemic pain for 10 minutes at rest and within past 48 hours and definite evidence of underlying ischemic heart disease (ECG changes during chest pain, history of prior MI, positive exercise test result, angiography with ≥ 50% stenosis).

    Exclusion Criteria: Included evolving Q-wave MI, left bundle branch block or permanent pacemaker, balloon angioplasty in prior 6 months, coronary bypass surgery in past 12 months, and contraindications to anticoagulation.

    Treatment: Aspirin 162.5 mg or aspirin plus heparin (100 U/kg bolus, then continuous infusion for 3–4 days), then aspirin plus warfarin [target international normalized ratio (INR) 2.0–3.0].

    Results: At 12 weeks, The non–Q-wave MI group had a higher incidence of MI (11% vs. 4%; $p < 0.01$) and death and MI (16% vs. 7%), whereas there was a trend toward more frequent recurrent angina in the unstable angina group (20% vs. 11%; $p = 0.10$).

    Comments: Subsequent analysis of 214 nonprior aspirin users showed that the combination therapy group had 61% fewer ischemic events at 14 days (10.5% vs. 27%; $p = 0.004$) and nonsignificant reduction at 12 weeks (13% vs. 25%; $p = 0.06$) (*see Circulation* 1994;89:81).

15. **Anand SS**, et al. The Organization to Assess Strategies for Ischemic Syndromes **(OASIS) Pilot Study** Investigators. Long-term oral anticoagulant therapy in patients with unstable or suspected non-Q wave MI. *Circulation* 1998;98:1064–1070.

    Design: Prospective, randomized, open, multicenter study. Primary end point was cardiovascular death, nonfatal MI, and refractory angina.

    Purpose: To evaluate the efficacy, feasibility, and safety of fixed-dose, low-intensity warfarin and moderate-intensity warfarin in patients with acute ischemic syndromes without ST-segment elevation.

    Population: Phase 1: 309 patients presenting within 12 hours of an episode of chest pain suspected to be due to unstable angina or MI without ST elevation. Phase 2: 197 patients presenting within 48 hours of onset of symptoms.

    Exclusion Criteria: Included major bleeding in previous 48 hours, requirement for coumadin, or CABG planned before or within 1 week of hospital discharge.

    Treatment: Phase 1: Fixed-dose warfarin for 180 days [started on days 5–7 (after 72 hours of heparin or hirudin) with 10-mg loading dose then 3 mg once daily]. Phase 2: Adjusted-dose warfarin for 3 months (started 24 hours after initiation or heparin or hirudin; target INR 2.0–3.0). Aspirin was recommended for all patients (actual rates 85%–87%).

Results: Phase 1: At 6 months, the fixed-dose warfarin group had nonsignificantly higher rates of cardiovascular death, MI, and refractory angina (6.5% vs. 3.9%, RR 1.66; p = 0.31), and death, new MI, and stroke (6.5% vs. 2.6%, RR 2.48; p = 0.10). The warfarin group had a significant excess of minor bleeds (RR 5.46; p = 0.001). Phase 2: Mean INR was 2.3. At 3 months, the warfarin group tended toward reductions in primary end points (5.1% vs. 12.1%, RR 0.42; p = 0.08), and death, MI, and stroke [5.1% vs. 13.1%, RR 0.39 (95% CI 0.14–1.05); p = 0.05]. The warfarin group did have significantly fewer rehospitalizations for unstable angina (7.1% vs. 17.2%, RR 0.42; p = 0.03) and more minor bleeding episodes (28.6% vs. 12.1%, RR 2.36; p = 0.004).

16. **Theroux P**, et al. Reactivation of unstable angina after the discontinuation of heparin. *N Engl J Med* 1992;327:141–145.

   This study demonstrated a clear rebound effect with discontinuation of heparin in patients not on aspirin. Four hundred three patients were randomized to intravenous heparin, aspirin, both, or neither and completed 6 days of treatment without refractory angina or MI. After discontinuation of therapy, heparin-only patients had more frequent reactivation of unstable angina or MI in the subsequent 96 hours: 14 of 107 patients versus only 5 patients in each of the other three groups (p < 0.01). Also, 11 of 14 of these reactivations required urgent interventions (thrombolysis, angioplasty, or bypass surgery) versus only 2 in the other groups combined (p < 0.01).

17. **Serneri GGN**, et al., Studio Eparina Sottocutanea nell Angina Instabile Refrattaria **(SESAIR)**. Randomised comparison of subcutaneous heparin, intravenous heparin and aspirin in unstable angina. *Lancet* 1995;345:1201–1204.

   This prospective, randomized trial was composed of 108 patients refractory to 24 hours of antianginal therapy. Patients received intravenous heparin (aPTT 1.5–2.0 times normal), subcutaneous heparin (5,000–7,500 U every 8 hours; goal aPTT 1.5–2.0 times normal), or aspirin 325 mg once daily for 3 days (after which treatment could be discontinued or dosage modified. Over the first 3 days, the heparin groups had a 91% reduction in frequency of angina, 46% fewer silent ischemic episodes, and 66% shorter overall duration of ischemia. In the subcutaneous group, reductions were 86%, 46%, and 61%, respectively. No significant effects were seen with aspirin. Favorable effects remained evident at 1 month.

Low-Molecular-Weight Heparins

18. **Wallentin L**, et al., Fragmin during Instability in CAD **(FRISC)**. Low molecular weight heparin during instability in coronary artery disease. *Lancet* 1996;347:561–568.

   Design: Prospective, randomized, double-blind, placebo-controlled, multicenter study. Primary end point was death or MI at 6 days.

   Purpose: To evaluate whether subcutaneous dalteparin provides an additive benefit to that provided by aspirin and antianginal drugs in patients with unstable angina or non–Q-wave MI.

   Population: 1,506 patients (men 40 years of age, women >1 year postmenopause) with chest pain in previous 72 hours. All had newly developed or increasing angina or angina at rest during previous 2 months or persisting chest pain with a suspicion of MI and ST depression ≥1 mm or T-wave inversion ≥1 mm in two adjacent leads without Q waves in ischemic leads.

Exclusion Criteria: Included increased bleeding risks (e.g., cerebral bleeding in previous 3 months, gastrointestinal bleeding in prior 5 years, platelet count <100,000, oral anticoagulation), creatinine >200 μM, new Q waves in ischemic leads, indications for thrombolysis, left bundle branch block or pacemaker, and PCI or bypass surgery planned before admission or in prior 3 months.

Treatment: Dalteparin 120 IU/kg subcutaneously twice daily for 6 days, then 7,500 IU daily for 35–45 days; or placebo.

Results: At 6 days, the dalteparin group had a 63% lower rate of death and new MI (1.8% vs. 4.8%; $p = 0.001$); a nonsignificant reduction was observed at 40 days (8% vs. 10.7%; $p = 0.07$).

Comments: Subsequent analysis showed the additive value of troponin T to predischarge ETT in providing risk stratification (*see Eur Heart J* 1997;18:762).

19. **Klein W**, et al. Fragmin in Unstable Coronary Artery Disease **(FRIC)**. Comparison of low molecular weight heparin with unfractionated heparin acutely and with placebo for 6 weeks in the management of unstable coronary artery disease. *Circulation* 1997; 96:61–68 (editorial pp. 3–5).

Design: Prospective, randomized, partially open-label, parallel, multicenter, study. Primary end point was death, MI, or recurrent angina.

Purpose: To compare the efficacy and safety of weight-adjusted subcutaneous dalteparin with unfractionated heparin in the acute treatment of unstable angina or non–Q-wave MI and the value of prolonged dalteparin compared with placebo in those initially anticoagulated.

Population: 1,482 patients with chest pain in preceding 72 hours and admission ECG with temporary or persistent ST depression ≥1 mV in at least two adjacent leads and/or temporary or persistent T-wave inversion ≥1 mm in two adjacent leads.

Exclusion Criteria: Included new Q waves, left bundle branch block, indication for thrombolytic therapy, oral anticoagulation, diastolic blood pressure (DBP) >120 mm Hg, bleeding diathesis or recent surgery, and history of cerebrovascular event.

Treatment: Phase 1 (open label, days 1–6): Dalteparin 120 IU/kg subcutaneously twice daily or intravenous unfractionated heparin. Phase 2 (double-blind, days 6–45): Dalteparin 7,500 IU subcutaneously once daily or placebo.

Results: In the first 6 days, no significant differences were observed between groups in death, MI, or recurrent angina [7.6% (heparin) vs. 9.3% (dalteparin), 95% CI 0.84–1.66]; death and MI (3.6% vs. 3.9%), or revascularization (5.3% vs. 4.8%). For days 6–45, similar incidences of composite end points (both 12.3%) and revascularization [14.2% (placebo) vs. 14.3%] were observed. Of note, the dalteparin group had a higher phase 1 mortality rate (11 vs. 3 deaths, RR 3.37, 95% CI 1.01–11.24).

Comments: Lack of benefit with dalteparin may be due to the low ratio of anti–Factor Xa to antithrombin activity (only 2.0).

20. **Cohen M**, et al. Efficacy and Safety of Subcutaneous Enoxaparin in Non-Q wave Coronary Events **(ESSENCE)**. A comparison of low molecular weight heparin with unfractionated heparin for unstable coronary artery disease. *N Engl J Med* 1997;337:447–452 (editorial pp. 492–494).

Design: Prospective, randomized, double-blind, placebo-controlled, parallel-group, multicenter study. Primary end point was death, MI, or recurrent angina at 14 days.

Purpose: To compare the efficacy and safety of enoxaparin with unfractionated heparin in patients with unstable angina or non–Q-wave MI.

Population: 3,171 patients with rest pain 10 minutes in preceding 24 hours accompanied by one of the following: (a) new ST depression ≥ 1 mm, transient ST elevation, or T-wave changes in at least two contiguous leads; (b) documented prior MI or revascularization procedure; or (c) noninvasive or invasive tests suggesting ischemic heart disease. Of note, only about one third had ST-segment changes on admission.

Exclusion Criteria: Included left bundle branch block or pacemaker, persistent ST elevation, angina with an established precipitating cause (e.g., heart failure), contraindications to anticoagulation, and creatinine clearance <30 mL/min.

Treatment: Enoxaparin 1 mg/kg subcutaneously twice daily or unfractionated intravenous heparin for 2–8 days (mean duration 2.8 days).

Results: Enoxaparin group had a 16% lower rate of death, MI, and recurrent angina at 14 days (16.6% vs. 19.8%; $p = 0.019$); at 30 days the benefit persisted (19.8% vs. 23.3%; $p = 0.016$). Enoxaparin also was associated with a lower 30-day revascularization rate (27% vs. 32.2%; $p = 0.001$). Similar rates of major bleeding were observed at 30 days (6.5% vs. 7.0%), but overall bleeding was higher in the enoxaparin group (18.4% vs. 14.2%; $p = 0.001$) due to injection site ecchymoses.

21. FRagmin and Fast Revascularization during InStability in coronary artery disease **(FRISC II)** Investigators. Long-term, low-molecular-mass heparin in unstable coronary artery disease: FRISC II prospective randomized multicenter study. *Lancet* 1999;354:701–707.

Design: Prospective, randomized, partially blinded parallel group, multicenter study. Primary end point was death or MI at 3 months.

Purpose: To assess the effects of long-term treatment with dalteparin compared with a placebo in patients undergoing a noninvasive treatment strategy.

Population: 2,267 patients (median age 67 years) with ischemic symptoms in previous 48 hours accompanied by ECG changes (ST depression or T wave inversion ≥ 0.1 mv) or elevated markers (e.g. CK-MB >6 mg/L, troponin T >0.10 mg/L).

Exclusion Criteria: Included angioplasty in previous 6 months, indication for or treatment with thrombolysis in past 24 hours, scheduled revascularization procedure.

Treatment: After 5 or more days of open-label dalteparin, patients randomized to subcutaneous dalteparin 120 IU/kg twice daily or placebo for 3 months.

Results: At 30 days, the dalteparin group had a significant reduction in death or MI (3.1% vs 5.9%, $p = 0.002$), but at 3 months the reduction was nonsignificant (6.7% vs 8.0%, $p = 0.17$). There was a significant reduction in the 3 month incidence of death, MI, or revascularization (29.1% vs 33.4%, $p = 0.031$), but this benefit did not persist at 6 months (38.4% vs 39.9%, $p = 0.50$).

22. **Antman E**, for the TIMI 11B Investigators. Enoxaparin prevents death and cardiac ischemic events in unstable angina/non–Q-wave MI: results of the TIMI II B trial. *Circulation* (in press).

 This prospective, randomized, double-blind, multicenter trial was composed of 3,910 patients with ischemic discomfort at rest within the past 24 hours and ST-segment deviation or positive CK-MB or troponin. Patients were randomized to enoxaparin [1 mg/kg subcutaneously twice daily (acute phase), then 60 mg (≥65 kg) or 40 mg (<65 kg) twice daily) during both acute (2–8 days) and chronic phases (through day 43), or to intravenous heparin (acute phase only). Preliminary results showed that the enoxaparin-treated patients had a significant 12% reduction in the primary composite end point of death, MI, or urgent revascularization at day 43 (17.3% vs. 19.7%; $p = 0.048$). This benefit was apparent by day 8 (12.4% vs. 14.5%; $p = 0.048$). Chronic enoxaparin treatment was associated with an increase in the rate of major hemorrhage (spontaneous and instrumented; 2.9% vs. 1.5%; $p = 0.021$). Bleeding rates during the acute phase were similar. When these results are pooled with the ESSENCE data, there is a significant reduction in death and MI at day 8 (4.1% vs. 5.3%), day 14 (5.2% vs. 6.5%), and day 43 (7.1% vs. 8.6%).

23. Fraxiparine in Ischemic Syndrome (FRAXIS). Preliminary results presented at the 20th Congress of the European Society of Cardiology in Vienna, Austria, August 1998.

 This prospective, randomized, controlled study was composed of 1,151 patients with unstable angina and non–Q-wave MI. Patients received fraxiparine for a short course (6 ± 2 days) or long course (14 days) or unfractionated heparin. At 14 days, the incidence of the primary composite end point, consisting of cardiovascular death, or recurrent angina, was similar in the three treatment groups (heparin, 15.1%; short-course fraxiparine, 17.8%; long-course fraxiparine, 20%). There was a higher incidence of hemorrhage in the long-course fraxiparine group (at 14 days, 3.5%).

β-*Blockers Calcium Antagonists and Nitrates*

24. **Gibson RS**, et al., Diltiazem Reinfarction Study Group. Diltiazem and reinfarction in patients with non–Q-wave MI. *N Engl J Med* 1986;315:423–429.

 Design: Prospective, randomized, double-blind, multicenter study. Primary end point was reinfarction at 14 days.

 Purpose: To determine whether diltiazem would reduce the incidence of early reinfarction in patients recovering from a non–Q-wave MI.

 Population: 576 patients with non–Q-wave MI [elevated CK-MB and either ischemic pain for 30 minutes or ST-segment deviation (elevation or depression ≥1 mm or T-wave inversions in at least two leads)].

 Exclusion Criteria: New Q-waves, advanced heart block, cardiogenic shock, and coronary bypass surgery in past 3 months.

 Treatment: Randomized at 24–72 hours to diltiazem 90 mg every 6 hours, or placebo.

Results: Diltiazem patients had a significantly lower 14-day re-infarction rate (5.2% vs. 9.3%; $p = 0.03$) and 50% less refractory angina. No significant difference was observed in mortality rates (3.1% vs. 3.8%). Mild adverse reactions were common in the diltiazem group.

25. **Gerstenblith G**, et al. Nifedipine in unstable angina. *N Engl J Med* 1982;306:885–889.

   This prospective, randomized, double-blind, placebo-controlled trial was composed of 138 patients with rest pain accompanied by ST or T-wave changes or arrhythmias. Patients received nifedipine 10–20 mg orally every 6 hours, and all were given nitrates and propranolol (unless contraindicated). At 4 months, nifedipine-treated patients had fewer events (coronary artery bypass surgery for persistent angina, MI, sudden cardiac death): 44% vs. 61% ($p = 0.03$). Nifedipine patients did have more side effects (hypotension, diarrhea), resulting in discontinuation of therapy in four patients versus one placebo patient.

26. **Gheorghiade M**, et al. Effects of propranolol in non–Q-wave acute MI in the β-blocker heart attack trial. *Am J Cardiol* 1990; 66:129–133.

   This retrospective analysis focused on the 601 β-Blocker Heart Attack Trial patients (17%) with a non–Q-wave MI. Patients in this trial were randomized to propranolol 180–240 mg/day or placebo. At follow-up (median 24.6 months), similar mortality, sudden death, and reinfarction rates were observed.

27. **Gobel EJA**, et al. Randomised, double-blind trial of intravenous diltiazem vs glyceryl trinitrate for unstable angina. *Lancet* 1995; 346:1653–1657 (editorial pp. 1644–1645).

   In this small study, 129 patients were randomized to diltiazem (25-mg intravenous bolus over 5 minutes, then 5–25 mg/h) or glyceryl trinitrate 1–5 mg/h for 48 hours. Diltiazem patients had less refractory angina (symptoms >1 hour on maximum dose; 6% vs. 17%; $p = 0.02$), better event-free survival, decreased heart rate and blood pressure, and fewer headaches requiring analgesia or dose adjustment (5% vs. 25%). However, 8% did have atrioventricular conduction disturbances and an intention-to-treat analysis showed nonsignificant differences. The accompanying editorial advocates using β-blockers first and as part of combination therapy.

Glycoprotein IIb/IIIa Inhibitors

28. Platelet Receptor Inhibition in Ischemic Syndrome Management in Patients Limited by Unstable Signs and Symptoms **(PRISM-PLUS)** Investigators. Inhibition of the platelet glycoprotein IIb/IIIa receptor with tirofiban in unstable angina and non–Q wave myocardial infarction. *N Engl J Med* 1998;338:1488–1497 (editorial pp. 1539–1541).

   Design: Prospective, randomized, double-blind, multicenter study. Primary end point was death, MI, or refractory ischemia at 7 days.

   Purpose: To investigate the clinical efficacy of tirofiban, a short-acting, nonpeptide glycoprotein IIb/IIIa inhibitor, in the prevention of acute ischemic events in patients with unstable angina and non–Q-wave MI.

Population: 1,915 patients presenting with prolonged anginal pain or repetitive episodes of angina at rest or during minimal exercise in the previous 12 hours and new ST-T changes [≥1 mm elevation or depression, ≥3 mm T-wave inversion on at least three limb leads or precordial leads [excluding V1], or pseudonormalization ≥? mm] or an elevated CK or CK-MB.

Exclusion Criteria: Included ST elevation >20 minutes, thrombolysis in previous 48 hours, angioplasty in past 6 months or coronary bypass surgery in previous month, stroke in prior year, active bleeding or high bleeding risk, history of thrombocytopenia or platelet count <150,000, and creatinine >2.5 mg/dL.

Treatment: 1) Tirofiban 0.6 μg/kg/min for 30 minutes, then 0.15 μg/kg/min and placebo heparin; 2) tirofiban 0.4 μg/kg/min for 30 minutes, then 0.1 μg/kg/min plus heparin; or 3) heparin plus placebo tirofiban.

Results: The tirofiban plus heparin group had a significant reduction compared with the heparin-alone group in the 7-day composite end points (12.9% vs. 17.9%, RR 0.68; $p = 0.004$). This difference persisted at 30-day and 6-month follow-up (18.5% vs. 22.3%, $p = 0.03$; 27.7% vs. 32.1%, $p = 0.02$). The tirofiban plus heparin group also had a significant reduction in death or MI at 7 days and 30 days (4.9% vs. 8.3%, $p = 0.006$; 8.7% vs. 11.9%, $p = 0.03$).

Comments: The entire benefit was achieved within the first 7 days. The event curves then remain parallel through later follow-up. Tirofiban alone group terminated prematurely due to excess mortality at 7 days [4.6% vs. 1.1% (heparin alone)].

29. Platelet Receptor Inhibition in Ischemic Syndrome Management **(PRISM)** Study Investigators. A comparison of aspirin plus tirofiban with aspirin plus heparin for unstable angina. *N Engl J Med* 1998;338:1498–1505 (editorial pp. 1539–1541).

Design: Prospective, randomized, multicenter study. Primary end point was death, MI, and refractory ischemia at 48 hours.

Purpose: To compare intravenous tirofiban with intravenous unfractionated heparin for the treatment of unstable angina in patients receiving aspirin.

Population: 3,232 patients with rest or accelerating chest pain within 24 hours of randomization and at least one of the following criteria: (a) ST depression ≥1 mm in at least two contiguous leads, transient (<20 minutes) ST elevation, or T-wave inversion; (b) elevated cardiac enzymes; and (c) history of MI, revascularization >6 months earlier, coronary surgery >1 month earlier, positive exercise or pharmacological stress test result, or >50% stenosis on prior angiogram.

Exclusion Criteria: Included thrombolytic therapy in previous 48 hours, creatinine >2.5 mg/dL, increased bleeding risks, history of thrombocytopenia, SBP >180 mm Hg, and DBP >110 mm Hg.

Treatment: Tirofiban 0.6 μg/kg/min for 30 minutes, then 0.15 μg/kg/min through 48 hours with placebo heparin, or unfractionated heparin (5,000-U bolus, then 1,000 U/h for 48 hours, adjusted if necessary based on aPTT at 6 and 24 hours). All patients were on aspirin 300–325 mg daily.

Results: Tirofiban group had a 32% reduction in the composite primary end points at 48 hours: 3.8% vs. 5.6% (RR 0.67; $p = 0.01$).

At 30 days, a similar frequency of composite end points was observed (15.9% vs. 17.1%; $p = 0.34$). At 7 days, the tirofiban group had a significantly lower mortality rate (2.3% vs. 3.6%; $p = 0.02$) and tended toward a reduction in death and MI (5.8% vs. 7.1%; $p = 0.11$). Tirofiban was associated with increased thrombocytopenia (1.1% vs. 0.4%; $p = 0.04$). Identical major bleeding rates were observed (0.4%).

30. Platelet IIb/IIIa Antagonism for the Reduction of Acute Coronary Syndrome Events in a Global Organization Network **(PARAGON)**. The PARAGON Investigators. International, randomized, controlled trial of lamifiban (a platelet glycoprotein IIb/IIIa inhibitor), heparin, or both in unstable angina. *Circulation* 1998;97: 2386–2395.

Design: Prospective, randomized, partial factorial (2×2), controlled (heparin alone), multicenter study. Primary end point was death or MI at 30 days.

Purpose: To evaluate the efficacy and safety of the glycoprotein IIb/IIIa inhibitor lamifiban alone, heparin alone, or both in unstable and non–Q-wave MI.

Population: 2,282 patients with chest discomfort in prior 12 hours associated with transient or persistent ST depression (≥ 0.5 mm) or T-wave inversion or transient (<30 minutes) ST elevation (≥ 0.5 mm).

Exclusion Criteria: Included anticoagulation or INR $<>1.5$, receiving heparin with an aPTT of >85 seconds, thrombolytic therapy within 24 hours, SBP 180 mm Hg, DBP 100 mm Hg despite treatment, creatinine >2.0 mg/dL, platelet count $<100,000$, stroke in prior year, angioplasty in prior week, and major trauma or surgery within 1 month.

Treatment: The patients were randomized to five groups: lamifiban placebo plus heparin (control); lamifiban (300-μg bolus then 1 μg/min), with and without heparin; and lamifiban (750-μg bolus then 5 μg/min), with and without heparin. Lamifiban was given for 3–5 days. (If the intervention was done on day 5, lamifiban was continued for 12–24 additional hours.) All patients received aspirin daily (160 mg recommended).

Results: A similar incidence of death and MI was observed at 30 days with heparin alone, low-dose lamifiban, and high-dose lamifiban (11.7%, 10.6%, 12.0%; $p = 0.668$). At 6 months, low-dose lamifiban was associated with fewer events compared with heparin alone [13.7% vs. 17.9%, $p = 0.027$; 16.4% (high-dose lamifiban), $p = 0.45$]. Low-dose lamifiban yielded the best results with heparin: the 6-month ischemic event rate was 12.6% vs. 17.9% without heparin ($p = 0.025$), and bleeding rates were similar.

Comments: The results suggest that the most favorable regimen is low-dose glycoprotein IIb/IIIa antagonism in conjunction with heparin.

31. Platelet Glycoprotein IIb/IIIa in Unstable Angina Receptor Suppression Using Integrelin Therapy **(PURSUIT)** Trial Investigators. Inhibition of platelet glycoprotein IIb/IIIa with eptifibatide in patients with acute coronary syndromes. *N Engl J Med* 1998; 339:436–443.

Design: Prospective, randomized, double-blind, placebo-controlled, multicenter study. Primary end point was death or nonfatal MI at 30 days.

Purpose: To determine if the addition of eptifibatide to heparin and aspirin provides additional benefit in patients with acute coronary syndromes without ST elevation.

Population: 10,948 patients with ischemic chest pain lasting 10 minutes in prior 24 hours (median 11 hours) and ECG changes (transient or persistent ST-segment depression >0.5 mm, transient ST-segment elevation >0.5 mm, or T-wave inversion >1 mm within 12 hours before or after chest pain), or serum CK-MB above the upper limit of normal.

Exclusion Criteria: Included persistent ST elevation >1 mm, SBP >200 mm Hg or DBP >100 mm Hg, major surgery within the prior 6 weeks, nonhemorrhagic stroke in the prior 30 days or any history of hemorrhagic stroke, renal failure, planned used of thrombolytic or glycoprotein IIb/IIIa inhibitors, and thrombolysis in the prior 24 hours.

Treatment: Eptifibatide 180 µg/kg bolus then 1.3 or 2.0 µg/ kg/min for 72 hours (up to 96 hours if intervention was near the end of a 72-hour period), or placebo; 1.3 µg/kg/min infusion was dropped after 3,218 patients enrolled. No protocol-mandated strategy of catheterization and revascularization was undertaken.

Results: Eptifibatide was associated with 9.6% lower rates of death and MI at 30 days (14.2% vs. 15.7%; $p = 0.04$); this effect was apparent by 72 hours. Among patients undergoing early PCI, eptifibatide was associated with a 32% benefit. Eptifibatide was associated with increased major bleeding (10.6% vs. 9.1%; $p = 0.02$) and higher transfusion rates (11.6% vs. 9.2%, RR 1.3; 95% CI 1.1–1.4). The eptifibatide group also had more cases of profound thrombocytopenia (platelet count <20,000): RR 5.0 (nine vs. two patients; 95% CI 1.3–32.4). Eptifibatide was not associated with increased incidence of bleeding in those undergoing CABG surgery. Stroke occurred in 79 patients (0.7%), 66 of which were nonhemorrhagic, and there were no significant differences in stroke rates between patients who received placebo and those assigned high-dose eptifibatide (*see Circulation* 1999;99:2371).

Comments: The finding of no extra bleeding risk in those undergoing CABG surgery is consistent with the short half-life of eptifibatide.

32. Orbofiban in Patients with Unstable Coronary Syndromes **(OPUS/ TIMI-16)** Preliminary Results presented by Cannon CP at the 48th ACC Scientific Session in New Orleans, LA, March 1999.

This prospective, randomized, multicenter, double-blind, placebo-controlled trial was composed of 10,302 patients with ECG changes or elevated cardiac markers (other lower risk inclusion criteria eliminated early in trial). Patients received orbofiban 50 mg twice daily for 1 month, then 30 or 50 mg twice daily; or placebo. This trial was stopped early because of excess mortality in the orbofiban 50/30 group. At 30 days, rates were 1.6% vs 2.3% vs 1.4%, respectively. Preliminary analysis of deaths in the first 30 days show more new thrombotic events in orbofiban-treated patients, suggesting a possible rebound phenomenon. Incidence of primary end point (death, MI, recurrent ischemia stroke) at 300 days was 19.5%, 20.2%, and 20.5%, respectively ($p = NS$). The incidence of severe bleeding, major bleeding, and thrombocytopenia was higher in orbofiban-treated patients.

33. **Cannon CP**, et al. The **TIMI-12** Investigators. Randomized trial of an oral glycoprotein IIb/IIIa antagonist, sibrofiban, in patients after an acute coronary syndrome. *Circulation* 1998;97; 340–349 (editorial pp. 312–314).

This phase II, double-blind, dose-ranging trial showed that effective sustained long-term platelet inhibition can be achieved with an oral glycoprotein IIb/IIIA inhibitor, but at the expense of significant minor bleeding. The pharmacokinetics/pharmaco-dynamics cohort consisted of 106 patients who were randomized to one of seven doses of sibrofiban (5 mg daily to 10 mg twice daily) for 4 weeks and a safety cohort of 223 patients who were randomized to one of four doses or aspirin for 4 weeks. Platelet inhibition (using 20 μmol of adenosine diphosphate) ranged from 47% to 97% at day 28. Major hemorrhage occurred in 1.5% and minor bleeding in 0%–32% (vs. 0% with aspirin alone). Minor bleeding was related to total daily dose ($p = 0.002$), once vs. twice daily dosing ($p < 0.0001$), renal function ($p < 0.0001$), and presentation with unstable angina ($p < 0.01$).

Direct Thrombin Inhibitors

34. **Topol EJ**, et al. Global Utilization of Strategies to Open Occluded Arteries **(GUSTO IIb)**. A comparison of recombinant hirudin with heparin for the treatment of acute coronary syndromes. *N Engl J Med* 1996;335:775–782.

Design: Prospective, randomized, double-blind, multicenter study. Primary end point was death or nonfatal MI (or reinfarction) at 30 days.

Purpose: To compare the clinical effectiveness of hirudin with that of heparin in patients with all types of acute coronary syndromes.

Population: 12,142 patients with chest pain in prior 12 hours accompanied by persistent ST elevation or depression ≥0.5 mm (n = 4,131) or T-wave inversion (n = 8,011).

Exclusion Criteria: Included oral anticoagulation, active bleeding, history of stroke, serum creatinine >2.0 mg/dL, contraindication to heparin, and SBP >200 mm Hg or DBP >110 mm Hg.

Treatment: Patients were randomized to heparin or hirudin [0.1 mg/kg intravenous bolus then 0.1 mg/kg/h (vs. 0.6 then 0.2 in GUSTO IIa)].

Results: At 30 days, the hirudin group had a nonsignificant 11% reduction in death and MI (8.9% vs. 9.8%; $p = 0.06$). Post hoc analysis showed that the hirudin group had a significant reduction in death and MI at 24 hours (1.3% vs. 2.1%; $p = 0.001$). Hirudin patients had more moderate (but not severe) bleeds (8.8% vs. 7.7%). Patients with ST elevation were younger and had fewer cardiac risk factors but a higher 30-day mortality rate (6.1% vs. 3.8%).

35. Organization to Assess Strategies for Ischemic Syndromes **(OASIS-2)** Investigators. Effects of recombinant hirudin (lepirudin) compared with heparin on death, MI, refractory angina, and revascularization procedures in patients with acute myocardial ischaemia without ST elevation: a randomised trial. *Lancet* 1999; 353:429–438 (editorial, pp. 423–424).

Design: Prospective, randomized, multicenter, double-blind, double-dummy study. Primary end point was cardiovascular death or new MI at 7 days.

Purpose: To evaluate whether hirudin is superior to heparin in reducing major cardiac events in patients with unstable angina or suspected non-STEMI.

Population: 10,141 patients 21–85 years of age with unstable angina (abnormal ECG required if <60 years of age) or suspected acute MI without ST elevation.

Exclusion Criteria: Included PTCA within prior 6 months, planned thrombolysis or primary PTCA, and history of stroke in prior year.

Treatment: Heparin 5,000-U bolus then 15 U/kg/h for 72 hours or hirudin 0.4 mg/kg bolus then 0.15 mg/kg/h for 72 hours.

Results: Hirudin group had a nonsignificant 16% RR reduction in cardiovascular death and MI at 7 days (3.6% vs. 4.2%; $p = 0.077$). The hirudin group also had a significant 18% RR reduction in cardiovascular death, MI, and refractory angina at 7 days (5.6% vs. 6.7%; $p = 0.0125$). Most of the differences between the groups were observed during the first 72 hours: cardiovascular death or MI RR 0.76 ($p = 0.039$), and cardiovascular death, MI, and refractory angina RR 0.78 ($p = 0.019$). The hirudin group had an excess of major bleeding (1.2% vs. 0.7%; $p = 0.01$) but no excess of life-threatening bleeds.

36. **Topol EJ**, et al. Recombinant hirudin for unstable angina pectoris: a multicenter, randomized angiographic trial. *Circulation* 1994; 89:1557–1566.

     This randomized, open label, multicenter, angiographic trial was composed of 163 patients with rest pain, abnormal ECG, and angiography demonstrating 60% stenosis of a major epicardial artery. Patients were randomized to one of two heparin groups (targeted aPTT of 65–90 or 90–110 seconds) or one of four hirudin groups (0.05, 0.1, 0.2, or 0.3 mg/kg/h) in a dose-escalating protocol. Repeat angiography was performed at 72–120 hours. A higher proportion of hirudin-treated patients had an aPTT within a 40-second range (71% vs. 16%). Hirudin patients tended to have a lower cross-sectional area of culprit lesion (primary efficacy variable; $p = 0.08$) and significant reduction in minimal luminal diameter ($p = 0.028$).

37. **Fuchs J**, et al. Thrombolysis in MI **(TIMI-7)**. Hirulog in the treatment of unstable angina: results of TIMI-7 trial. *Circulation* 1995;92:727–733.

     In this prospective, randomized trial, 410 patients were randomized to aspirin (325 mg daily) plus hirulog for 72 hours at one of four dosages (0.02, 0.25, 0.5, or 1.0 mg/kg/h). Fewer deaths and nonfatal MIs through hospital discharge were observed in the three higher dose groups (3.2% vs. 10%; $p = 0.008$). Only two patients experienced a major hemorrhage.

38. **Andersen K**, et al. on behalf of the Thrombin Inhibition in Myocardial Ischemia **(TRIM)** Study Group. Heparin is more effective than inogatran, a low-molecular weight thrombin inhibitor in suppressing ischemia and recurrent angina in unstable coronary disease. *Am J Cardiol* 1998;81:939–944.

     This randomized study was composed of 324 patients with chest pain in the prior 24 hours. Patients received inogatran (one of three doses) or heparin for 72 hours. Continuous ECG monitoring was performed during the first 24 hours. Heparin patients had fewer ischemic episodes (ST-vector magnitude 1 ± 2.6 vs. 2 4. ±

4.5, $p < 0.001$; ST-vector magnitude change 3 ± 4.7 vs. 6 ± 7.6, $p < 0.001$) and less death, MI, and refractory or recurrent angina at 7 days (35% vs. 50%; $p < 0.05$).

Thrombolytics

39. **Bar FW**, et al. Unstable Angina Study Using Eminase **(UNASEM)**. Thrombolysis in patients with unstable angina improves the angiographic but not clinical outcome—results of UNASEM, a multicenter, randomized, placebo-controlled, clinical trial with anistreplase. *Circulation* 1992;86:131–137.

Design: Prospective, randomized, double-blind, placebo-controlled, multicenter study.

Purpose: To evaluate the safety and efficacy of thrombolytic therapy in unstable angina.

Population: 159 patients 30 to 70 years of age with angina of recent onset (<4 weeks) or of the crescendo type with the last episode within 12 hours of admission and ischemic ST changes (ST depression ≥1 mm, T-wave inversion ≥2 mm).

Exclusion Criteria: Included previous MI, previous coronary angioplasty, left bundle branch block or pacemaker, valvular disease, SBP >190 mm Hg or DBP >110 mm Hg, streptokinase or anistreplase in past year, bleeding diathesis, gastrointestinal or genitourinary bleeding in prior 3 months, oral anticoagulation, pregnancy, and recent trauma or cardiopulmonary resuscitation.

Treatment: After angiography, patients were randomized to anistreplase 30 U over 5 minutes or placebo. Repeat angiography was performed at 12–28 hours. All patients received intravenous nitroglycerin (started prior to catheterization), heparin, and aspirin 300 mg/day (started after second catheterization).

Results: Anistreplase group had a significant decrease in stenosis diameter between the first and second angiograms [11% (from 70% to 59%) vs. 3% (from 66% to 63%); $p = 0.008$]. However, no difference was observed in clinical outcome (e.g., infarct size, MI rate), and more bleeding complications were observed with anistreplase (32% vs. 11%; $p = 0.001$).

40. Thrombolysis in Myocardial Ischemia **(TIMI IIIA)** Investigators. Early effects of tissue-type plasminogen activator added to conventional therapy on the culprit coronary lesion in patients presenting with ischemic cardiac pain at rest. Results of the TIMI IIIA Trial. *Circulation* 1993;87:38–52.

Design: Prospective, randomized, open, parallel-group, multicenter study. Primary end point was 10% reduction of stenosis and improvement of two TIMI flow grades.

Purpose: To evaluate the effects of tPA added to conventional therapy on the culprit coronary lesion in patients with unstable angina or non—Q-wave MI

Population: 306 patients 22–75 years of age with chest pain at rest lasting 5 minutes to 6 hours and accompanied by ECG changes or documented CAD.

Exclusion Criteria: Included coronary bypass surgery, MI in prior 21 days, PTCA in prior 6 months, cardiogenic shock, and oral anticoagulation requirement.

Treatment: Front-loaded tPA (maximum 80 mg) or placebo plus conventional antianginal therapy. All patients received heparin

(5,000-U bolus and infusion for 18–48 hours) and aspirin 325 mg daily.
Results: tPA group had more frequent improvement of TIMI flow by two grades or reduction of stenosis by 20% on repeat angiography at 18–48 hours (15% vs. 5%; $p = 0.003$). The tPA benefit was most marked in patients with thrombus-containing lesions (36% vs. 15%; $p < 0.01$) and non–Q-wave MI (33% vs. 8%; $p < 0.005$).
Comments: Only modest angiographic improvement was observed.

41. **Ambrose JA**, et al. Thrombolysis and Angioplasty in Unstable Angina **(TAUSA)**. Adjunctive thrombolytic therapy during PTCA for ischemic rest angina. *Circulation* 1994;90:69–77.
Design: Prospective, randomized, double-blind, multicenter study.
Purpose: To assess the role of intracoronary urokinase during angioplasty for unstable angina or postinfarction rest angina.
Population: 469 patients ≤80 years of age with ischemic rest pain accompanied by ST-segment or T-wave changes and an angiogram demonstrating 70% stenosis.
Exclusion Criteria: Included normal baseline ECG, blood pressure >180/ 110, prior stroke, recent (within <10 days) major surgery, bleeding diathesis, active gastrointestinal or genitourinary bleeding.
Treatment: Intracoronary urokinase (250,000 or 500,000 U) or placebo; all patients received aspirin and heparin (target activated clotting time >300 seconds).
Results: No significant differences in incidence of post-PTCA thrombi were observed [13.8% (urokinase) vs. 18%; $p = $ NS], but the urokinase group had a higher acute closure rate (10.2% vs. 4.3%, $p < 0.02$; most of difference in 500,000 U group) and more adverse outcomes (ischemia, MI, coronary artery bypass surgery; 6.3% vs. 2.9%, $p < 0.02$).
Comments: Possible explanations of adverse effects of urokinase include increased hemorrhagic dissection, lack of intimal sealing, and procoagulant or platelet-activating effects.

42. Thrombolysis in MI **(TIMI IIIB)**. Effects of tissue plasminogen activator and a comparison of early invasive and conservative strategies in unstable angina and non–Q-wave MI. *Circulation* 1994;89:1545–1556.
Design: Prospective, randomized (2 × 2 factorial design), double-blind, placebo-controlled, multicenter study. Primary end point was death, MI, or failure of treatment at 6 weeks (for tPA comparison) and death, MI, or positive ETT (for strategy comparison).
Purpose: To evaluate the use of thrombolytic therapy in unstable angina and non–Q-wave MI and to compare an early invasive with a conservative strategy.
Population: 1,473 patients 21–76 years of age presenting within 24 hours of ischemic discomfort at rest consistent with unstable angina or non–Q-wave MI.
Exclusion Criteria: Included treatable cause of unstable angina, MI in prior 21 days, coronary angiography in prior 30 days, PTCA within 6 months, history of CABG, SBP >180 mm Hg or DBP >100 mm Hg, and contraindication to thrombolysis.
Treatment: tPA 0.8 mg/kg over 90 minutes (maximum 80 mg, mean 63 mg), including one third of dose as an intravenous bolus

(up to 20 mg); or placebo. The early invasive strategy involved catheterization 18–48 hours after randomization and revascularization if feasible. Early conservative strategy allowed for catheterization if patient had recurrent ischemia at rest with ECG changes or other failure of medical therapy.

Results: No difference was observed between invasive and conservative strategies in combined primary end points (16.2% vs. 18.1%), but the early invasive strategy was associated with a shorter hospital stay and lower incidence of rehospitalization. tPA was not shown to be beneficial and may be harmful (e.g., four intracranial hemorrhages vs. none with placebo; $p = 0.06$).

Comments: One-year results (*see J Am Coll Cardiol* 1995; 26:1643) showed similar death and nonfatal reinfarction rates between tPA and placebo (12.4% vs. 10.6%; $p = 0.24$) and early invasive versus early conservative groups (10.8% vs. 12.2%; $p = 0.42$). The early invasive group had a higher revascularization rate (64% vs. 58%; $p < 0.001$), primarily due to more PTCAs [39% vs. 32%), but fewer readmissions (26% vs. 33%; $p < 0.001$). Subsequent analysis showed that the optimal aPTT range was 45–60 seconds (71).

Invasive versus Conservative Management

43. **Boden WE**, et al. for the Veteran Affairs Non–Q-Wave Infarction Strategies in Hospital **(VANQWISH)** Trial Investigators. Outcomes in patients with acute non–Q-wave MI randomly assigned to an invasive as compared with a conservative strategy. *N Engl J Med* 1998;338:1785–1792 (editorial pp. 1838–1839).

Design: Prospective, randomized, controlled, multicenter study. Primary end point was death or MI.

Purpose: To compare a conservative with an invasive strategy on the incidence of clinical outcomes in non–Q-wave MI.

Population: 920 patients with an evolving MI characterized by no Q waves on serial ECGs and CK-MB >1.5 times the upper limit of normal.

Exclusion Criteria: Included persistent or recurrent ischemia at rest despite intensive medical therapy, severe heart failure despite intravenous diuretics and/or vasodilators, and serious coexisting conditions.

Treatment: Patients were assigned within 24–72 hours to invasive strategy (routine angiography followed by revascularization, if feasible) or conservative strategy (medical therapy, noninvasive testing, and invasive procedures only in setting of spontaneous or inducible ischemia). All patients received aspirin (325 mg daily) and diltiazem (180–300 mg/day).

Results: Only 9% excluded secondary to high-risk ischemic complications. Only 29% of the conservative group (vs. 64% in TIMI-IIIB) underwent catheterization within 30 days. At follow-up (average 23 months), the two groups had a similar incidence of death and MI [152 events (invasive, 32.9%) vs. 139 (conservative, 30.3%); $p = 0.35$]. The conservative group showed a nonsignificant trend toward lower mortality (hazard ratio 0.72, 95% CI 0.51–1.01). Fewer patients treated conservatively had death plus MI or death at hospital discharge (36 vs. 15 patients, $p = 0.004$; 21 vs. 6, $p = 0.007$), at 1 month (48 vs. 26, $p = 0.012$; 23 vs. 9, $p = 0.021$), and at 1 year (111 vs. 85, $p = 0.05$; 58 vs. 36, $p = 0.025$). Of note, the

invasive group had a higher coronary bypass surgery mortality rate [11.6% vs. 3.4% (11 vs. 3 patients in conservative group)].
Comments: No subgroup benefited from an invasive strategy (e.g., anterior MI, low ejection fraction, ST-segment depression on entry ECG).

44. **McCullough PA**, et al. Medicine vs. Angioplasty in Thrombolytic Exclusion (**MATE**). A prospective, randomized trial of triage angiography in acute coronary syndromes ineligible for thrombolytic therapy. *J Am Coll Cardiol* 1998;32:596–605.
Design: Prospective, randomized, controlled, multicenter study. Primary composite end point was death and recurrent ischemic events.
Purpose: To determine if early triage with revascularization, if indicated, favorably affects clinical outcomes in patients with suspected acute MI who are ineligible for thrombolysis.
Population: 201 patients presenting within 24 hours with an acute chest syndrome consistent with acute MI (high clinical suspicion with or without immediate enzymatic confirmation) and considered ineligible for thrombolysis because of lack of ECG changes (68% without ST elevation), symptoms for >6 hours, or increased bleeding or stroke risks.
Exclusion Criteria: Included symptoms for >24 hours or an absolute indication or contraindication to cardiac catheterization.
Treatment: Early triage angiography and subsequent therapies based on the angiogram versus conventional medical therapy consisting of aspirin, intravenous heparin, nitroglycerin, β-blockers, and analgesics.
Results: Acute MI was confirmed in 51% and 54% of triage angiography and conservative patients, respectively. The triage angiography group had a significant reduction in the primary end points of recurrent ischemic events and death (13% vs. 34%, risk reduction 45%, 95% CI 27%–59%; $p = 0.0002$). In the triage angiography group, 58% received revascularization, whereas in the conservative group, 60% subsequently underwent nonprotocol angiography due to recurrent ischemia and 37% received revascularization ($p = 0.004$). The mean time to revascularization was substantially shorter in the triage angiography group (27 vs. 98 hours; $p = 0.0001$). No differences were seen in length of stay or hospital costs. At long-term follow-up (median 21 months), no significant differences in late revascularization, recurrent MI, or all-cause mortality were observed.
Comments: This was a low-risk study group (in-hospital mortality rate only 2%) and was not powered to show reduction in long-term recurrent MI and death. Troponin testing was not used in making the decision to use early angiography.

45. FRagmin and Fast Revascularization during InStability in coronary artery disease (**FRISC II**) Investigators. Invasive compared with noninvasive treatment in unstable coronary artery disease: FRISC II prospective randomized multicenter study. *Lancet* 1999;354:708–715.
Design: Prospective, randomized, partially open (strategy assignment), multicenter study. Primary end point was death or MI at 6 months.
Purpose: To compare an early invasive with a noninvasive strategy in patients with unstable coronary disease in addition to optimum background antithrombolic medication.

Population: 2,457 patients with ischemic symptoms in previous 48 hours accompanied by ECG changes (ST depression or T wave inversion ≥0.1 mv) or elevated markers (e.g. CK-MB > 6 mg/L, troparin T >0.10 mg/dL).
Exclusion Criteria: see reference 21.
Treatment: Early invasive or noninvasive treatment strategy (coronary angiography within 7 days performed in 96% and 10%, and revascularization in first 10 days in 71% and 9%). Patients also received dalteparin or placebo for 3 months.
Results: The invasive group had a significantly lower incidence of death or MI at 6 months (9.4% vs 12.1% [noninvasive group], $p = 0.031$). There was a significant decrease in MI alone (7.8% vs 10.1%, $p = 0.045$), while the reduction in mortality was nonsignificant (1.9% vs 2.9%, $p = 0.10$). Subgroup analysis showed these benefits were restricted to men (risk ratios of death or MI at 6 months 0.64 and 1.26 in men and women, respectively). Invasive strategy was also associated with 50% lower recurrent angina and hospital readmission rates.

Miscellaneous

46. **Gurfinkel E**, et al. for the **ROXIS** Study Group. Randomised trial of roxithromycin in non–Q-wave coronary syndromes: ROXIS pilot study. *Lancet* 1997;350:404–407 (editorial pp. 378–379).

    This prospective, randomized, double-blind, placebo-controlled, multicenter study was composed of 202 patients with rest pain lasting >10 minutes in the previous 48 hours and ischemic ECG changes (ST depression, transient ST elevation ≥1 mm, T-wave inversion in at least two contiguous leads). Patients received roxithromycin 150 mg twice daily or placebo for 30 days. The antibiotic group had fewer primary events (death, MI, recurrent angina) from 72 hours to 31 days (2% vs. 9%; adjusted $p = 0.032$). There was no significant difference in incidence of death or MI (0% vs. 2%). The accompanying editorial points out that the study also failed to measure markers of inflammation, thrombogenesis, and endothelial dysfunction and did not report response based on *Chlamydia* seropositivity (48%). Preliminary results from the large ACADEMIC study show no benefit on clinical end points associated with antibiotic therapy.

Prognosis and Assessment
Clinical or General Analyses

47. **Cannon CP**, et al. Predictors of non–Q-wave MI in patients with acute ischemic syndromes: an analysis from the TIMI III trials. *Am J Cardiol* 1995;75:977–978.

    This analysis focused on 1,473 TIMI IIIB patients who had rest pain and ECG changes or documented CAD. One third of patients had a non–Q-wave MI. There were four independent predictors of non–Q-wave MI: no history of PTCA (odds ratio 3.3; $p < 0.001$), pain ≥60 minutes (odds ratio 2.9; $p < 0.001$), ST-segment deviation on initial ECG (odds ratio 2.0; $p < 0.001$), and recent-onset angina (odds ratio 1.7; $p < 0.002$). For all TIMI 3 patients, with zero risk factors, 7% had non–Q-wave MI; with one risk factor, 19.6%; two risk factors, 24.4%; three risk factors, 49.9%; all four risk factors, 70.6%.

48. **Schreiber TL**, et al. Cardiologist vs internist management of patients with unstable angina: treatment patterns and outcomes. *J Am Coll Cardiol* 1995;26:577–582 (editorial pp. 583–584).

This study showed that cardiologists more frequently prescribe appropriate medications and order more invasive testing compared with internists. The study population was composed of 890 consecutive unstable angina patients (225 treated by internists, 665 by cardiologists) at community-based Michigan hospitals. Internists used less aspirin, heparin, and β-blockers (68% vs. 78%; 67% vs. 84%; 18% vs. 30%). They also ordered more exercise tests (37% vs. 22%) but fewer catheterizations and angioplasties (27% vs. 61%; 7% vs. 40%). The cardiologist-treated group showed a trend toward lower mortality (4% vs. 1.8%; $p = 0.06$), despite being higher risk patients (increased prior MI, balloon angioplasty, and bypass surgery). The accompanying editorial points out that fewer studies by internists could be secondary to less prior cardiac disease (53% vs. 80%). Also, more studies do not guarantee better outcome, as seen in TIMI III.

49. **Armstrong PW**, et al. Acute coronary syndromes in the GUSTO-IIb trial. Prognostic insights and impact of recurrent ischemia. *Circulation* 1998;98:1860–1868.

Recurrent ischemia was ~50% more common in non–ST-elevation patients than in ST-elevation patients (35% vs. 23%; $p <$ 0.001). This may explain why the non–ST-elevation group had a lower mortality rate at 30 days (3.8% vs. 6.1%; $p < 0.001$) but a similar rate by 1 year (8.8% vs. 9.6%). Compared with unstable angina patients, non-STEMI patients had higher rates of reinfarction at 6 months (9.8% vs. 6.2%) and higher 6-month and 1-year mortality rates (8.8% vs. 5.0%; 11.1% vs. 7.0%).

50. **Farkouh ME**, et al. A clinical trial of a chest-pain observation unit for patients with unstable angina. *N Engl J Med* 1998;339: 1882–1888.

This community-based, prospective study of 424 unstable angina patients showed that a chest pain observation unit located in the emergency department can be safe, effective, and result in cost savings. Patients with rest angina lasting >20 minutes, new-onset angina on exertion meeting criteria for CCS class 3 or higher, and postinfarction were eligible. High-risk patients, such as those with ST-segment depression in several ECG leads, were excluded. Eligible patients were randomized to routine hospital admission (monitored bed on cardiology service) or admission to the chest pain observation unit. There was no significant difference in rate of cardiac events between the two groups (odds ratio for chest pain observation unit group 0.50, 95% CI 0.20–1.24). At 6 months, chest pain observation unit patients had used less resources ($p = 0.003$ by rank-sum test).

51. **Stone PH**, et al. Influence of race, sex and age of management of unstable angina and non–Q-wave MI (TIMI III registry). *JAMA* 1996;275:1104–1112.

This prospective analysis of 3,318 patients showed disparities in care among blacks, women, and the elderly. Compared with non-blacks, blacks were less likely to be treated with intensive antiischemic therapy and undergo invasive procedures (risk ratio 0.65; $p < 0.001$). However, of those who had angiography (45% of blacks and 61% of nonblacks), blacks had less extensive and severe coronary stenoses. Also, blacks had less recurrent ischemia. Women were also less likely to receive intensive antiischemic therapy and undergo angiography (risk ratio 0.71; $p < 0.001$) and had less severe and extensive coronary disease; however, they had a similar risk of experiencing an adverse cardiac event by 6 weeks. Elderly patients (>75 years of age) received less aggressive therapy and had less frequent angiography (risk ratio 0.65; $p < 0.001$) and fewer revascularization procedures (risk ratio 0.79; $p = 0.002$) despite having more extensive disease. At 6 weeks, the elderly had a higher incidence of adverse cardiac events (risk ratio 1.91; $p < 0.001$).

52. **Calvin JE**, et al. Risk stratification in unstable angina: prospective validation of Braunwald classification. *JAMA* 1995;273:136–141.

This prospective analysis focused on 393 consecutive patients admitted with unstable angina. Multiple logistic regression analysis identified four clinical factors used in the Braunwald classification that predicted in-hospital complications (death, MI after 24 hours, congestive heart failure, ventricular tachycardia, or fibrillation): (a) recent MI (<14 days earlier; odds ratio 5.72); (b) need for intravenous nitroglycerin (odds ratio 2.33); (c) lack of β-blocker or calcium-channel blocker prior to admission (odds ratio 3.83); and (d) baseline ST-segment depression (odds ratio 2.81). Two other clinical factors not utilized in the Braunwald classification, age and diabetes, were also significant predictors.

53. **Zaacks SM**, et al. Unstable angina and non–Q-wave MI: does the clinical diagnosis have therapeutic implications? *J Am Coll Cardiol* 1999;33:107–118.

This review of published literature asserts that the distinction between unstable angina and non–Q-wave MI is no longer adequate to identify high-risk patients. Instead, such individuals are best identified using patients' characteristics (e.g., age), specific ECG changes, newer biochemical markers (e.g., troponins), and angiographic findings.

54. **Alexander JH**, et al. Prior aspirin use predicts worse outcomes in patients with non-ST elevation acute coronary syndromes. *Am J Cardiol* 1999;83:1147–1151.

This analysis of 9,461 PURSUIT trial patients found that prior aspirin users had a higher rate of death or MI at 30 days and 6 months (16.1% vs. 13.0%, $p = 0.001$; 19.9% vs. 15.9%, $p = 0.001$) despite a lower incidence of an index MI (vs. unstable angina) (43.9% vs. 48.8%; $p = 0.001$). After adjustment for all significant, independent baseline predictors, prior aspirin users remained less likely to have an index MI (odds ratio 0.88; 95% CI 0.79–0.97) and more likely to suffer death or MI at 30 days (odds ratio 1.16, 95% CI 1.00–1.33) but not at 6 months (odds ratio 1.14; 95% CI 0.98–1.33).

Troponins

55. **Hamm CW**, et al. The prognostic value of serum troponin T in unstable angina. *N Engl J Med* 1992;327:146–150 (editorial pp. 192–194).

This prospective, multicenter analysis focused on 109 consecutive unstable angina patients (84 with rest angina and 25 with accelerated or subacute angina) who had CK, CK-MB, and troponin T sampled every 8 hours for 2 days after hospital admission. Troponin T was detected (range 0.20–3.64 μg/L) in 39% of the

84 patients with rest angina; only 3 of these patients had an elevated CK-MB (1 of 3 with negative troponin T). Positive troponin T patients had high event rates, with MI occurring in 30% and in-hospital death in 15%. In contrast, only 1 of 51 patients with rest angina and a negative troponin T had an MI ($p < 0.001$), and this patient died ($p = 0.03$). Troponin T was not detected in any of the 25 patients with accelerated or subacute angina.

56. **Lindahl B**, et al. Relation between troponin T and the risk of subsequent cardiac events in unstable coronary artery disease. *Circulation* 1996;93:1651–1657.

    This prospective analysis of 976 FRISC patients showed that 5-month rates of cardiac death and MI correlate with troponin T. In the first quintile (maximum troponin T in first 24 hours <0.06 µg/L), the incidence of death and MI was 4.3%; second quintile (0.06–0.18 µg/L), 10.5%; top three quintiles, 16.1%. In multivariate analysis, independent predictors of death and MI included troponin T (other predictors were age, hypertension, number of antianginal drugs, and rest ECG changes). A subsequent analysis (*see J Am Coll Cardiol* 1997;29:43) showed that the dalteparin group had a lower rate death and MI only if troponin T was ≥0.1 µg/L (7.4% vs. 14.2%; $p < 0.01$).

57. **Antman E**, et al. Cardiac-specific troponin I levels to predict the risk of mortality in patients with acute coronary syndromes. *N Engl J Med* 1996;335:1342–1349 (editorial pp. 1388–1389).

    This analysis focused on 1,404 TIMI IIIB patients. Troponin I was elevated (≥0.4 ng/mL) in 573 patients and associated with a significantly increased 42-day mortality rate (3.7% vs. 1.0%; $p < 0.001$). Each 1 ng/mL increase in troponin I was associated with a mortality increase: ≤0.4, 1%; 0.4–0.9, 1.7%; 1–1.9, 3.4%; 2–4.9, 3.7%; 5–8.9, 6%; and ≥9, 7.5%. If no CK-MB elevation was present (948 patients), a troponin I elevation was still associated with increased mortality: 2.5% vs. 0.8% (RR 3.0; 95% CI 0.97–9.2).

58. **Hamm CW**, et al. Benefit of abciximab in patients with refractory unstable angina in relation to serum troponin T levels. *N Engl J Med* 1999;340:1623–1629.

    This analysis focused on 890 CAPTURE trial patients with unstable angina who had serum samples drawn at the time of randomization to abciximab or placebo. Patients with postinfarction angina were excluded. Among placebo-treated patients, the incidence of death and nonfatal MI at 6 months was threefold higher in patients with elevated troponin T levels (>0.1 ng/mL, 23.9% vs. 7.5%; $p < 0.001$), whereas there was no difference among abciximab-treated patients (9.5% vs. 9.4%). The lower incidence of death or MI in elevated troponin T patients receiving abciximab compared with placebo (RR 0.32, $p = 0.002$) was due to the significant reduction in MI rate (odds ratio 0.23; $p < 0.001$). In patients without elevated troponin T levels, no significant benefit was associated with abciximab treatment.

59. **Galvani M**, et al. Prognostic influence of elevated values of cardiac troponin I in patients with unstable angina. *Circulation* 1997; 95:2053–2059.

    This prospective cohort study was composed of 91 patients with rest chest pain within 48 hours of admission and ECG changes but normal CK in the first 16 hours. Seven patients had an elevated troponin I level on admission, compared with 15 at 8 hours.

The elevated troponin group had an increased 30-day rate of death and MI (27.3% vs. 5.8%; $p = 0.02$) and an increased 1-year event rate (32% vs. 10%; $p = 0.01$).

60. **Luscher MS**, et al. Applicability of cardiac troponin T and I for early risk stratification in unstable coronary artery disease. *Circulation* 1997;96:2578–2585.

    This analysis of 516 TRIM study patients with suspected unstable CAD showed that troponins independently predict cardiac death. Elevated troponin T (≥ 0.10 µg/L was associated with increased risk of cardiac death at 30 days compared with patients with normal levels (3.2% vs. 0.4%; $p = 0.014$). Similarly, elevated of troponin I (>2.0 µg/L was associated with increased cardiac death (3.2% vs. 0.7%; $p = 0.026$).

Inflammatory Markers

61. **Haverkate F**, et al. Production of C-reactive protein and risk of coronary events in stable and unstable angina. *Lancet* 1997; 349:362–366.

    This analysis focused on 2,121 outpatients with angina (1,030 unstable, 743 stable, 348 atypical); all had baseline angiography. At 2-year follow-up, patients with CRP in the fifth quintile (>3.6 mg/L) had a twofold higher risk of a coronary event. Thus, acute phase responses are probably not due to myocardial necrosis.

62. **Toss H**, et al. Prognostic influence of increased fibrinogen and C-reactive protein levels in unstable coronary artery disease. *Circulation* 1997;96:4204–4210.

    This analysis of 965 FRISC study patients with unstable angina or non–Q-wave MI showed the independent predictive value of fibrinogen and CRP. Fibrinogen and CRP were measured at inclusion and related to outcomes at 5 months. Fibrinogen by tertiles (<3.38, 3.38–3.99, and >4.0 g/L) was associated with death in 1.6%, 4.6%, and 6.9% ($p = 0.005$) and death and MI in 9.3%, 14.2%, and 19.1% of patients ($p = 0.002$). CRP by tertiles (<2, 2–10, and >10 mg/L) was associated with death in 2.2%, 3.6%, 7.5% of patients ($p = 0.003$). In multiple logistic regression analysis, increased fibrinogen levels were independently associated with death and death and/or MI ($p = 0.013$) and CRP was independently associated with death ($p = 0.012$).

63. **Morrow DA**, et al. C-reactive protein is a potent predictor of mortality independently of and in combination with troponin T in acute coronary syndromes: a TIMI-11 substudy. *J Am Coll Cardiol* 1998;31:1460–1465.

    A total of 437 unstable angina/non–Q-wave MI patients had quantitative CRP and rapid troponin T assays performed. CRP was higher among patients who died than in survivors (7.2 vs. 1.3 mg/dL; $p = 0.0038$). Patients with CRP ≥ 1.55 mg/dL and an early positive troponin T assay result (≥ 10 minutes) had the highest mortality rates, followed by those with either CRP ≥ 1.55 or early positive troponin T assay results, whereas those with a low CRP and negative troponin T assay results were at very low risk (9.10% vs. 4.65% vs. 0.36%; $p = 0.0003$).

64. **Montalescot G**, et al. Early increase of von Willebrand factor predicts adverse outcome in unstable coronary artery disease. *Circulation* 1998;98:294–299 (editorial pp. 287–289).

C-reactive protein, fibrinogen, von Willebrand factor antigen, endothelin-1, and troponin I were measured on admission and at 48 hours in 68 ESSENCE patients. All five markers showed high levels at admission that rose further at 48 hours. Multivariate analysis demonstrated that the rise of von Willebrand factor over 48 hours was a significant and independent predictor of the composite end points (death, MI, recurrent angina, and revascularization) at both 14 and 30 days. The other four markers did not predict outcome. The early increase in von Willebrand factor was more frequent and severe with unfractionated heparin than with enoxaparin ($p < 0.0001$). Thus, enoxaparin may achieve its additional protection via its effects on von Willebrand factor. Potential mechanisms for this effect include enoxaparin being more efficient than unfractionated heparin in binding to the heparin-binding domain of von Willebrand factor; enoxaparin's greater anti-Xa activity, resulting in less thrombin generation and subsequently less platelet activation and less released von Willebrand factor; and enoxaparin decreasing the rate of von Willebrand factor synthesis by endothelial cells.

65. **Liuzzo G**, et al. The prognostic value of C-reactive protein and serum amyloid A protein in severe unstable angina. *N Engl J Med* 1994;331:417–424 (editorial pp. 468–469).

This small study was composed of 32 patients with chronic stable angina, 31 with severe unstable angina, and 29 with acute MI. CK and troponin T levels were normal in all patients (on admission), but elevated CRP (>0.3 mg/dL) was seen in 13%, 65%, and 76%, respectively. Unstable angina patients (with elevated levels) had more ischemic episodes (4.8 vs. 1.8; $p = 0.004$), more MIs (five vs. zero), and more immediate revascularization (12 vs. 2). The accompanying editorial suggests that these findings may explain why many MIs occur from thrombin on lesions that are not highly stenotic (i.e., inflammatory state more important).

66. **Becker RC**, et al. Prognostic value of plasma fibrinogen concentration in patients with unstable angina and non–Q-wave MI (TIMI IIIB). *Am J Cardiol* 1996;78:142–147.

Analysis of 1,473 unstable angina patients showed no association between baseline levels of fibrinogen and in-hospital MI. However, in unstable angina patients, concentration ≥300 mg/dL was associated with a 61% increased rate of death, MI, and spontaneous ischemia ($p = 0.04$).

67. **Biasucci LM**, et al. Elevated levels of C-reactive protein at discharge in patients with unstable predict recurrent instability. *Circulation* 1999;99:855–860.

In this single center study, 53 patients were admitted to CCU for Braunwald class IIIB unstable angina. Plasma levels of CRP, serum amyloid A, fibrinogen, total cholesterol, and *Helicobacter pylori* and *Chlamydia pneumoniae* antibody titers were measured at admission, at discharge, and at 3 months. At discharge, 49% of patients had elevated CRP levels (>3 mg/L). At 1-year follow-up, the readmission rate for recurrent instability or new MI was more than four times higher in patients with elevated CRP at discharge (68% vs. 15%; $p < 0.001$). Serum amyloid A levels had similar prognostic value to CRP, whereas fibrinogen levels were not predictive. *Chlamydia pneumoniae* but not *Helicobacter pylori* antibody titers corresponded significantly with CRP levels.

Specific Tests: Laboratory, Noninvasive, and Invasive

68. **Dewood MA**, et al. Coronary arteriographic findings soon after non-Q wave MI. *N Engl J Med* 1986;315:417–423.

    In this angiography study, 341 non–Q-wave MI patients were divided into three groups: angiography at ≤24 hours, 24–72 hours, ≥72 hours for 7 days. Frequency of total occlusion and visible collateral vessels both increased with time [26% at ≤24 hours vs. 42% at ≥72 hours ($p < 0.05$); 27% vs. 42% ($p < 0.05$)]. The subtotal occlusion rate decreased with time.

69. **Silver MT**, et al. A clinical rule to predict preserved left ventricular ejection fraction in patients after MI. *Ann Intern Med* 1994; 121:750–756.

    This retrospective analysis focused on 314 consecutive MI patients undergoing one of following tests: transthoracic echocardiography, contrast left ventriculography, or radionuclide ventriculography, and gated blood pool scan. Multivariate analysis showed left ventricular ejection fraction to be >40% in those with an interpretable ECG, no previous Q-wave MI, no history of congestive heart failure, and an index event that is not a Q-wave anterior MI. The positive predictive value was >98% in both derivation and validation sets. Results suggest that assessment of left ventricular function is not necessary in all MI patients.

70. **Becker RC**, et al. Relation between systemic anticoagulation as determined by activated thromboplastin and heparin measurements and in-hospital clinical events in unstable angina and non–Q-wave MI. *Am Heart J* 1996;131:421–433.

    This prospective observational study of 1,473 TIMI IIIB patients showed a lower than expected optimal aPTT range. No differences were observed between treatment groups in median aPTTs for the 72- to 96-hour infusion period. Time-dependent covariate analyses failed to identify changes in aPTT or heparin levels between patients with and without in-hospital events ($p = 0.27$). Also, no difference in events was observed between those with optimal anticoagulation (all aPTTs >60 seconds and heparin levels >0.2 U/mL) and those with values below these thresholds. Thus, this study suggests that the optimal aPTT range is 45–60 seconds.

71. **Langer A**, et al. Late assessment of thrombolytic efficacy (LATE) study: prognosis in patients with non–Q-wave MI. *J Am Coll Cardiol* 1996;27:1327–1332 (editorial pp. 1333–1334).

    This post hoc analysis focused on 4,759 of 5,711 patients with documented MI, 1,309 with a non–Q-wave MI. Non–Q-wave MI versus Q-wave MI was associated with a lower 1-year mortality rate (13.3% vs. 17.1%; $p = 0.001$) and a similar reinfarction rate (8.6% vs. 7.9%; $p = 0.7$). Overall, no difference in rt-PA versus placebo was observed in patients with ST elevation, but rt-PA patients treated at <3 hours after admission had a lower 1-year mortality rate (15.8% vs. 19.6%; $p = 0.028$). Patients with >2 mm ST depression demonstrated a significant benefit from thrombolysis (20.1% vs. 31.9%; $p = 0.006$). The accompanying editorial points out the need for more detailed analysis of LATE to see if any subgroup at >6 hours benefits from thrombolysis. It is unclear what percentage of ST depression >2 mm occurred in anterior leads, which could represent reciprocal changes from posterior MI due to an occluded left circumflex artery.

72. **Cannon CP**, et al. The electrocardiogram predicts one year out-
    come of patients with unstable angina and non–Q-wave MI:
    results of TIMI III Registry Ancillary Study. *J Am Coll Cardiol*
    1997;30:133–140.

    This prospective study focused on 1,416 patients, 14.3% with
    new ST deviation ≥1 mm, 21.9% had isolated T-wave inversion,
    and 9% had left bundle branch block. The incidence of death and
    MI at 1 year was 11% in the group with ST changes [$p < 0.001$ (vs.
    no ST deviation)], 6.8% with T-wave inversion, and 8.2% without
    ECG changes. Two high-risk groups were identified: one with left
    bundle branch block [22.9%; RR 2.80 (multivariate analysis)] and
    the other with 0.5-mm ST changes (16.3%; RR 2.45).

Myocardial Infarction

EPIDEMIOLOGY

In the United States, approximately 1.5 million patients develop acute myocardial infarction (MI) each year; 40% to 50% are accompanied by ST-segment elevation. Between 25% and 30% of nonfatal MIs are unrecognized by the patient and are discovered by routine electrocardiography or at postmortem examination. The overall associated mortality rate ranges from 5% to 30%, depending on patient characteristics, with half of the deaths (most of them due to ventricular fibrillation) occurring before the patient receives medical attention. Among those who arrive at a hospital, approximately 25% of deaths occur in the first 48 hours. Men typically experience a first MI 10 years earlier in life than women.

PATHOPHYSIOLOGY

ST elevation MI is the result of thrombotic coronary artery occlusion in approximately 90% of patients. Non-ST elevation MIs are typically the result of nonocclusive thrombus over an underlying stenosis (see Chapter 3). Approximately two thirds of MIs occur in plaques with less than 50% underlying stenosis. Inflammation appears to play a role in plaque rupture (*see Circulation* 1988;78:1157).

DIAGNOSIS (see page 199)

Even with a strong clinical suspicion of MI based on history and physical examination, MI is subsequently confirmed in only 85% to 90% of patients (21). Also, MI is not diagnosed by the first electrocardiogram (ECG) or creatine kinase (CK)/CK-MB in 25% to 35% of patients; serial testing is needed.

Pain (see page 194)

The pain of MI typically lasts for more than 30 minutes. In one study, the probability of MI (or unstable angina) was very low if (a) the pain was sharp or stabbing, (b) the pain was reproducible by palpation or was pleuritic or positional, and (c) the patient had no history of angina or MI (5).

Electrocardiography (see pages 196, 264–266)

Early ECG may show only hyperacute T waves. ST elevation 1 mm in two contiguous leads is highly sensitive, but can also be seen in left ventricular hypertrophy, Wolff-Parkinson-White syndrome, and pericarditis. New left bundle branch block should raise strong clinical suspicion of MI.

With right ventricular infarction, ST elevation is seen in the V4R lead with a sensitivity of approximately 90% and specificity approximately 80% (197). With posterior infarction, precordial depression and ST elevation are usually seen in leads V7 to V9 (12,204,205; *see* also *Am J Cardiol* 1999;83:323).

Echocardiography

Echocardiography is useful if the ECG results have been non-diagnostic and in those with suspected aortic dissection. Areas of abnormal wall motion are typically observed in patients with acute MI, especially those with transmural involvement.

Serum Markers (see pages 197, 198)

CK-MB and troponin I (TnI) and troponin T (TnT) exceed normal ranges within 4 to 8 hours and levels peak at 24 hours (CK-MB peak occurs sooner with successful thrombolysis). CK-MB levels normalize by 48 to 72 hours, whereas TnI remains elevated for up to 10 days. Of note, TnI and TnT are cardiac specific and levels strongly correlate with mortality (17). Myoglobin peak levels are reached earlier (within 1–4 hours), with a rapid rise indicative of successful reperfusion (19). Myoglobin also has an excellent negative predictive value (14).

TREATMENT

Aspirin (see page 201)

In the second International Study of Infarct Survival (ISIS-2) (29), aspirin (162 mg chewed, to ensure rapid therapeutic blood levels) use was associated with a 23% lower mortality rate, as well as fewer reinfarctions and strokes. Importantly, aspirin and thrombolytic therapy have an additive benefit (42% lower mortality rate in ISIS-2). If a patient has an aspirin allergy, clopidogrel (75 mg daily) could be substituted because it showed a slight benefit compared with aspirin in more than 8,000 patients with a recent MI (CAPRIE trial, *see* Chapter 1, ref. 191), although its onset of action is not immediate (Table 4-1).

β-Blockers (see pages 210–214)

Metoprolol 5 mg may be administered intravenously every 2 to 5 minutes for three doses along with 25 mg orally, then, if tolerated, up to 50 mg every 6 hours (ultimately converted to twice

Table 4-1. Treatment of ST elevation MI

Beneficial	Limited Data or No Benefit	Special Situations	Harmful
Aspirin	Heparin	Coumadin	Nifedipine
β-blockers	Nitrates	Vasopressors	Lidocaine
Thrombolytics	Magnesium	Intraaortic balloon pump	
Primary PCI	Verapamil	Surgery	
ACE inhibitors	Amiodarone	Diuretics	
	GP IIb/IIIa inhibitors	Insulin	
	Direct thrombin inhibitors		

daily dosing); alternatively, atenolol 5 to 10 mg may be administered intravenously, then 100 mg/day orally. Early randomized trials showed mortality benefits with timolol, propranolol, and metoprolol (50,51,56). In the large ISIS-1 trial (53), use of atenolol (5–10 mg intravenously then 100 mg/day orally) was associated with a 15% mortality benefit. In the Thrombolysis in MI (TIMI IIB) trial (54), immediate initiation of β-blockade was shown to be superior to delayed initiation (at 6–8 days). A meta-analysis of randomized trials (most completed before the widespread use of thrombolysis and aspirin) showed a 13% mortality reduction with early initiation of a β-blocker agent. However, even delayed therapy provides substantial benefit, as shown in the early placebo-controlled trials (50,51). β-blockade was also associated with a decreased incidence of cardiac rupture and ventricular fibrillation (57). One analysis showed that the benefits of β-blockade are independent of thrombolytic and angiotensin-converting enzyme (ACE) inhibitor use (59).

A newer agent, carvedilol (β and α antagonist), has shown promise in one small study of MI patients, reducing cardiac events by 45% (60).

Contraindications include hypotension, bradycardia/heart block, severe chronic obstructive pulmonary disease (COPD), and rates 10cm above the diaphragm. If β-blockade is still desired, the clinician should consider using esmolol (500 μg/kg/min for 1 minute, then 50–200 μg/kg/min).

Thrombolytic Therapy (see pages 215, 228)

Thrombolytic therapy confers a 20% to 25% mortality benefit. Time to treatment is important: a 6.5% absolute mortality benefit if given in first hour versus 2% to 3% if given after 1 to 6 hours (63) (Fig. 4-1). No benefit results if thrombolytic therapy is given after 12 hours (94). The largest benefit is seen in those with left bundle branch block and anterior MI (Fig. 4-2).

Indications for Thrombolysis

Thrombolysis should be considered if ST elevation is ≥1 mm in contiguous precordial leads in anatomically related limb leads, or if new left bundle branch block is present. Thrombolysis is underused, given to only 65% to 70% of eligible patients.

Contraindications (see pages 227, 228)

Contraindications include substantial gastrointestinal bleeding, aortic dissection (known or suspected), prolonged cardiopulmonary resuscitation (CPR), intracranial neoplasm/aneurysm/arteriovenous malformation, trauma or surgery in prior 2 weeks, pregnancy, prior hemorrhagic stroke, or any stroke within the prior year.

Relative contraindications include non-hemorrhagic stroke more than 1 year earlier, active peptic ulcer disease, coumadin use, bleeding diathesis, prolonged CPR, systolic blood pressure (SBP) ≥180 mm Hg, or diastolic blood pressure (DBP) ≥110 mm Hg.

Advanced age is not a contraindication. These patients have increased complications (especially intracranial hemorrhage) but highest absolute mortality reduction.

Prehospital administration has been shown to confer a benefit in several trials (92, 93). A systematic overview showed a signifi-

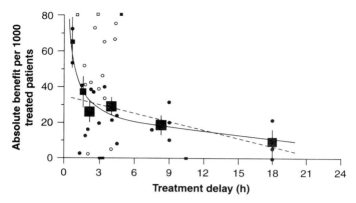

FIG. 4-1. Absolute 35-day mortality reduction versus treatment delay. •, Information from trials included in Fibrinolytic Therapy Trialists (FTT) analysis, which found a linear relationship between treatment delay and absoluted mortality benefit (dotted line); ○, information from additional trials; □, data beyond scale of x/y cross. ■, average effects in six time-to-treatment groups. (Areas of squares are inversely proportional to variance of absolute benefit described.) Analysis by Boersma et al., of randomized trials with ≥100 (50,246 patients) yielded a nonlinear regression curve (solid line), suggesting greatest benefit with time saved early after symptom onset. (Adapted from Boersma E, et al. (63), with permission.)

cant 17% mortality reduction. The magnitude of benefit correlates with time saved.

Common Agents

Streptokinase (see pages 216–226)

Intravenous streptokinase regimens proved superior to placebo in the trial of the Gruppo Italiano per lo Studio della Sopravvivenza nell' Infarto Miocardico (GISSI-1; 18% lower mortality) (87) and ISIS-2 (25% lower mortality) (88). Streptokinase was comparable with tissue plasminogen activator (tPA) in GISSI-2 and ISIS-3 (67,68), but was inferior to it in the Global Utilization of Strategies to Open Occluded Arteries (GUSTO I) study (69; *see* tPA section below).

Anistreplase (see pages 219–231)

Early studies with anistreplase [anisoylated plasminogen streptokinase activator complex (APSAC)] showed a mortality benefit compared with placebo and heparin [APSAC Intervention Mortality Study (AIMS) and German Multicenter Trial (100, 101)]. The second Thrombolytic Trial of Eminase in Acute MI (TEAM-2) showed similar benefits compared with streptokinase (78), but the rt-PA-APSAC Patency Study (TAPS) and Thrombolysis in MI (TIMI-4) study showed lower patency and more in-hospital deaths compared with tPA (71,79).

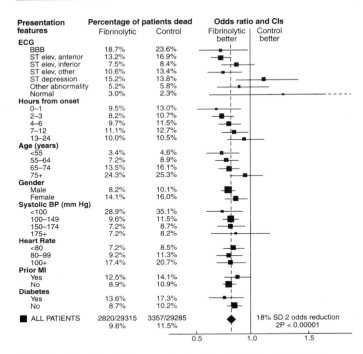

Presentation features	Percentage of patients dead		Odds ratio and CIs	
	Fibrinolytic	Control	Fibrinolytic better	Control better
ECG				
BBB	18.7%	23.6%		
ST elev, anterior	13.2%	16.9%		
ST elev, inferior	7.5%	8.4%		
ST elev, other	10.6%	13.4%		
ST depression	15.2%	13.8%		
Other abnormality	5.2%	5.8%		
Normal	3.0%	2.3%		
Hours from onset				
0–1	9.5%	13.0%		
2–3	8.2%	10.7%		
4–6	9.7%	11.5%		
7–12	11.1%	12.7%		
13–24	10.0%	10.5%		
Age (years)				
<55	3.4%	4.6%		
55–64	7.2%	8.9%		
65–74	13.5%	16.1%		
75+	24.3%	25.3%		
Gender				
Male	8.2%	10.1%		
Female	14.1%	16.0%		
Systolic BP (mm Hg)				
<100	28.9%	35.1%		
100–149	9.6%	11.5%		
150–174	7.2%	8.7%		
175+	7.2%	8.2%		
Heart Rate				
<80	7.2%	8.5%		
80–99	9.2%	11.3%		
100+	17.4%	20.7%		
Prior MI				
Yes	12.5%	14.1%		
No	8.9%	10.9%		
Diabetes				
Yes	13.6%	17.3%		
No	8.7%	10.2%		
■ ALL PATIENTS	2820/29315	3357/29285	18% SD 2 odds reduction	
	9.6%	11.5%	2P < 0.00001	

0.5   1.0   1.5

FIG. 4-2. Mortality differences during days 0 to 35 subdivided by presentation features in a collaborative overview of nine thrombolytic trials. Absolute mortality rates are shown for the fibrinolytic and control groups in the center portion of the figure for each of the clinical features at presentation listed on the left side of the figure. The ratio of the odds of death in the fibrinolytic group to that in the control group is shown for each subdivision (■), along with its 99% confidence interval (*horizontal line*). The summary odds ratio at the bottom of the figure corresponds to an 18% proportional reduction in 35-day mortality and is highly statistically significant. The absolute reduction is 9 deaths per 1,000 patients treated with thrombolytic agents. (Adapted from Fibrinolytic Therapy Trialists' Collaborative Group (62), with permission.)

Tissue Plasminogen Activator (see pages 217–231)

A clear mortality benefit with tPA compared with placebo was shown in the Anglo-Scandinavian Study of Early Thrombolysis (ASSET) (90). When compared with streptokinase in the large GISSI-2 and ISIS-3 trials, mortality rates were similar. However, the front-loaded tPA regimen was not used, and tPA was given without heparin or with subcutaneous heparin. Of note, the now widely used front-loaded regimen (15-mg bolus, then 50 mg over 30 minutes and 35 mg over final 60 minutes) was shown to achieve earlier patency with better TIMI grade 3 flow at 60 and 90 minutes (102). This was also demonstrated in TIMI-4 (71) and the GUSTO Angiography substudy (70).

In the GUSTO I trial (69) (Table 4-2), the tPA and intravenous heparin group had the best outcome: 6.3% 30-day mortality versus 7.2% and 7.4% in the streptokinase groups ($p < 0.001$). The greatest benefit was seen in those patients with large anterior MIs.

In the Continuous Infusion versus Double-Bolus Administration of Alteplase (COBALT) study (96), a double-bolus regimen (50 mg $\times$ 2 [30 minutes apart]) yielded clinically worse outcomes compared with a front-loaded tPA regimen (mortality +0.44%, intracranial hemorrhage +0.3%). Statistically, outcomes also were not equivalent to those with front-loaded tPA.

Reteplase (see pages 221, 222)

A double-bolus regimen of reteplase (rPA) was approved for use by the U.S. Food and Drug Administration (FDA) based on demonstrated equivalence to streptokinase in the International Joint Efficacy Comparison of Thrombolytics (INJECT) trial (73). In the RAPID II angiographic trial (74), rPA showed better TIMI grade 3 flow at 90 minutes compared with front-loaded tPA (60% vs. 45%; $p = 0.01$); however, mortality was similar to tPA in the large GUSTO III study (75) (Table 4-3).

New Agents

The following agents have not been approved by the FDA for the treatment of MI (as of October 1999).

Lanoteplase (see pages 222, 224)

In intravenous nPA for treatment of infarcting myocardium early (InTIME I), an angiographic trial, high-dose lanoteplase (nPA; single bolus of 120 U/kg) was associated with better patency (TIMI grade 2 or 3 flow) compared with front-loaded tPA (83% vs. 71%; $p < 0.05$) (85). The InTIME II trial compared nPA with tPA in approximately 15,000 patients and found similar 30-day mortality rates. nPA was associated with a higher ICH rate (1.13% vs. 0. 62%; $p = 0.003$), whereas there was a trend toward lower rates of several secondary cardiac endpoints (76).

One potential benefit of bolus administration is ease of administration. [In GUSTO I, incorrect dosing of tPA was associated with higher mortality (7.7% vs. 5.5% for correct dosing; $p < 0.0001$)].

TNK-tPA (see pages 222, 225)

TNK-tPA is another single-bolus thrombolytic that achieves TIMI grade 3 flow similar to that of tPA alone (86; *see also Circulation* 1997;95:351). The Assessment of the Safety and Efficacy of a New Thrombolytic: TNK-tPA (ASSENT II) trial enrolled nearly 17,000 patients and showed TNK-tPA to be equivalent to tPA alone (30-day mortality rates 6.17% and 6.15%) (77).

Staphylokinase (see page 224)

In one small study, a 20-mg dose of staphylokinase demonstrated TIMI grade 3 flow in 74% of the patients (82).

Saruplase (see page 224)

A mortality rate similar to that of streptokinase was associated with the use of saruplase in the Comparative Trial of Saruplase versus Streptokinase (COMPASS) (84).

Table 4-2.   Results from the Global Utilization of Streptokinase and t-PA for Occluded coronary arteries trial

	Streptokinase and Subcutaneous Heparin	Streptokinase and Intravenous Heparin	Front-loaded t-PA and Intravenous Heparin	t-PA and Streptokinase and Intravenous Heparin	p Value (t-PA vs Both Streptokinase Regimens)
Patients (n)	9,796	10,377	10,344	10,328	
30-day mortality (%)	7.2	7.4	6.3	7.0	0.005
Net clinical benefit (death or disabling stroke %)	7.7	7.9	6.9	7.6	0.006
24-h mortality (%)	2.8	2.9	2.3	2.8	0.005
Intracranial hemorrhage	0.5	0.5	0.7	0.9	0.03
Congestive heart failure	17.5	16.8	15.2	16.8	<0.001
Cardiogenic shock	6.9	6.3	5.1	6.1	<0.001
Angiographic substudy Patients (n)	293	283	292	299	
Infarct-related artery patency (TIMI grade 2 or 3 flow) at 90 min (%)	54	60	81	73	<0.001
TIMI grade 3 flow at 90 min (%)	29	32	54	38	<0.001

Data from the GUSTO Investigators (69) and the GUSTO Angiographic Investigators (70).
TIMI, Thrombolysis in Myocardial Infarction; t-PA, tissue plasminogen activator.

Table 4-3.

Agent	Dosage	90-Minute TIMI Grade 3 Flow	Heparin	Allergy	Cost
SK	1.5 million U over 60 min	30%–35%	No	Yes	Low
Anistreplase	30-U bolus over 3–5 min	~40%	No	Yes	Moderate
t-PA	15-mg bolus, 0.75 mg/kg over 30 min, then 0.5 mg/kg over 60 min (max 100 mg)	54%–60%	Yes	No	High
r-PA	10 U + 10 U given 30 min apart	~60%	Yes	No	High

TIMI, thrombolysis in myocardial infarction; t-PA, tissue plasminogen activator; r-PA, reteplase. (From refs. 70, 71, 74.)

Prognostic Indicators (see pages 215, 274–284)

1. Early infarct-related artery (IRA) patency. Ninety-minute patency (TIMI grade 2 or 3 flow) correlates strongly with outcome: greater than twofold higher 1-year mortality rate in those with persistent occlusion at 90 minutes in TIMI 1 and similar findings in subsequent studies (243). Subsequent analyses showed TIMI grade 3 flow to be associated with significantly better outcomes than TIMI grade 2 flow (243, 245,248). The corrected TIMI frame count, which treats flow as a continuous variable, appears to provide an even more accurate prognostic assessment (253).
2. Time to treatment. Lower mortality is achieved with early thrombolysis, especially within the the first "golden" hour (63).
3. Reocclusion. A 10% to 15% incidence is observed by approximately 2 weeks, which increases to approximately 30% at 1 year. Although approximately 50% of cases are not accompanied by clinical reinfarction or ischemia (i.e., silent), reocclusion is associated with a more than twofold higher mortality rate (290). Revascularization appears to be helpful (*see N Engl J Med* 1992;327:1825).
4. Reinfarction is associated with a two- to threefold higher mortality rate (2.6-fold in TIMI II).
5. Smoking. Active smokers have better outcomes, but this appears to be attributable to their younger age, higher frequency of inferior MI, and less three-vessel disease (262).

Percutaneous Coronary Intervention

Angioplasty

Primary Angioplasty versus Thrombolysis (see pages 231–234)

Percutaneous transluminal coronary angioplasty (PTCA) had a lower associated mortality rate in the Primary Angioplasty in MI (PAMI) trial (2.6% vs. 6.5%) (108), and a nonsignificant trend toward lower mortality was observed in the larger GUSTO IIb trial (110). However, there was no mortality difference in a recent study of 19 Seattle hospitals (109). A recent meta-analysis shows a significant mortality benefit of primary angioplasty compared with thrombolysis: odds ratio 0.66 [95% confidence interval (CI) 0.46–0.94] (104). Thus, PTCA is likely to yield a better outcome with a clear benefit when performed at experienced centers that can achieve a short door-to-balloon time.

Rescue Angioplasty

Rescue angioplasty (i.e., after failed thrombolytic therapy) reduces postinfarct angina, and pooled data from two small randomized trials showed a trend toward lower mortality (odds ratio 0.38; 95% CI 0.13–1.06) (*see Circulation* 1999;91:476).

Routine Immediate PTCA (after Thrombolysis) versus Delayed PTCA or Conservative Management (see pages 236–239)

Most trials show immediate PTCA to be associated with increased bleeding and an overall trend toward increased mortality [Thrombolysis and Angioplasty in MI (TAMI), TIMI-2A, and European Cooperative Study Group (ECSG-4)] (118,119,123).

Routine Delayed PTCA (after Thrombolysis)
versus Conservative Management (see page 238)

Similar mortality and reinfarction rates and ejection fractions have been reported [TIMI II-B and the Should We Intervene Following Thrombolysis (SWIFT) study] (121). Of note, in TIMI IIB the subgroup with a prior MI did have a lower 6-week mortality rate.

Cardiogenic Shock (see page 240)

Results of the Should We Emergently Revascularize Occluded Coronaries for Cardiogenic Shock (SHOCK) trial showed that emergent revascularization (balloon angioplasty or bypass surgery) did not result in improved 30 day survival compared with aggressive medical management [e.g., thrombolysis, intraaortic balloon pump (IABP)]. However, at 6 months, mortality was lower (50.3% vs 63.1%, p = 0.027) with emergent revascularization compared with medical therapy (129).

Stenting (see pages 241–243)

Excellent outcomes have been achieved with stenting used after angioplasty yields suboptimal results. In a recent small randomized study comparing primary stenting with angioplasty (with bailout stenting only if prolonged balloon inflation was unsuccessful), the stented group had fewer reinfarctions and better cardiac event-free survival (130–133).

ACE Inhibitors (see pages 243–247)

Captopril 6.25 to 50 mg three times daily (rapidly titrated) and lisinopril 5 to 20 mg daily are used most commonly (likely a class effect with these agents). Early initiation of ACE inhibition was found to decrease mortality in two large placebo-controlled trials. In GISSI-3 (140), use of lisinopril (5–10 mg daily) was associated with a 12% mortality reduction, whereas in ISIS-4 (142), use of captopril (initially 6.25 mg titrated to maximum 50 mg) was associated with a 7% mortality reduction (greatest benefit in those with anterior MI). Among patients with left ventricular dysfunction, mortality was reduced by approximately 20% to 30% by oral ACE inhibition [Survival and Ventricular Enlargement (SAVE), Acute Infarction Ramipril Efficacy (AIRE), and Trandolapril Cardiac Evaluation (TRACE) trials (137,139,144)]. Intravenous administration was used in the Cooperative New Scandinavian Enalapril Survival Study (CONSENSUS II) and was deemed harmful (136). A meta-analysis of 15 trials with more than 100,000 patients showed a 7% risk reduction, with the majority of benefit seen in anterior MIs (1.2% absolute mortality benefit vs. 0.1% for inferior MIs) (135). Approximately one third of the benefit of ACE inhibition is seen in the first few days after MI.

The HOPE trial evaluated the effects of ACE inhibition in patients with CAD or risk factors but without left ventricular dysfunction (ejection fraction ≥40%). Cardiac death, MI, or stroke at 5 years was significantly reduced with ramipril versus placebo (13.9% vs 17.5%, p < 0.001) [see Chapter 1, ref. 68].

Heparin (see pages 200, 216–217)

Intravenous heparin should be used in conjunction with tPA, or rPA or TNK-tPA, (GUSTO data show the optimal partial thromboplastin time range to be 50–70 seconds (*see Circulation* 1996; 93:870). Heparin is optimal if the patient is not also receiving a thrombolytic agent. A meta-analysis of prethrombolytic trials showed an approximately 20% mortality benefit (27). Another meta-analysis of trials comprising approximately 70,000 patients showed borderline benefit when used with thrombolytics (6% lower mortality; $p = 0.03$) (28).

Subcutaneous administration showed no benefit in reducing death or reinfarction (ISIS-3 and GISSI-2) (67,68).

Low-Molecular-Weight Heparins (see pages 202, 203)

Low-molecular-weight heparins require further evaluation in ST elevation MI (benefits have been clearly shown in patients with unstable angina and non-ST elevation MI; see Chapter 3). Results from a small pilot study found that dalteparin in conjunction with streptokinase resulted in higher IRA TIMI grade 3 flow (35), whereas the preliminary results of another study found that enoxaparin given for 4 days after thrombolysis was associated with a significant reduction in death, MI, and hospital readmission due to chest pain at 3 months without any increased bleeding (*see J Am Coll Cardiol* 1999;31:191A). The Fragmin in Acute MI (FRAMI) trial showed that dalteparin reduced left ventricular thrombus formation and rate of arterial embolism (34), but at the expense of increased minor and major bleeding.

Direct Thrombin Inhibitors (see pages 203, 204)

Trials using hirudin showed no significant advantage (TIMI-5 and TIMI-9B) (36,37). In the Hirulog Early Perfusion/Occlusion (HERO) trial (38), hirulog showed better TIMI grade 3 flow compared with streptokinase, but outcomes were similar (larger HERO-2 trial is underway).

Warfarin (see pages 205–206, 285)

Warfarin yields similar outcomes when compared with aspirin but is associated with increased bleeding [Aspirin/Anticoagulants Following Thrombolysis with Eminase in Recurrent Infarction (AFTER) trial (43)]. Thus, warfarin should be considered if the patient is aspirin intolerant; a 24% lower mortality rate versus placebo was observed in the Warfarin Reinfarction Study (WARIS) (41) and a 25% lower mortality rate among non–aspirin-treated patients was observed in a more recent meta-analysis. Warfarin also should be considered in patients at high risk of left ventricular thrombus formation (large anterior MI, ejection fraction <20%). In an analysis of 11 studies, anticoagulation was associated with 68% lower rate of embolization (296).

Nitrates (see pages 246–250)

Nitrates are indicated for relief of persistent pain (sublingual nitroglycerin 0.4 mg every 5 minutes for three doses or intravenous nitroglycerin 10–200 µg/min). Nitrates also are useful as a vasodilator in patients with left ventricular dysfunction. In the large GISSI-3 and ISIS-4 trials (141,150), routine use of intravenous and oral nitrates after MI conferred no mortality benefit. Another trial showed that nitropatch therapy prevents remodeling in patients with an ejection fraction less than 40% (152).

Nitrates should not be used in patients with inferior MI complicated by right ventricular involvement (reduces preload).

Calcium-Channel Blockers (see pages 250–258)

Nifedipine has been associated with increased mortality [Trial of Early Nifedipine in Acute MI (TRENT), and Secondary Prevention Reinfarction Israel Nifedipine Trials I and II (SPRINT-I and-II) (153,156,160)]. In the Multicenter Diltiazem Post-Infarction Trial (MDPIT) (154), diltiazem was deemed harmful in those with pulmonary congestion and low ejection fraction (41% increase in cardiac events). Verapamil was believed to be safe (meta-analysis showed a significant 19% lower reinfarction rate and nonsignificant 7% mortality reduction) (157). A meta-analysis of 24 trials of all types of calcium-channel blockers showed a nonsignificant 4% increase in mortality (175). These agents should be considered only in patients with clear contraindication(s) to β-blockade and good left ventricular function (153–160).

Magnesium (see pages 253, 254)

Magnesium use is controversial. Initial studies suggested a mortality benefit [second Leicester Intravenous Magnesium Intervention Trial (LIMIT-2) (161)], and a meta-analysis showed 54% lower mortality (163). However, in the ISIS-4 megatrial (163), magnesium had no mortality benefit and was associated with excess hypotension. Of note, more ISIS-4 patients received thrombolysis [70% vs. 36% (LIMIT-2)], and magnesium was started 1 hour after thrombolytic administration (vs. concomitantly in LIMIT-2). Proponents of magnesium argue that it is beneficial in high-risk patients and perhaps when given prior to thrombolysis therapy, which may prevent reperfusion injury (163,164). The NHLBI-sponsored MAGIC trial will examine these hypotheses (161–166).

Antiarrhythmics (see pages 255–258)

Prophylactic use of lidocaine appears to be harmful, with a meta-analysis showing a 12% higher mortality rate (168–176). However, lidocaine (1–3 mg/min) can be used in patients who have had ventricular tachycardia or ventricular fibrillation.

In the Cardiac Arrhythmia Suppression Trials (CAST I and II) (169,170), the routine use of type I agents (e.g., encainide, flecainide, moricizine) was associated with significantly higher all-cause mortality rates.

In the Basel Antiarrhythmic Study of Infarct Survival (BASIS) (168), amiodarone (1 g for 5 days, then 200 mg daily) in patients with complex ventricular ectopy was associated with 61% lower 1-year mortality rates ($p < 0.05$). However, in two large trials [the European MI Amiodarone Trial (EMIAT) and Canadian Amiodarone MI Arrhythmia Trial (CAMIAT) (172,173)], when given to patients with frequent ventricular ectopy and left ventricular dysfunction, amiodarone (vs. placebo) showed no overall mortality benefit, although arrhythmic deaths were decreased.

The Survival with Oral d-sotalol (SWORD) trial showed 65% increased mortality with d-sotalol (171).

Intravenous Glycoprotein IIb/IIIa Inhibitors

Abciximab (see pages 208–210)

Abciximab alone (i.e., heparin but no thrombolytic) achieves limited TIMI grade 3 flow (32% in TIMI-14) (47). Abciximab in conjunction with percutaneous coronary interventions (PCIs) has been shown to reduce subsequent ischemic events. The Reopro and Primary PTCA Organization and Randomized Trial (RAPPORT) showed that abciximab use in conjunction with primary PTCA resulted in a significant reduction in death, MI, and urgent revascularization at 30 days (46). [*See* also EPIC and GUSTO III subgroup analyses (*J Am Coll Cardiol* 1998;31:191A).] The Abciximab before Direct Angiography and Stenting in MI Regarding Acute and Long-term Follow-up (ADMIRAL) trial showed that abciximab use in conjunction with stenting resulted in a nearly 50% reduction in the incidence of death, MI, and urgent revascularization (49). Abciximab started before PCI achieved TIMI grade 2 or 3 flow in 40% of patients in the small Glycoprotein Receptor Antagonist Patency Evaluation (GRAPE) pilot study (48), but whether this translates into improved outcomes requires evaluation in larger studies.

Eptifibatide (Integrelin) (see page 207)

In IMPACT-AMI (45), the highest dose of integrelin (180 µg/kg intravenous bolus then 0.75 µg/kg/min) with full-dose tPA was associated with better TIMI grade 3 flow at 90 minutes compared with full-dose tPA alone. When used in conjunction with full-dose streptokinase, modestly higher TIMI grade 3 flow was achieved, but at the expense of increased bleeding (*see J Am Coll Cardiol* 1998; 94:842–843).

Reduced-dose thrombolysis in conjunction with intravenous glycoprotein IIb/IIIa administration is being evaluated in several trials. TIMI-14 found that a combination of abciximab and tPA (15-mg bolus then 35 mg over 60 minutes) resulted in better TIMI grade 3 flow at 60 and 90 minutes than tPA alone (72% vs. 43%, p = 0.0009; 77% vs. 62%, p = 0.02). Ongoing trials include SPEED (abciximab plus reteplase), GUSTO IV (abciximab plus reteplase), INTRO-AMI (integrelin plus tPA), the final phase of TIMI-14 (abciximab plus reteplase), and others with TNK-tPA.

OTHER MODES OF TREATMENT

Oxygen

Oxygen may be used initially, but may not be necessary if the patient is not hypoxic.

Analgesia

Morphine sulfate may be administered 2 to 5 mg intravenously, repeated every 5 to 15 minutes (some patients require up to 30 mg for adequate pain relief). It is particularly helpful in patients with pulmonary edema.

Diuretics

Intravenous lasix is indicated in severe congestive heart failure (CHF) but should be avoided if right ventricular infarct is present.

Vasopressors/Inotropes

Vasopressors/Inotropes are useful in the treatment of cardiogenic shock (SBP < 90 mm Hg, cardiac index ≤2.2 L/kg/m^2). Initial choices include dopamine (5–20 µg/kg/min) and dobutamine (2.5–20 µg/ kg/min; ideal agent if blood pressure is adequate but cardiac output is poor). If SBP is less than 60 mm Hg, norepinephrine should be considered.

Insulin (see page 261)

Aggressive serum glucose control in diabetics via insulin drip resulted in a significant mortality benefit in the Diabetic Insulin-Glucose Infusion in Acute MI (DIGAMI) trial (185).

Intraaortic Balloon Pump (see pages 259, 260)

Using a balloon pump appears useful in the treatment of cardiogenic shock (trend toward lower mortality in GUSTO I) (182) and after emergent catheterization [IABP Trial (177)]. Contraindications include the presence of aortic regurgitation and severe peripheral vascular disease. Vascular complications occur in 5% to 20% of cases (177–181).

Emergent CABG/Surgery

Emergent CABG should be considered if PTCA fails to result in persistent pain or hemodynamic instability, left main disease, acute mitral regurgitation, and ventricular septal defect.

New Agents

Angiotensin II receptor inhibitors and clopidogrel need further evaluation. The role of antibiotics is currently being assessed (ACADEMIC trial showed no significant benefit; *see* Chapter 1).

SPECIAL CASE

Right Ventricular Infarction (see pages 264, 265)

Right ventricular infarction is typically caused by right coronary artery occlusion proximal to the acute marginal branch and is associated with 20% to 50% of inferior MIs (196–203). If the right coronary artery is occluded, right ventricular infarction is six times more likely in the absence of preinfarction angina (203).

Diagnosis

1. Triad of hypotension, clear lung fields, and elevated jugular venous pressure is highly specific, but only 25% sensitive.
2. Hemodynamics. Right atrial pressure is more than 10 mm Hg and within 1 to 5 mm Hg of pulmonary capillary wedge pressure (73% sensitivity, 100% specificity).
3. ECG. ST elevation is present in lead V4R (sensitivity 80%–100%, 80%–100% specificity) and resolves quickly. In one study, ST elevation resolved in 48% of patients within 10 hours (*see Br Heart J* 1983;49:368). Right bundle branch block and complete heart block may be observed.
4. Echocardiography. Typical features are right ventricular dilatation, right ventricular wall asynergy, and abnormal interventricular septal motion. Tricuspid regurgitation, ventricular septal defect, and/or early pulmonary valve opening also may be seen.

Complications

High-degree atrioventricular block is present in up to 50% of patients and atrial fibrillation in up to one third. A high incidence of pericarditis is seen, mostly due to transmural involvement of the thin-walled right ventricle.

Treatment (see pages 264, 265)

Diuretics and nitrates should be avoided (i.e., to not decrease preload). Beneficial measures include:

1. Volume loading (2–4 liters of normal saline is commonly needed)
2. Inotropic support (dobutamine) if volume does not improve cardiac output
3. Temporary wire placement if complete heart block develops and atrioventricular sequential pacing if hemodynamics are poor
4. Cardioversion if atrial fibrillation is present
5. Thrombolysis significantly reduces mortality (199)
6. Unsuccessful PTCA is associated with high mortality [58% vs. 2% in one study (200)]

COMPLICATIONS

Early (see pages 269, 270)

1. Pump failure: incidence approximately 5%; most common if more than 40% of myocardium involved
2. Post-infarct angina: more frequent after thrombolysis than primary PTCA
3. Reinfarction: more frequent after thrombolysis and if non–Q-wave MI; should be treated with intravenous heparin, or repeat thrombolysis if ST elevation MI
4. Arrhythmias (Table 4-4)
   a. Ventricular tachycardia: incidence 5% to 20%; associated with larger infarcts/left ventricular dysfunction; nonsustained ventricular tachycardia occurring beyond several hours after MI also may portend poorer prognosis [relative mortality risk 7.5 at 24 hours in one study (223)]
   b. Ventricular fibrillation: declining incidence (now <1%); primary ventricular fibrillation occurs in 85%–90% of cases in the first 24 hours, 60% in first 6 hours; secondary ventricular fibrillation occurs at 1–4 days; poor prognosis (25% survival)
   c. Asystole: associated with high mortality; transcutaneous or transvenous pacing is indicated
   d. Atrial fibrillation (219): incidence 5%–15%; treated with anticoagulation, rate control (β-blockers, calcium-channel blockers, digoxin), cardioversion if hemodynamically unstable, amiodarone if multiple episodes occur
   e. Heart block: common with inferior MI (increased vagal tone, atrioventricular node ischemia): first-degree heart block typically progresses to Mobitz I and then to third degree; anterior MI (His Purkinje system affected): bundle branch block progresses to Mobitz II and then third degree (advanced block associated with mortality rate of >40%); temporary pacer indicated for high-degree block that develops via Mobitz II mechanism or bifascicular block
   f. Accelerated idioventricular rhythm: occurs more frequently in patients with early reperfusion; temporary pacing is not indicated
   g. Premature ventricular contractions: incidence approximately 75%; routine suppression with lidocaine associated with increased mortality
   h. Sinus tachycardia: if it persists, may signify evolving CHF

Table 4-4.   Cardiac arrhythmias and their management during acute MI

Category	Arrhythmia	Objective of Treatment	Therapeutic Options
Electrical instability	Ventricular premature beats	Correction of electrolyte deficits and increased sympathetic tone	Potassium and magnesium solutions, β-blocker
	Ventricular tachycardia	Prophylaxis against ventricular fibrillation, restoration of hemodynamic stability	Antiarrhythmic agents; cardioversion/defibrillation
	Ventricular fibrillation	Urgent reversion to sinus rhythm	Defibrillation;
	Accelerated idioventricular rhythm	Observation unless hemodynamic function is compromised	Increase sinus rate (atropine, atrial pacing); antiarrhythmic agents
	Nonparoxysmal atrioventricular junctional tachycardia	Search for precipitating causes (e.g., digitalis intoxication); suppress arrhythmia only if hemodynamic function is compromised	Atrial overdrive pacing; antiarrhythmic agents; cardioversion relatively contraindicated if digitalis intoxication present
Pump failure/ excessive sympathetic stimulation	Sinus tachycardia	Reduce heart rate to diminish myocardial oxygen demands	Antipyretics; analgesics; β-blocker unless CHF present; treat latter if present with anticongestive measures (diuretics, afterload reduction)

(continued)

Table 4-4.   Continued

Category	Arrhythmia	Objective of Treatment	Therapeutic Options
	Atrial fibrillation and/or atrial flutter	Reduce ventricular rate; restore sinus rhythm	Verapamil, digitalis glycosides; anticongestive measures (diuretics, afterload reduction); cardioversion; rapid atrial pacing (for atrial flutter)
	Paroxysmal supraventricular tachycardia	Reduce ventricular rate; restore sinus rhythm	Vagal maneuvers; verapamil, cardiac glycosides, β-adrenergic blockers; cardioversion; rapid atrial pacing
Bradyarrhythmias and conduction disturbances	Sinus bradycardia	Increase heart rate only if hemodynamic function is compromised	Atropine; atrial pacing
	Junctional escape rhythm	Acceleration of sinus rate only if loss of atrial "kick" causes hemodynamic compromise	Atropine; atrial pacing
	High-degree atrioventricular block and intraventricular block		Insertion of pacemaker

CHF, congestive heart failure. Modified from Braunwald EB. *Heart Disease.* Philadelphia: W.B. Saunders, 1997;1245 (with permission).

5. Cholesterol embolization: more common with thrombolytic therapy (*see Circulation* 1990;81:477)

Intermediate (see pages 281, 285)
1. Left ventricular thrombus: incidence 4% to 20%; most common in anterior MI; treatment: anticoagulation (usually warfarin for 3 months); decreases the risk of embolization (295); primary prevention: consider anticoagulation if ejection fraction is less than 30% to 35%
2. Rupture: causes a higher percentage of deaths in patients undergoing thrombolysis [12% vs. 6% (276)]; risk factors include first MI, female gender, age over 60 years, no left ventricular hypertrophy, hypertension, and possibly thrombolysis after 12 hours
   a. Free wall: incidence approximately 5%; lower risk after thrombolysis and with use of β-blockers; although most die immediately, treatment includes emergency pericardiocentesis and fluids followed by immediate surgical repair
   b. Septum: incidence 0.5% to 2.0%; new murmur with palpable thrill in 50%; surgical mortality 30% (higher if inferior MI) versus 80% to 90% with medical therapy
   c. Papillary muscle: incidence approximately 1%; primarily occurs with inferior MIs; posteromedial papillary muscle affected; best treatment is surgery (mortality ~10%)
3. Fibrinous pericarditis: most common after Q-wave MI; treated with aspirin and analgesics [nonsteroidal antiinflammatory drugs NSAIDs) may impair healing]

Late
1. Ventricular aneurysm: usually do not rupture, but often complicated by mural thrombi and severe CHF; treated by surgical resection if complicated by CHF, severe arrhythmias, thromboemboli; primary prevention is early ACE inhibition
2. Pseudoaneurysm: contained rupture of myocardium; surgical resection usually recommended
3. Dressler's syndrome: incidence approximately 1%; treated with NSAIDs (if they fail, steroids)

POST-MI RISK STRATIFICATION (see pages 269–279)

The majority of hospitalized patients with MI are at low-risk for adverse outcomes. Age is a strong predictor of outcome. In a multivariate analysis of GUSTO I data, mortality ranged from 1.1% in those under 45 years of age to 20.5% in those over 75 (263). Other factors associated with mortality included lower systolic blood pressure, higher Killip class, elevated heart rate, and anterior infarct. These five factors contributed to approximately 90% of prognostic information (Fig. 4-3). Another analysis of 3,339 TIMI-2 patients identified a low-risk group (26%, zero of eight risk factors) that had a 6-week mortality rate of 1.5%. Patients with one risk factor (age 70 years, female gender, diabetes, prior MI, anterior MI, atrial fibrillation, SBP <100 mm Hg, heart rate >100 beats/min) had a 6-week mortality rate of 5.3% ($p < 0.001$), whereas those with four risk factors had a 17.2% mortality rate (Table 4-5). Numerous other studies have examined specific risk factors associated with poor outcome, including diabetes (264), both left and

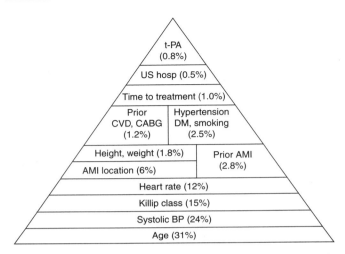

FIG. 4-3. **Influence of clinical characteristics on 30-day mortality after myocardial infarction (MI) in patients treated with thrombolytic agents based on GUSTO I data.** Although much attention has been paid to optimizing thrombolytic regimens, the choice of the agent is far less important than are certain clinical variables with respect to mortality. This pyramid depicts the importance of such clinical characteristics as calculated from a regression analysis in the GUSTO trial. Numbers in parentheses represent the proportion of risk for 30-day mortality associated with the particular characteristics. *AMI*, acute myocardial infarction; *BP*, blood pressure; *CVD*, cardiovascular disease; *DM*, diabetes mellitus; *t-PA*, tissue-type plasminogen activators; *US Hosp*, patients treated in a United States hospital. (Modified from Braunwald EB. *Heart Disease*. Philadelphia: W.B. Saunders, 1997;1218, with permission.)

right bundle branch block (222; *see* also *Circulation* 1997;96:1139), and atrial fibrillation (219). Psychosocial predictors of adverse outcomes include depression (267) and living alone (266). Finally, an analysis of more than 8,000 Medicare patients showed that MI patients treated by cardiologists fared better than those treated by other types of physicians (268).

Uncomplicated Course (see page 238)

For a large MI, the clinician should consider obtaining an echo-cardiogram, especially with a high clinical suspicion of left ventricular dysfunction. Catheterization should be considered if the ejection fraction is below 40%. If the ejection fraction is 40% or above, the patient usually should perform the exercise treadmill test (ETT). If the result of the ETT is positive for ischemia, or patient has rest pain, the patient should be catheterized (Fig. 4-4).

For a small MI, the patient should usually have an ETT. If results of this test are negative, medical therapy should be contin-

Table 4-5. Mortality 6 weeks following thrombolytic therapy for each of eight risk factors in 3,261 patients

Risk Factor	Deaths by 6 Weeks (%)
None	1.5
Age ≥70 yr	11.2
Previous infarction	7.9
Anterior infarction	5.6
Atrial fibrillation	10.6
Rales in more than one third of lung fields	1.24
Hypotension and sinus tachycardia	10.1
Female gender	7.1
Diabetes mellitus	8.5

Seventy-eight patients with cardiogenic shock or pulmonary edema were excluded.
Data from analysis of patients enrolled in phase II of the Thrombolysis in Myocardial Infarction (TIMI) Trial (259).

ued, with repeat symptom-limited ETT after several weeks. If the results are positive, catheterization is usually warranted (122).

Complicated Course

Examples of a complicated course include severe heart failure, cardiogenic shock, failed thrombolysis, recurrent ischemia, and ventricular tachycardia or ventricular fibrillation after 48 hours (*see* Fig. 4-4).

Treatment is composed of catheterization and PTCA or coronary artery bypass graft (CABG) surgery as indicated; for late ventricular tachycardia/ventricular fibrillation, electrophysiologic testing with possible defibrillator implantation should be considered.

Specific Tests (see pages 270, 271)

1. ETT has an excellent safety record: 0.03% mortality in one review of 151,949 tests (225). The strongest predictors of poor outcome are limited exercise duration and hypotension. ST depression was predictive of death in only 43% of studies in one large overview. If no pre-discharge ETT is performed, it portends a poor prognosis (226).
2. ETT with nuclear imaging may be used to detect multiple perfusion defects associated with multivessel disease and poor outcomes (228). The predictive value for mortality is lowered to approximately 40% to 50% by posttest treatment. Positive test results lead to angiography and revascularization, which lowers the future cardiac event rate.
3. Echocardiography is useful in the assessment of left ventricular function, which often guides decisions about the need for catheterization, coronary bypass surgery (mortal-

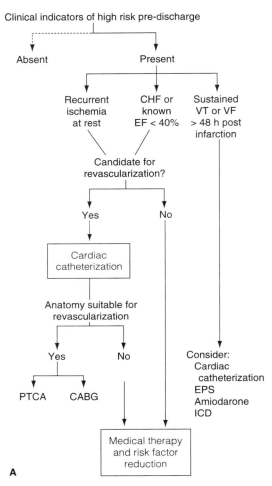

FIG. 4-4. Management algorithm for risk stratification following acute MI. A: Patients with clinical indicators of high-risk at hospital discharge such as recurrent ischemia at rest or depressed left ventricular function should be considered candidates for revascularization and referral to cardiac catheterization for ultimate triage to either angioplasty/CABG surgery or medical therapy and risk factor reduction. Patients with life-threatening arrhythmias such as sustained ventricular tachycardia (*VT*) or ventricular fibrillation (*VF*) should be considered for diagnostic cardiac catheterization, electrophysiology study (*EPS*), and management with either amiodarone or an implantable cardioconverter-defibrillator (*ICD*) or both. **B:** Patients without indicators of high risk at hospital discharge can be evaluated either with a submaximal exercise test prior to discharge or with a symptom-limited exercise test at 14 to 35 days. Patients with either a markedly abnormal exercise test or evidence of reversible ischemia on an exercise imaging study should be referred for cardiac catheterization. Patients with a negative exercise test result or no evidence of reversible ischemia on an exercise imaging study can be managed with medical therapy and risk factor reduction. (Adapted from Braunwald EB. *Heart Failure.* Philadelphia: W.B. Saunders, 1997;1262, with permission.)

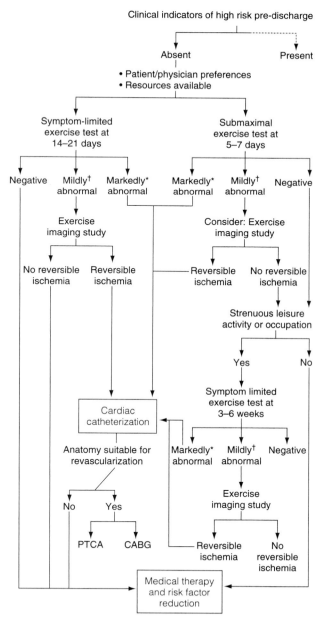

Clinical indicators of high risk pre-discharge

Absent — Present

- Patient/physician preferences
- Resources available

Symptom-limited exercise test at 14–21 days

Submaximal exercise test at 5–7 days

Negative   Mildly† abnormal   Markedly* abnormal

Markedly* abnormal   Mildly† abnormal   Negative

Exercise imaging study

Consider: Exercise imaging study

No reversible ischemia   Reversible ischemia

Reversible ischemia   No reversible ischemia

Strenuous leisure activity or occupation

Yes   No

Symptom limited exercise test at 3–6 weeks

Cardiac catheterization

Markedly* abnormal   Mildly† abnormal   Negative

Anatomy suitable for revascularization

Exercise imaging study

No   Yes

PTCA   CABG

Reversible ischemia   No reversible ischemia

Medical therapy and risk factor reduction

*High risk (≥ 2mm ST segment depression, hypotension at peak exercise, low working capacity)
† Positive, not high risk (≤1 mm ST segment depression, good working capacity)

B

Table 4-6. Mortality 6 weeks following thrombolytic therapy according to number of risk factors present initially

No. of Risk Factors	No. of Patients	No. of Deaths Within 6 Weeks	Mortality Rate (%)
0	864	13	1.5
1	1,384	32	2.3
2	689	48	7.0
3	231	30	13.0
≥4	93	16	17.2

Seventy-eight patients with cardiogenic shock or pulmonary edema were excluded.
Possible risk factors listed in Table 4-5.
Data from analysis of patients enrolled in phase II of the Thrombolysis in Myocardial Infarction (TIMI) Trial (259).

ity benefit if ejection fraction <35% and three-vessel disease is present), chronic ACE inhibition therapy, and long-term anticoagulation.
4. Pharmacologic stress echocardiography is performed using agents such as dobutamine, adenosine, and dipyridamole and typically is performed in higher risk patients. Thus, even a negative test result has been associated with subsequent moderate event rate.
5. Signal-averaged ECG is highly specific but modestly sensitive.
6. Ambulatory monitoring is used to detect frequent premature beats and nonsustained ventricular tachycardia, which are associated with increased risk.

REFERENCES

General Review Articles

1. **Lieu TA**, et al. Primary angioplasty and thrombolysis for acute myocardial infarction: an evidence summary. *J Am Coll Cardiol* 1996;27:737–750.
   This article provides a tabular summary (without commentary) of published trials on primary angioplasty and/or thrombolysis. Tables are organized to address the following questions: exclusion criteria, in-hospital mortality, other end points, and stroke rates.
2. **Ryan TJ**, et al. ACC/AHA Guidelines for the management of patients with acute myocardial infarction: a report of the American College of Cardiology/American Heart Association Task Force on Practice Guidelines (updated: *Circulation* 1999;100: 1016–1030). *J Am Coll Cardiol* 1996;28:1328–1428.
3. **Hennekens CH**, et al. Adjunctive drug therapy of acute MI: evidence from clinical trials. *N Engl J Med* 1996;335:1660–1667.
   This article is an overview of trials that have addressed the use of β-blockers, ACE inhibitors, nitrates, calcium-channel blockers, antiarrhthmic agents, and magnesium.

4. **Collins R**, et al. Aspirin, heparin and fibrinolytic therapy in suspected acute MI. *N Engl J Med* 1997;336:847–860.

The authors present evidence supporting their controversial recommendations to avoid the routine use of heparin in acute MI and that subcutaneous heparin (vs. intravenous heparin) is adequate in conjunction with tPA administration. Also, using questionable statistical analyses of the GISSI-2, ISIS-3, and GUSTO I data, they argue that there are no clear differences between different fibrinolytic regimens (i.e., streptokinase is equivalent to tPA).

Diagnosis

Chest Pain and Symptoms

5. **Lee TH**, et al. Acute chest pain in the emergency room: identification and examination of low-risk patients. *Arch Intern Med* 1985;145:65–69.

This analysis of 596 emergency department patients showed that no one variable could identify low-risk patients as efficiently as an ECG. However, a combination of three variables defined a group of patients (8%) in whom ECGs did not add accuracy, and the probability of MI/unstable angina was 0%: (a) sharp or stabbing pain; (b) pain that was reproducible by palpation or was pleuritic or positional; and (c) no history of angina or MI (if just the first two variables, 3% probability of unstable angina, 0% of MI).

6. **Edmondstone WM**. Cardiac chest pain: does body language help the diagnosis? *BMJ* 1995;311:1660–1661.

This study was composed of 203 consecutive patients with chest pain. Among the patients in whom a cardiac etiology was established (68%), 80% used three types of hand movements—Levine's sign (clenched fist to middle of chest), flat hand to center of chest, both hands placed flat in middle of chest and drawn outwards—versus only 51% with noncardiac etiology ($p < 0.01$). Overall, sensitivity was 80%, specificity 49%, positive predictive value 77%, and negative predictive value 53%.

7. **Douglas PS,** Ginsburg GS. The evaluation of chest pain in women. *N Engl J Med* 1996;334:1311–1315.

This review article discusses the major determinants of coronary artery disease (CAD) in women [chest pain (quality and incidence), hormonal status, diabetes, peripheral vascular disease], as well as intermediate determinants (hypertension, smoking, lipoproteins) and minor determinants (age >65 years, obesity, sedentary life-style, family history). The review concludes with a discussion of diagnostic testing.

8. **Goldman L**, et al. Prediction of the need for intensive care in patients who come to emergency departments with chest pain. *N Engl J Med* 1996;334:1498–1504.

This study was composed, in part, of a derivation set (10,682 patients) used to identify clinical predictors of major complications: ST elevation or Q waves, other ECG changes indicating myocardial ischemia, low SBP, pulmonary rales above bases, or an exacerbation of known ischemic heart disease. The validation set (4,676 patients) stratified patients into four groups with risk of major complications ranging from 0.15% to 8%. After 12 hours, the probability was updated based on whether the patient had a complication or confirmed MI. Of note, patients with intermediate events (e.g., heart block, pulmonary edema without hypotension, recurrent ischemia not requiring CABG or PTCA within 72 hours) or confirmed MI had 3.5%–7.5% risk of a major event per 24-hour period. Authors recommended ICU admission in this group. Of note, echocardiographic, serum marker, or stress imaging data were not incorporated into this risk stratification algorithm.

9. **Panju AA**, et al. Is this patient having a myocardial infarction? *JAMA* 1998;280:1256–1263.

Case-based discussion of the numerous history, physical, and ECG findings that are suggestive of diagnosis of MI. Likelihood ratios are provided for these features; the most powerful predictors (or nonpredictors) of MI include new ST elevation (likelihood ratio range 5.7–53.9), new Q wave (5.3–24.8), chest pain radiating to both arms simultaneously (7.1), positional chest pain (0.3), chest pain reproduced by palpation (0.2–0.4), pleuritic chest pain (0.2), and a normal ECG (0.1–0.3).

Electrocardiography

10. **Edmunds JJ**, et al. Significance of anterior ST depression in inferior wall acute MI. *Am J Cardiol* 1994;73:143–148.

This small study was composed of 39 patients with chest pain of >30 minutes' duration, inferior ST elevation, and early sestamibi imaging. Anterior ST depression patients had more myocardium at risk (23% vs. 15%; $p = 0.008$) and much greater lateral extent of defect.

11. **Sgarbossa EB**, et al. Electrocardiographic diagnosis of evolving acute MI in the presence of left bundle branch block. *N Engl J Med* 1996;334:481–487 (editorial pp. 528–529).

Three ECG criteria were derived from an analysis of 131 GUSTO patients: (#1) ST elevation of 1 mm concordant with QRS complex; (#2) ST depression of 1 mm in V1, V2, or V3; and (#3) ST elevation of 5 mm discordant with QRS. Odds ratios for confirmed MI were 25.2, 6.0, and 4.3. If the index score was 3 (#1, n = 5 patients; #2, n = 3 patients; #3, n = 2 patients), sensitivity was 78% and specificity 90%. However, sensitivity was only 36% in the validation group of 45 patients. The authors assert that the low sensitivity is an intrinsic property of ST elevation. Of note, the reported sensitivity and specificity depend on a 50% prevalence of MI (i.e., high index of suspicion of MI necessary). A retrospective cohort analysis of 83 patients presenting with left bundle branch block and symptoms suggestive of MI found that the sensitivity of the above algorithm was only 10% (*see JAMA* 1998;281:714).

12. **Casas RE**, et al. Value of leads V7–V9 in diagnosing posterior wall acute MI and other causes of tall R waves in V1–V2. *Am J Cardiol* 1997;80:508–509.

This large retrospective analysis found that 250 of ~17,000 hospital patients had leads V7 to V9 assessed because of a tall R in V1 and/or suspicion of posterior MI. Among this selected group, 110 patients had evidence of new or old posterior MI, and in 25% of cases, V7 to V9 were the only leads diagnostic of MI.

Serum Markers

13. **Puleo PR**, et al. Use of rapid assay of subforms of CKMB to diagnosis or rule out acute MI. *N Engl J Med* 1994;331:561–566 (editorial pp. 607–608).

This prospective analysis focused on 1,110 evaluated patients with chest pain in the preceding 24 hours. Diagnosis of MI was confirmed in 121 patients. If $CK-MB_2$ was ≥ 1.0 U/L and $CK-MB_2/CK-MB_1$ was ≥ 1.5 in the first 6 hours, then sensitivity was 95.7% (vs. 48% for CK-MB) and specificity 93.9% (vs. 94%). The test requires 6 minuted to perform.

14. **deWinter RJ**, et al. Value of myoglobin, troponin T and CK-MB in ruling out an acute MI in the emergency room. *Circulation* 1995;92:3401–3407.

    This prospective analysis focused on 309 consecutive patients with chest pain. At 3–6 hours after symptoms, myoglobin yielded the best negative predictive value (89% at 4 hours). The negative predictive value of CK-MB reached 95% at 7 hours. Of note, the markers were found to rise fastest with large MIs.

15. **Stubbs P**, et al. Prognostic significance of admission troponin T concentration in patients with MI. *Circulation* 1996;94: 1291–1297.

    This prospective study was composed of 240 patients showing any detectable TnT on admission associated with worse prognosis (median follow-up 3 years). Admission TnT of 0.2 ng/mL was associated with a higher risk of subsequent cardiac death ($p = 0.0002$) and death plus MI ($p = 0.00006$). Most of this excess risk was confined to those with ST-segment elevation on admission ECG.

16. **Ohman EM**, et al. Cardiac troponin T levels for risk stratification in acute myocardial ischemia. *N Engl J Med* 1996;335:1333–1341.

    This analysis focused on 801 GUSTO IIa patients, of whom 72% had a MI. An elevated TnT (>1 ng/ml) was associated with a threefold higher 30-day mortality rate (11.9% vs. 3.9%; $p < 0.001$). Overall, the top mortality predictors were an elevated TnT (chi-square 21, $p < 0.001$), ECG category (ST change or T-wave inversion; chi-square 14, $p = 0.003$), and CK-MB (chi-square 11, $p = 0.004$). TnT was still predictive in a model incorporating all three of these factors (chi square 9.2, $p = 0.027$). Proposed explanations of the increased mortality with elevated TnT included (a) later presentation; (b) higher in cases of reocclusion, which is known to be associated with increased mortality; and (c) patients who died had larger infarcts (also earlier release). Also, TnT had predictive prognostic value even in patients with ST elevation.

17. **Antman E**, et al. Cardiac-specific TnI levels to predict the risk of mortality in patients with acute coronary syndromes. *N Engl J Med* 1996;335:1342–1349 (editorial pp. 1388–1389).

    This analysis focused on 1,404 TIMI IIIB patients. TnI was elevated (≥ 0.4 ng/mL) in 573 patients and associated with a significantly increased 42-day mortality rate (3.7% vs. 1.0%; $p < 0.001$). Even after adjustments for ST depression and age ≥ 65 years (the two independent mortality predictors), each 1 ng/mL increase in TnI was associated with a mortality increase: ≤ 0.4, 1%; 0.4–0.9, 1.7%; 1–1.9, 3. 4%; 2–4.9, 3.7%; 5–8.9, 6%; and 9, 7.5%. TnI provided more prognostic information in patients with a late presentation (> 6 hours to 24 hours): mortality 4% (TnI ≥ 0.4 ng/mL) vs. 0.4% (relative risk 9.5). In contrast, in patients presenting early, the relative risk was only 1.8 (3. 1% vs. 1.7%; $p = $ NS). If no

CK-MB elevation was present (948 patients), a TnI elevation was still associated with increased mortality: 2.5% vs. 0.8% (relative risk 3.0; 95% CI 0.97–9.2). Of note, the elevated TnI group had more ST deviation and less stenosis on angiography at 18–48 hours post symptom onset. However, few had angiography within hours of symptom onset. The accompanying editorial points out that in the Fragmin during Instability in CAD (FRISC) trial (unstable angina patients), an elevated TnT in the first 24 hours was associated with an increased death and MI, and low-molecular-weight heparin treatment in this group was associated with a 48% decreased mortality (see Chapter 3). Unresolved questions include the role of serial measurements and bedside assays and the sensitivity/specificity. Prospective studies are ongoing to evaluate the role of troponins in patient selection for revascularization procedures (e.g. TACTICS-TIMI 18).

18. **Newby LK**, et al. Value of serial TnT measures for early and late risk stratification in patients with acute coronary syndromes. *Circulation* 1998;98:1853–1859 (editorial pp. 1831–1833).

    This GUSTO IIa substudy of 734 patients showed the usefulness of the addition of later cardiac TnT (cTnT) samples. All patients had cTnT samples drawn at baseline, 8 hours, and 16 hours. At baseline, 260 patients were cTnT positive (>0.01 ng/mL), 323 became positive later, and 151 remained negative. The mortality rates were 10% in the baseline-positive group, 5% in the late-positive group, and 0% in negative patients. Thus, late positive patients are at intermediate risk. After adjustment for baseline characteristics, any positive cTnT result predicted 30-day mortality. Only age and ST-segment elevation were stronger predictors than baseline cTnT. Most of the mortality difference between cTnT-positive and -negative patients occurred in the first 30 days. The accompanying editorial stresses the need for large-scale clinical trials to evaluate whether early treatment of high-risk patients as identified by diagnostic markers results in improved outcomes.

19. **Tanasijevic MJ**, et al. Myoglobin, creatine-kinase-MB and cardiac troponin I 60-minute ratios predict infarct-related artery patency after thrombolysis for acute MI: results from TIMI 10B. *J Am Coll Cardial* 1999;34:739–747.

    This study was composed of 442 TIMI 10B patients who had CK-MB and cTnI measured immediately before and 60 minutes after TNK-tPA administration. Patent IRA (TIMI grade 2 or 3 flow) at 60 minutes was demonstrated in 77.8%. The diagnostic performance of the 3 assays was similar–area under receiver-operating characteristic (ROC) curve for diagnosis of occlusion was 0.71, 0.70, and 0.71 for myoglobin, cTnI, and CK-MB. Sixty minute ratios (concentration at 60 minutes/concentration at baseline) of ≥ 4.0 for myoglobin, ≥ 3.3 for CK-MB, and >2.0 for cTnI yielded probabilities of patency of 90%, 88%, and 87%, respectively. We assert that early invasive interventions to establish IRA patency may not be needed in these patients with high 60-minute ratios.

Emergency Room Evaluation

20. **Goldman L**, et al. A computer protocol to predict MI in emergency department patients with chest pain. *N Engl J Med* 1988; 318:797–803.

4. Myocardial Infarction 199

This prospective study was composed of 4,770 MI patients. Treatment decisions based on computer protocol had a higher specificity (74% vs. 71%) and similar sensitivity (88% vs. 87.8%) than those based on physician judgment. Computer protocol–based decisions would have resulted in 11.5% fewer cardiac care unit admissions without MI (thus, cost savings). Of note, whether physicians who are aided by the protocol would perform better than unaided physicians was not assessed.

21. **Karlson BW**, et al. Early prediction of acute MI from clinical history, examination and electrocardiogram in the emergency room. *Am J Cardiol* 1991;68:171–175.

This retrospective analysis focused on 7,157 Swedish patients with suspected MI, 13% with confirmed MI. Among patients with a normal ECG (34%) but no signs of acute ischemia, 14% had a confirmed MI. Among those with an abnormal ECG plus acute ischemia, 51% had MI. Among those with a clinically obvious MI, only 88% actually had an MI. Among those with a strong clinical suspicion of MI (30%), 34% actually had an acute MI; vague suspicion (54%), 8%; no suspicion (10%), 1%.

22. **Gibler WB**, et al. A rapid diagnostic and treatment center for patients with chest pain in the emergency department. *Ann Emerg Med* 1995;25:1–8.

This analysis focused on 1,010 patients with possible acute ischemic heart disease (patients directly admitted if known CAD, hemodynamic instability, ST-segment changes >1 mm, or ongoing chest pain). Serial CK-MB sampling was done at 0, 3, 6, and 9 hours, and continuous ECG monitoring was done for 9 hours. Two-dimensional echocardiography was performed at 9 hours if these tests were negative. If the echocardiogram was then negative, the patient underwent a graded exercise test. Overall, 82% of patients were discharged from the emergency department. Of the admitted patients, a substantial portion (34%) were found to have cardiac causes.

23. **Jesse RL, Kontos MC**. Evaluation of chest pain in the emergency department. *Curr Probl Cardiol* 1997;22:154–236.

This thorough review discusses the differential diagnosis of chest pain, presenting symptoms, and ECG analysis, and the role of serum markers and noninvasive testing. It concludes with a discussion of the role of guidelines, protocols, and pathways.

24. **Hilton TC**, et al. Technetium-99m sestamibi myocardial perfusion imaging in the emergency room evaluation of chest pain. *J Am Coll Cardiol* 1994;23:1016–1022.

This study was composed of 102 patients with typical angina and a normal or nondiagnostic ECG who underwent sestamibi imaging during symptoms. Among the 70 patients with a normal perfusion scan, only 1 patient (1.4%) had a subsequent cardiac event (follow-up 3 months), compared with 13% and 71% rates in those with equivocal or abnormal scans, respectively. Multivariate regression analysis identified an abnormal perfusion image as the only independent predictor of adverse cardiac events ($p = 0.009$).

25. **Gomez MA**, et al. for the Rapid Rule-Out of Myocardial Ischemia Observation (**ROMIO**) study group. An emergency department-based on protocol for rapidly ruling out myocardial ischemia reduces hospital time and expense: resulting of a randomized study (ROMIO). *J Am Coll Cardiol* 1996;28:25–33.

This study randomized 100 low-risk patients to emergency department rule-out or hospital care. The emergency department protocol consisted of enzyme tests at 0, 3, 6, and 9 hours, serial ECGs with continuous ST-segment monitoring, and, if results were negative, predischarge exercise testing. The protocol group had a shorter hospital stay and incurred fewer costs. The routine care group included more MI and unstable angina patients, but among patients ruled out, the protocol still was associated with decreased stay and cost (12 vs. 23 hours, p = 0.0001; initial stay: $890 vs. $1,350, 30 days: $900 vs. $1,520, p < 0.0001).

26. **Kontos MC**, et al. Comparison of myocardial perfusion imaging and cardiac troponin I in patients admitted to the emergency department with chest pain. *Circulation* 1999;99:2073–2078.

This study was composed of 620 patients considered low to moderate risk for acute coronary syndromes who underwent gated single-photon emission Tc sestamibi imaging and serial measurements of CK, CK-MB, and TnI over 8 hours. The incidence of MI was 9%, significant CAD was demonstrated in 13%, and revascularization was performed in 9%. Perfusion imaging was more sensitive but less specific than TnI in identifying patients who were revascularized [sensitivity 81% vs. 26% (TnI 1.0 ng/ml), specificity 74% vs. 96%].

Treatment

General Meta-Analysis

27. **Lau JL**, et al. Cumulative meta-analysis of therapeutic trials for MI. *N Engl J Med* 1992;327:248–254.

This overview showed that significant mortality reduction was associated with aspirin (19,077 patients; odds ratio 0.77, p < 0.001), β-blockers (31,669 patients; odds ratio 0.88, p = 0. 024), thrombolytics (odds ratio 0.75, p < 0.001), intravenous vasodilators (2,170 patients; odds ratio 0.57, p < 0.001), magnesium (only 1,304 patients; odds ratio 0.44, p < 0.001), and anticoagulation (4,975 patients; odds ratio 0.78, p < 0.001). Calcium-channel blockers and prophylactic lidocaine were both associated with a nonsignificant increase in mortality (6,420 patients, odds ratio 1.12; 8,745 patients, odds ratio 1.15). For secondary prevention, a protective effect was seen with β-blockers (20,138 patients; odds ratio 0.81, p < 0.001), anticoagulation (4,975 patients; odds ratio 0.78, p < 0.001), cholesterol-lowering drugs (10,775 patients; odds ratio 0.86, p < 0.001), and antiplatelet agents (18,411 patients; odds ratio 0.90, p = 0.051). Rehabilitation programs also were beneficial (5,022 patients; odds ratio 0.80, p = 0.012). No benefit was seen with calcium-channel blockers (13,114 patients, odds ratio 1.10), whereas class I antiarrhythmics were shown to be harmful (4,336 patients; odds ratio 1.28, p = 0.03).

Antithrombotic Agents

General Reviews

28. **Collins R**, et al. Clinical effects of anticoagulation therapy in suspected acute MI: systemic overview of randomised trials. *BMJ* 1996;313:652–659.

This analysis focused on 26 randomized studies (GUSTO not included). Of note, no aspirin was used in 5,000 patients, whereas routine aspirin was given in ~68,000 patients. In the absence of aspirin, anticoagulation reduced mortality by 25% (and fewer strokes occurred). With aspirin use, heparin was associated with 6% lower mortality (5 deaths/1,000; $2p$ = 0.03) but excess bleeding (+3/1,000). It was unclear whether heparin provides benefit if no thrombolytic agent is administered.

Aspirin

29. Second International Study of Infarct Survival (**ISIS-2**). Randomised trial of intravenous streptokinase, oral, both, or neither among 17,187 cases of suspected acute MI. *Lancet* 1988;332: 349–360.

     This large trial clearly demonstrated the additive benefit of thrombolytic therapy and aspirin administration. Patients were randomized to streptokinase 1.5 million U over 60 minutes and/or aspirin 162.5 mg; or placebo. The streptokinase and aspirin alone groups had 25% and 23% lower 5 week vascular mortality, respectively [9.2% vs. 12.0% (placebo), p < 0.00001; 9.4% vs. 11.8%, p < 0.00001). The streptokinase and aspirin group had a larger 42% mortality reduction (8% vs. 13.2%). Combination therapy was also effective in patients with left bundle branch block (mortality 14% vs. 27.7 %). Aspirin reduced nonfatal reinfarction and stroke rates (1.0% vs. 2.0%; 0.3% vs. 0.6%).

30. **Roux S**, et al. Effect of aspirin on coronary reocclusion and recurrent ischemia after thrombolysis: a meta-analysis. *J Am Coll Cardiol* 1992;19:671–677 (editorial pp. 678–680).

     This analysis of 32 studies (19 randomized, 13 nonrandomized) from 1980 to 1990 showed the impressive benefits of aspirin. In these studies, 3,209 of 4,930 patients were treated with aspirin. Among the 1,022 patients who underwent angiography, aspirin use was associated with a 56% lower reocclusion rate (11% vs. 25%; p < 0.001) and fewer recurrent ischemic events (25% vs. 41%; p < 0.001). This protective effect of aspirin was similar in trials with either streptokinase or recombinant tissue-type plasminogen activator (rt-PA).

Heparin

31. **Hsia J**, et al. for the Heparin Aspirin Reperfusion Trial (**HART**) Investigators. A comparison between heparin and low-dose aspirin as adjunctive therapy with tissue plasminogen activator for acute MI. *N Engl J Med* 1990;323:1433–1437 (editorial pp. 1483–1485).

     Design: Prospective, randomized, open-label, multicenter study. Primary end point was IRA patency at 7–24 hours and 7 days.
     Purpose: To compare the effects of heparin with aspirin after rt-PA in patients with acute MI.
     Population: 205 patients ≤75 years of age with acute ST-elevation MI (≥0.1 mm in at least two contiguous leads).
     Exclusion Criteria: Severe hypotension, cerebrovascular disease, bleeding disorders, left bundle branch block, prior CABG, recent surgery, and prolonged CPR.
     Treatment: rt-PA 100 mg intravenously over 6 hours (6-mg bolus, 54 mg during 1st hour, 20 mg in 2nd hour, 5 mg/h for 4 hours) plus either aspirin 80 mg/day or heparin 5,000 U intravenous bolus then 1,000 U/h [adjusted to keep activated partial thromboplastin time (aPTT) within 1.5–2.0 times control]. Coro-

nary angiography was performed 7–24 hours after rt-PA infusion was started and again at 7 days.

Results: Heparin group had higher patency (TIMI grade 2 or 3 flow) at initial angiography (82% vs. 52%; $p < 0.0001$), but no significant difference was seen by the time of the second angiograms (88% vs. 95%). No significant differences were seen in hemorrhagic or recurrent ischemic events.

Comments: A retrospective analysis showed that patients with open arteries at early angiography had a higher mean PTT (81 vs. 54 seconds; $p < 0.02$). However, patients with a PTT of >100 at 8 hours had a higher rate of access-related hemorrhage (*see J Am Coll Cardiol* 1992;20:513).

32. **O'Connor CM**, et al. for the Duke University Clinical Cardiology Study (**DUCCS**) Group. A randomized trial of intravenous heparin in conjunction with anistreplase (anisoylated plasminogen streptokinase activator complex) in acute MI: the DUCCS 1. *J Am Coll Cardiol* 1994;23:11–18.

Design: Prospective, randomized, open, single center study. Primary composite end points were death, reinfarction, recurrent ischemia, and IRA patency.

Purpose: To evaluate if complications are reduced by not using heparin following APSAC administration in patients with acute MI.

Population: 250 patients ≤85 years with ≥1 mm ST elevation in at least two contiguous ECG leads.

Exclusion Criteria: Prior streptokinase or APSAC treatment, need for chronic heparin or warfarin therapy, history of bleeding diathesis, history of cerebrovascular disease, SBP >180 mm Hg or DBP >110 mm Hg, and cardiogenic shock.

Treatment: Heparin 15 U/kg/h intravenous bolus given 4 hours after APSAC (30 U over 2–5 minutes) and infusion adjusted to keep PTT at 50–90 seconds (stopped 18–24 hours prior to day 5 catheterization); or no heparin. All patients were given aspirin 325 mg once daily.

Results: Addition of heparin was not helpful and was possibly harmful. No difference was observed in combined primary end points (42% vs. 43%), infarct-related patency (80% vs. 73%), or left ventricular function at day 5 ventriculography (52% vs. 50.5%), whereas more bleeding complications were noted (32% vs. 17%; $p = 0.006$).

33. **Gueret P**, et al. Effects of full-dose heparin anticoagulation on the development of left ventricular thrombosis in acute transmural MI. *J Am Coll Cardiol* 1986;8:419–426.

This small prospective study showed that thrombi occur frequently in anterior MIs. Ninety patients (46 anterior, 44 inferior) presenting an average 5.2 hours after onset of symptoms were randomized to heparin or no heparin. No thrombi were detected on first echocardiograms (done at 10.3 ± 8 hours). In the anterior MI group, 46% had thrombi at 4.3 ± 3.0 days [38% (heparin) vs. 52% (no heparin); $p = 0.76$]. No thrombi formed in the inferior group.

Low-Molecular-Weight Heparin

34. **Kontny F**, et al. on behalf of the Fragmin in Acute MI (**FRAMI**) Study Group. Randomized trial of low molecular weight heparin (dalteparin) in prevention of left ventricular thrombus formation

and arterial embolism after acute anterior MI: the FRAMI study. *J Am Coll Cardiol* 1997;30:962–969.

Design: Prospective, randomized, multicenter study. Primary outcomes were thrombus formation (echocardiography at 9 ± 2 days) and arterial embolism.

Purpose: To evaluate the efficacy and safety of dalteparin in the prevention of left ventricular thrombus formation and arterial embolism after acute anterior MI.

Population: 776 patients presenting at ≤15 hours after symptom onset with ≥2 mm ST elevation in ECG leads V1 to V6 or ≥1 mm in leads I and aVL.

Exclusion Criteria: Prior anterior MI, ongoing treatment with or indication for heparin or warfarin, SBP >210 mm Hg or DBP >115 mm Hg, recent cerebrovascular events (≤2 months), and increased bleeding risks.

Treatment: Dalteparin 150 IU/kg every 12 hours or placebo; 91.5% of patients received a thrombolytic agent.

Results: Only 517 patients had echocardiograms available for analysis. The dalteparin group had a lower rate of thrombus formation and arterial embolism: 14.2% vs. 21.9% (p = 0.03). Regarding individual end points, left ventricular thrombus-relative risk was 0.63 (p = 0.02), arterial embolism six vs. five patients (p = NS), and reinfarction eight vs. six patients (p = NS). In both groups, 23 patients died. However, dalteparin was associated with increased major and minor hemorrhage rates (2.9% vs. 0.3%, p = 0.006; 14.8% vs. 1.8%, p < 0.001).

35. **Forstfeldt G**, et al. Low molecular weight heparin (dalteparin) as adjuvant treatment to thrombolysis in acute myocardial infarction—a pilot study: biochemical markers in acute coronary syndromes (**BIOMACS II**). *J Am Coll Cardiol* 1999;33:627–633.

    A total of 101 patients presenting within 12 hours of onset of symptoms with ST elevation or new left bundle branch block were randomized to dalteparin 100 IU/kg or placebo. The first dose was given prior to streptokinase, and a second injection was given 12 hours later. Coronary angiography was performed at 20–28 hours. There was a trend toward higher IRA TIMI grade 3 flow in the dalteparin group (68% vs. 51%; p = 0.10). Continuous ECG monitoring revealed a lower incidence of ischemic episodes after the start of treatment in the dalteparin group (16% vs. 38%; p = 0.04). The authors recognize the need for larger studies and suggest evaluation of low-molecular-weight regimens using an initial intravenous dose.

Direct Thrombin Inhibitors

36. **Cannon CP**, et al. for the Thrombolysis in MI Trial (**TIMI-5**) Investigators. A pilot trial of recombinant desulfatohirudin compared with heparin in conjunction with tissue-type plasminogen activator and aspirin for acute MI: results of the TIMI 5 trial. *J Am Coll Cardiol* 1994;23:993–1003.

    Design: Prospective, randomized, open, dose escalation, multicenter study. Primary end point was IRA TIMI grade 3 flow at 90 minutes and 18–36 hours.

    Purpose: To evaluate the effectiveness of recombinant desulfatohirudin (hirudin) as adjunctive therapy to thrombolysis in acute MI.

Population: 246 patients 21–75 years of age with ischemic pain lasting ≥30 minutes and ≥1 mm ST elevation in at least two contiguous ECG leads or new left bundle branch block.

Exclusion Criteria: Prior coronary artery bypass surgery, angiography, or PTCA; thrombolytic therapy for acute MI in prior 2 weeks; cardiogenic shock; and current anticoagulation.

Treatment: Hirudin intravenously at one of four ascending doses: 0.15 mg/kg bolus then 0.05 mg/kg/h, 0.1 mg/kg bolus then 0.1 mg/kg/h, 0.3 mg/kg bolus then 0.1 mg/kg/h, 0.6 mg/kg bolus then 0.2 mg/kg/h; or heparin 5,000-U intravenous bolus then 1,000 U/h (with adjustments to keep aPTT at 60–90 seconds). All patients received front-loaded tPA and aspirin 160 mg/day.

Results: A trend toward better IRA TIMI 3 grade 3 flow was observed at 90 minutes and 18–36 hours with hirudin: 61.8% vs. 49.4%, $p = 0.07$ (at 90 minutes only, 64.8% vs. 57.1%, $p =$ NS; 18–36 hours, 97.8% vs. 89%, $p = 0.01$). Hirudin groups also showed a trend toward less IRA reocclusion (1.6% vs. 6.7%, $p = 0.07$) and significant reduction in in-hospital death or reinfarction (6.8% vs. 16.7%, $p = 0.02$). All four hirudin doses yielded similar angiographic and clinical and point results. No significant differences were seen in major spontaneous hemorrhage (1.2% vs. 4.7%, $p = 0.09$) or instrumented site bleeding (16.3% vs. 18.4%).

37. **Antman EM**, et al. for the **TIMI-9B** Investigators. Hirudin in AMI. *Circulation* 1996;94:911—921 (editorial pp. 863–865).

    Design: Prospective, randomized, double-blind, parallel-group, multicenter study. Primary end point was 30-day incidences of death, nonfatal MI, severe CHF, and cardiogenic shock.

    Purpose: To compare the safety and effectiveness of hirudin with heparin in patients undergoing thrombolysis for acute MI.

    Population: 3,002 patients within 12 hours of onset of symptoms and with ≥1 mm ST elevation in at least two contiguous ECG leads; mean age 60 ± 12 years.

    Exclusion Criteria: Contraindications to thrombolytic therapy, serum creatinine >2.0 mg/dL, cardiogenic shock, therapeutic anticoagulation (prothrombin time ≥14 seconds, aPTT ≥60 seconds).

    Treatment: Heparin 5,000 intravenous bolus then 1,000 U/h, or hirudin 0.1 mg/kg intravenous bolus then 0.1 mg/kg/h (maximum 15 mg/h) for 96 hours. Infusions were started before or immediately following thrombolysis (front-loaded tPA or streptokinase) and adjusted to keep aPTT at 55–85 seconds. All patients were thrombolyzed.

    Results: No significant difference in primary end points was observed: 12.9% (hirudin) vs. 11.9%. Nor were any differences observed in hemorrhage and intracranial hemorrhage rates (4.6% vs. 5.3; 0. 4% vs. 0.9%). Target aPTT was achieved more frequently with hirudin.

38. **White HD**, et al. on behalf of the Hirulog Early Perfusion/Occlusion (**HERO**) Trial Investigators. Randomized, double-blind comparison of hirulog versus heparin in patients receiving streptokinase and aspirin for acute MI (HERO). *Circulation* 1997; 96:2155–2161 (editorial pp. 2118–2120).

    Design: Prospective, randomized, double-blind, multicenter study. Primary outcome was TIMI grade flow at 90–120 minutes.

    Purpose: To evaluate and compare the safety and efficacy of two hirulog regimens with heparin in acute MI patients receiving streptokinase.

Population: 412 patients presenting within 12 hours of symptom onset and with ≥1 mm ST elevation in at least two contiguous limb leads and/or V4 to V6 or ≥2 mm in V1 to V3.

Exclusion Criteria: Prior streptokinase; recent (≤3 months) bleeding, trauma, or surgery; recent stroke or transient ischemic attack (≤6 months); severe uncontrolled hypertension (not defined); and cardiogenic shock.

Treatment: Heparin 5,000-U intravenous bolus then 1,000–1,200 U/h, low-dose hirulog (0.125 mg/kg intravenous bolus, 0.25 mg/kg/h for 12 hours, then 0.125 mg/kg/h), or high-dose hirulog (0.25 mg/kg intravenous bolus, 0.5 mg/kg/h for 12 hours, then 0.25 mg/kg/h).

Results: Hirulog groups had better TIMI grade 3 flow at 90–120 minutes (primary outcome): 46% and 48% vs. 35% (heparin vs. hirulog. $p = 0.023$; heparin vs. high-dose hirulog, $p = 0.03$). However, no significant difference in rates of reocclusion was observed at 48 hours (5% and 1% vs. 7%) or death, shock, and reinfarction at 35 days (14% and 12.5% vs. 17.9%). Hirulog also was associated with less major bleeding: 14% and 19% vs. 28% (low-dose hirulog vs. heparin, $p < 0.01$).

39. **ARGAMI-2.** Preliminary results. Presented at the 47th American College of Cardiology (ACC) Scientific Session in Atlanta, GA, March 1998.

   This study randomized 1,001 patients to argatroban (60-μg intravenous bolus then 2 μg/kg/min, or 120-μg bolus then 4 μg/kg/min) or heparin. Enrollment into the low-dose argatroban arm was terminated early (after 609 patients) due to lack of efficacy. There was no significant difference in 30-day mortality between the high-dose argatroban and heparin groups (5.5% vs. 5.4%). The argatroban group did show a trend toward fewer major bleeding events.

40. **Lee LV**, et al. for the **TIMI-6** Investigators. Initial experience with hirudin and streptokinase in acute MI: results of TIMI-6. *Am J Cardiol* 1995;75:7–13.

   This dose-ranging study randomized 193 patients to hirudin (at one of three doses: 0.15 mg/kg intravenous bolus then 0.05 mg/kg/h, 0.3 mg/kg intravenous bolus then 0.1 mg/kg/h, or 0.6 mg/kg intravenous bolus then 0.2 mg/kg/h) or heparin (5,000-U bolus then 1,000 U/h and adjusted to an aPTT of 65–90 seconds) in conjunction with streptokinase and aspirin. All treatment groups had similar hemorrhage rates. The two higher dosing regimens of hirudin yielded the best results. At hospital discharge, they were associated with a lower rate of death, nonfatal reinfarction, CHF, and cardiogenic shock (9.7% and 11.4%), compared to lower dose hirudin (21.6% [heparin: 17.6%]).

Coumadin

41. **Smith P**, et al. Warfarin Reinfarction Study (**WARIS**). The effect of warfarin on mortality and reinfarction after MI. *N Engl J Med* 1990;323:147–152.

   Design: Prospective, randomized, double-blind, placebo-controlled, multicenter study. Mean follow-up period was 37 months. Primary end point was all-cause mortality and reinfarction.

Purpose: To evaluate the effects of warfarin on mortality, reinfarction, and cerebrovascular events in post-MI patients.

Population: 1,214 patients ≤75 years of age; mean time since index MI 27 days.

Exclusion Criteria: Required anticoagulant use and significant bleeding risk (e.g., peptic ulcer disease and hemorrhagic diathesis).

Treatment: Warfarin dose adjusted to achieve target international normalized ratio (INR) of 2.8–4.8; or placebo.

Results: Warfarin group had 24% lower all-cause mortality (15.5% vs. 20.3%; $p = 0.03$), 34% fewer reinfarctions (13.5% vs. 20.4%; $p < 0.001$), and 55% fewer cerebrovascular accidents (3.3% vs. 7.2%; $p = 0.0015$). The serious bleeding rate in the warfarin group was 0.6%/yr (intracranial hemorrhage rate 0.2%/yr).

42. Anticoagulants in Secondary Prevention of Events in Coronary Thrombosis (**ASPECT**) Research Group. Effect of long-term anticoagulant treatment on mortality and cardiovascular morbidity after MI. *Lancet* 1994;343:499–503.

Design: Prospective, randomized, double-blind, placebo-controlled, multicenter study. Mean follow-up period was 37 months. Primary end point was all-cause mortality.

Purpose: To evaluate the impact of long-term anticoagulation in the secondary prevention of morbidity and mortality after acute MI.

Population: 3,404 patients with cardiac serum marker evidence of an acute MI (at least twice the upper limit of normal).

Exclusion Criteria: Need for chronic anticoagulation, anticoagulation therapy in prior 6 months, increased bleeding tendency, and anticipated coronary revascularization procedure.

Treatment: Phenprocoumon or nicoumalone started within 6 weeks of hospital discharge to achieve an INR of 2.8–4.8; or placebo.

Results: No significant mortality difference was observed between groups [10% (anticoagulation) vs. 11.1%]. Anticoagulation was associated with a reduction in two secondary end points: >50% fewer recurrent MIs (6.7% vs. 14.2%) and ~40% fewer cerebrovascular events (2.2% vs. 3.6%). The anticoagulation group did have more major bleeding complications (4.3% vs. 1.1%).

Comments: A post hoc analysis showed that the optimal INR was 3–4. The rate of major bleeding plus thromboembolic complications was 3.2 per 100 patient years (INR <2, 8.0; 2–3, 3.9; 4–5, 6.6; >5, 7.7) (*see J Am Coll Cardiol* 1996;27:1349).

43. **Julian DG**, et al. for the Aspirin/Anticoagulants Following Thrombolysis with Eminase in Recurrent infarction (**AFTER**) Study Group. A comparison of aspirin and anticoagulation following thrombolysis for MI (the AFTER study): a multicentre unblinded randomised clinical trial. *BMJ* 1996;313:1429–1431.

Design: Prospective, randomized, unblinded, multicenter study. Follow-up period was 1 year. Primary end point was cardiac death and nonfatal MI at 30 days.

Purpose: To compare aspirin with heparin followed by oral anticoagulation therapy in MI patients undergoing thrombolysis with anistreptlase.

Population: 1,036 patients treated with anistreptlase within 6 hours of onset of symptoms (ECG criteria: ≥2 mm ST elevation in at least two adjacent precordial leads or ≥1 mm in at least two limb leads).

Exclusion Criteria: Contraindication to anistreplase or treatment with aspirin, nonsteroidals, or oral anticoagulation prior to qualifying event.

Treatment: Aspirin 150 mg/day or heparin 1,000 U/h for 24 hours (started 6 hours after anistreplase 30 U) followed by oral anticoagulation to achieve a target INR of 2.0–2.5. Therapy was discontinued after 3 months.

Results: Similar 30 day incidences of cardiac death and reinfarction were observed [11.2% (aspirin) vs. 11%]. The anticoagulation group did have more severe bleeding and strokes: at 3 months, 3.9% vs. 1.7% (*p* = 0.04).

Comments: Slowing patient recruitment led to early termination of the trial.

44. Coumadin Aspirin Reinfarction Study (**CARS**) Investigators. Randomised double-blind trial of fixed low-dose warfarin with aspirin after MI. *Lancet* 1997;350:389–396.

Design: Prospective, randomized, double-blind, multicenter study. Median follow-up period was 14 months. Primary end point was MI, stroke, and cardiovascular death.

Purpose: To compare chronic administration of aspirin alone with lower dose aspirin in combination with fixed low-dose regimens of oral anticoagulation in acute MI patients.

Population: 8,803 patients 21–85 years of age with a documented MI 3–21 days prior to enrollment.

Exclusion Criteria: Cardiogenic shock, rest angina refractory to medical therapy, stroke (without full recovery or prior hemorrhage), thrombocytopenia (platelet count <100,000), and SBP >180 mm Hg or DBP >100 mm Hg.

Treatment: Aspirin 160 mg/day, aspirin 80 mg/day and warfarin 1 mg/day, or aspirin 80 mg/day and warfarin 3 mg/day

Results: Average measured INRs at week 4 were 1.02 (aspirin alone), 1.05 (aspirin and warfarin 1 mg/day), and 1.27 (aspirin and warfarin 3 mg/day). No significant difference in primary end points (MI, stroke, or cardiovascular death) was observed (1-year rates 8.6% [aspirin], 8.8% [aspirin and warfarin 1 mg/day], 8.4% [aspirin and warfarin 3 mg/day]). However, the warfarin 3 mg/day group had a higher rate of spontaneous major hemorrhage versus aspirin alone: 0.74%/yr vs. 1.4%/yr (*p* = 0.014).

44a. **Meijer A**, et al. Antithrombotics in the Prevention of Reocclusion in Coronary Thrombolysis (**APRICOT**) study. Aspirin versus coumadin in the prevention of reocclusion and recurrent ischemia after successful thrombolysis: a prospective placebo-controlled angiographic study. *Circulation* 1993;87:1524–1530.

A total of 300 patients with patent artery at angiography (<48 hours) were randomized to aspirin 325 mg daily or coumadin (heparin until INR was 2.8–4.0). At 3 months, no change in reocclusion rates was observed (25%, 30% [placebo], 32% [coumadin]). However, aspirin showed decreased reinfarction vs. placebo [3% vs. 11% (coumadin 8%)], best event-free course [93% vs. 82% vs. coumadin (76%); *p* < 0.05) and increased ejection fraction (+4.6%).

Glycoprotein IIb / IIIa Inhibitors

45. **Ohman EM**, et al. for the **IMPACT-AMI** Investigators. Combined accelerated tissue plasminogen activator and platelet gly-

coprotein IIb/IIIa integrin receptor blockade with integrelin in acute MI. *Circulation* 1997;95:846–854 (editorial pp. 793–795).
Design: Prospective, randomized, placebo-controlled, partially open (first 132 patients), partially blinded (last 48 patients), dose-ranging, multicenter study. Primary end point was TIMI grade 3 flow at 90 minutes.
Purpose: To determine the safety and efficacy of eptifibatide in conjunction with aspirin, heparin, and accelerated alteplase in acute MI.
Population: 180 patients presenting within 6 hours of onset of symptoms with chest pain lasting ≥30 minutes, ST elevation ≥1 mm in at least two inferior or precordial leads or leads I and aVL, ST depression in V1 to V6 consistent with posterior injury, or left bundle branch block.
Exclusion Criteria: Weight >125 kilograms, bleeding diathesis, SBP >200 mm Hg or DBP >100 mm Hg, prior stroke, oral anticoagulation, recent (<6 weeks) bleeding, prolonged CPR (>10 minutes), platelets <100,000, and creatinine >4.0 mg/dL.
Treatment: 132 patients assigned in 2:1 fashion to one of six doses of eptifibatide (36–180 µg/kg intravenous bolus followed by 0.2–0.75 µg/kg/min); or placebo. All patients were given front-loaded tPA, heparin [40 U/kg intravenous bolus (except two highest integrelin dose groups) then 15 U/kg/h], and aspirin 325 mg/day and front-loaded tPA. The final 48 patients were randomized in 3:1 fashion to high-dose eptifibatide (180 µg/kg bolus then 0.75 µg/kg/min); or placebo.
Results: Highest dose group had better 90 TIMI grade 3 flow [66% vs. 39% (placebo); $p = 0.006$] and shorter time to ST-segment recovery (65 vs. 116 minutes; $p = 0.05$). However, no significant difference was observed in in-hospital composite end points of death, reinfarction, stroke, revascularization, new CHF, and pulmonary edema (43% vs. 42%). Similar bleeding complication rates were observed (4% vs. 5%).
Comments: Study was weakly powered. The accompanying editorial points out that the open and double-blind data were inappropriately pooled. If only the double-blind data were analyzed, 90-minute TIMI grade 3 flow was actually better with placebo (77% vs. 64%).

46. **Brener SJ**, et al. on behalf of the Reopro And Primary PTCA Organization and Randomized Trial (**RAPPORT**) Investigators. Randomized, placebo-controlled trial of primary glycoprotein IIb/IIIa blockade with primary angioplasty for acute MI. *Circulation* 1998;98:734–741.
Design: Prospective, randomized, double-blind, placebo-controlled, multicenter study. Primary end point (at 6 months) was death, MI, and any target vessel revascularization (TVR).
Purpose: To evaluate whether platelet IIb/IIIa receptor blockade with abciximab reduces ischemic events in acute MI patients undergoing primary angioplasty.
Population: 483 patients presenting within 12 hours of onset of symptoms with ischemic chest pain lasting >20 minutes accompanied by significant ST elevation in at least two contiguous leads or new left bundle branch block.
Exclusion Criteria: Severe thrombocytopenia, ongoing internal bleeding or recent major surgery, previous stroke, severe uncon-

trolled hypertension, PTCA of IRA in prior 3 months, cardiogenic shock, and prior abciximab or thrombolytic therapy.

Treatment: Abciximab 0.25 mg/kg bolus then 0.125 µg/kg/min (maximum 10 µg/min) for 12 hours. All patients received aspirin and heparin 100 U/kg bolus before PTCA (with further boluses as needed to keep activated clotting time >300 seconds). Stenting was discouraged but was allowed for residual dissection with >50% restenosis and for abrupt or threatened closure.

Results: No difference was observed between the two groups in incidence of 6-month primary end points (28.1% vs. 28.2%). However, the abciximab group had lower rates of death, MI, and urgent TVR at 7 days (3.3% vs. 9.9%; $p = 0.003$), 30 days (5.8% vs. 11.2%; $p = 0.03$), and 6 months (11.6% vs. 17.8%; $p = 0.05$). The abciximab group had 42% less bailout stenting (11.9% vs. 20.4%; $p = 0.008$). Abciximab was associated with increased major bleeding (defined as hematocrit drop of >5; 16.6% vs. 9.5%, $p = 0.02$), mostly at the arterial access site. On-treatment analysis showed that abciximab was associated with decreased death and MI at 7 days (1.4% vs. 4.7%; $p = 0.047$) with a trend at 6 months (6.9% vs. 12%; $p = 0.07$).

Comments: The low-risk population (30 day mortality rates ~2%) may have an attenuated impact of abciximab. Increased bleeding with abciximab was likely due to double-blind design, as the investigators were unwilling to discontinue heparin immediately after procedure(s) for early sheath removal.

47. **Antman EM**, et al. for the **TIMI-14** Investigators. Abciximab facilitates the rate and extent of thrombolysis. *Circulation* 1999; 99:2720–2732 (editorial pp. 2714–2716).

Design: Prospective, randomized, dose-ranging, multicenter study. Primary end point was IRA TIMI grade 3 flow at 90 minutes.

Purpose: To determine if abciximab is an effective and safe addition to reduced-dose thrombolytic regimens for ST elevation MI.

Population: 888 patients 18–75 years of age presenting within 12 hours of symptom onset with ≥1 mm ST elevation in at least two contiguous ECG leads.

Exclusion Criteria: Left bundle branch block, 6,000 U heparin in the hour prior to randomization, prior CABG surgery, percutaneous intervention or thrombolytic therapy in prior 7 days, and history of stroke or transient ischemic attack.

Treatment: (a) 100 mg of accelerated dose alteplase (control). (b) Abciximab (0.25 mg/kg bolus then 0.125 µg/kg/min for 12 hours) plus reduced-dose streptokinase (500,000 to 1.5 million U). (c) Abciximab plus reduced-dose alteplase (20–65 mg). (d) Abciximab alone. All patients received aspirin. Control patients received standard weight-based heparin (70 U/kg bolus, initial infusion 15 U/kg/h), whereas abciximab groups received low-dose heparin (60 U/kg bolus then 7 U/kg/h). Very low-dose heparin also was tested in the dose confirmation phase (30 U kg/ bolus then 4 U/kg/h).

Results: Abciximab alone achieved TIMI grade 3 flow at 90 minutes in only 32% and abciximab plus streptokinase 500,000 to 1.25 million U in only 34%–46%. Higher rates of TIMI grade 3 flow at 60 and 90 minutes were seen with increasing duration of alteplase infusion, progressing from bolus alone to bolus and 30- or 60-minute infusion ($p < 0.02$). Best regimen was abciximab and alteplase 50 mg (15-mg bolus, 35 mg over 60 minutes), which produced TIMI 3 flow in 77% at 90 minutes (vs. 62% with alteplase alone; $p = 0.02$). TIMI 3 flow at 60 minutes was also significantly better with this regimen [72% vs. 43% (alteplase alone); $p = 0.0009$]. Major hemorrhage occurred in 3% receiving abciximab alone, 6% with alteplase alone, 10% with streptokinase plus abciximab, 7% with 50 mg alteplase plus abciximab plus low-dose heparin, 1% with 50 mg alteplase plus abciximab plus very low-dose heparin.

Comments: Accompanying editorial suggests that glycoprotein IIb/IIIa inhibition in conjunction with reduced-dose thrombolysis provides a regimen that will likely prove to be equivalent or superior to mechanical perfusion therapy. Future studies that directly compare the two strategies will obviously be needed to evaluate this hypothesis.

48. **van den Merkhof**, et al. Glycoprotein Receptor Antagonist Patency Evaluation (**GRAPE**) Pilot Study. Abciximab in the treatment of acute MI eligible for primary percutaneous transluminal coronary angioplasty. *J Am Coll Cardiol* 1999;33:1528–1532.

This study was composed of 60 patients presenting within 6 hours of onset of symptoms who had abciximab (250 µg/kg bolus then 10 µg/min for 12 hours) started before proceeding to the catheterization laboratory for possible primary angioplasty. Median time from initiation of abciximab to contrast injection of the IRA was 45 minutes. TIMI grade 3 flow was observed in 18%, and TIMI 2 flow in 22%. These numbers are higher than those seen in primary angioplasty trials without abciximab pretreatment.

49. Abciximab before Direct Angiography and Stenting in MI Regarding Acute and Long-term Follow-up (**ADMIRAL**) study. Preliminary results presented at the 48th ACC Scientific Session in New Orleans, LA, March 1999.

This prospective, randomized, multicenter, double-blind, placebo-controlled trial was composed of 300 patients with ≥1 mm ST elevation in at least two leads who presented within 12 hours of onset of symptoms. Patients underwent angioplasty or stenting (85% of patients) and were randomized to abciximab or placebo. The abciximab group had a 46.5% lower incidence of the primary composite end point, consisting of death, MI, and ischemia requiring urgent TVR (10.7% vs. 20.0%; $p < 0.03$). Abciximab patients also had better TIMI grade 3 flow at 24 hours (85.6% vs. 78.4%; $p < 0.05$), lower incidence of any revascularization (18.8% vs. 29.3%; $p < 0.04$), and a better ejection fraction at 30 days (62.6% vs. 55.3%). Abciximab use was associated with more frequent major and minor bleeding (4.0% vs. 2.6%, 6.7% vs. 1.3%).

β-Blockers

50. Norwegian Multicenter Group. Timolol-induced reduction in mortality and reinfarction in patients surviving acute MI. *N Engl J Med* 1981;304:801–807.

Design: Prospective, randomized, double-blind, placebo-con-trolled, multicenter study. Mean follow-up period was 17 months. Primary end point was all-cause mortality.

Purpose: To evaluate the efficacy of long-term β-blockade after MI.

Population: 1,884 patients randomized at 7–28 days after acute MI meeting at least two of the following criteria: (a) chest pain >15 minutes, acute pulmonary edema, or cardiogenic shock; (b) pathologic Q waves and/or ST elevation followed by T-wave inversion in at least two leads; or (c) elevated serum markers.

Exclusion Criteria: Resting heart rate <50 beats/min, severe CHF, second- or third-degree atrioventricular block, SBP <100 mm Hg, and severe comorbidity.

Treatment: Timolol 10 mg twice daily or placebo.

Results: Timolol group had a 39% lower mortality rate (13.3% vs. 21.9%; $p < 0.001$) and a 28% lower reinfarction rate (14.4% vs. 20.1%; $p < 0.001$).

Comments: Six-year follow-up showed a persistent mortality benefit of timolol (26.4% vs. 32.3%; $p = 0.003$).

51. β-blocker Heart Attack Trial (**BHAT**) Research Group. A ran-domized trial of propranolol in patients with acute MI. *JAMA* 1982;247:1707–1714.

Design: Prospective, randomized, double-blind, placebo-controlled, multicenter study. Mean follow-up period was 25 months. Primary end point was all-cause mortality.

Purpose: To evaluate if long-term propranolol administration after MI reduces mortality.

Population: 3,837 patients <70 years of age enrolled 5–21 days after an acute MI.

Exclusion Criteria: Marked bradycardia, current β-blocker ther-apy, history of severe heart failure or asthma, and planned car-diac surgery.

Treatment: Propranolol 60–80 mg three times daily, or placebo.

Results: Propranolol group had 26.5% lower mortality (7.2% vs. 9.8%; $p < 0.005$), 28% fewer sudden cardiac deaths (3.3% vs. 4.6%; $p < 0.05$), and 23% fewer major cardiac events (nonfatal MI plus fatal coronary disease). Serious side effects were infrequent.

Comments: Post hoc analysis showed that the benefit of propra-nolol was restricted to a high-risk group of 383 patients: 43% mortality reduction ($p < 0.01$).

52. The Metoprolol in Acute MI (**MIAMI**) Trial Research Group. Metoprolol in Acute MI (MIAMI): a randomised placebo-controlled international trial. *Eur Heart J* 1985;6:199–226.

Design: Prospective, randomized, double-blind, placebo-con-trolled, multicenter study. Primary end point was all-cause mortality.

Purpose: To evaluate if metoprolol administration after MI re-duces mortality.

Population: 5,728 patients <75 years of age presenting within 24 hours of onset of symptoms (average 7 hours).

Exclusion Criteria: Current treatment with β-blockers or cal-cium antagonists, and heart rate ≤65 beats/min.

Treatment: Metoprolol 15 mg intravenously then 200 mg/day orally, or placebo.

Results: Metoprolol group had a nonsignificant 13% mortality reduction at 15 days (4.3% vs. 4.9%). The high-risk subgroup (meeting at least three of the following criteria: >60 years of age, prior MI, ECG consistent with MI, previous angina, CHF, diabetes, on digoxin or diuretics) had 29% lower mortality.

53. **ISIS-1** Collaborative Group. Randomised trial of intravenous atenolol among 16,107 cases of suspected acute MI. *Lancet* 1986; 328:57–65.

Design: Prospective, randomized, open, parallel-group, multicenter study. Primary end point was vascular mortality at 7 days.

Purpose: To determine the effects of atenolol in MI patients on 7-day vascular mortality.

Population: 16,107 patients presenting within 12 hours (average 5 hours) of an acute MI who were not on a β-blocker or verapamil.

Exclusion Criteria: Heart rate <50 beats/min, SBP <100 mm Hg, second- or third-degree heart block, severe heart failure, and bronchospasm.

Treatment: Atenolol 5–10 mg intravenously over 5 minutes followed by 100 mg/day orally for 7 days. No placebo was given to controls.

Results: Atenolol group had a 15% lower 7-day vascular mortality rate (3.89% vs. 4.57%; $p < 0.04$). Of note, most of mortality difference occurred in the first 24 hours. At 1 year, the benefit persisted, with an 11% vascular mortality reduction (10.7% vs. 12.0%; $p < 0.01$). After year 1, there was a nonsignificant excess of vascular deaths in the atenolol group (179 vs. 145; $p = 0.07$).

Comments: A later analysis showed that the benefit of atenolol in the first 24 hours was primarily due to a lower rate of pulseless electrical activity, reflecting less cardiac rupture (*see Lancet* 1988;331:921).

54. **Roberts R**, et al. for the TIMI-IIB Investigators. Immediate vs. deferred beta-blockade following thrombolytic therapy in patients with acute MI: results of TIMI II-B. *Circulation* 1991; 83:422–437.

Design: Prospective, randomized, open, parallel-group, multicenter study. Primary end point was pre-discharge left ventricular ejection fraction (LVEF).

Purpose: To compare immediate intravenous versus deferred (started on day 6) β-blocker in acute MI patients treated with rt-PA.

Population: 1,434 patients ≤75 years of age presenting within 4 hours of chest pain and with ≥1 mm ST elevation in at least two contiguous ECG leads and having no contraindications to β-blockade. Low risk subgroup is defined as an absence of all the following: history of MI, anterior ST elevation, rates greater than one-third up lung fields, SBP <100 mmHg or cardiogenic shock, HR >100 bpm, atrial fibrillation or flutter age ≥70 years.

Exclusion Criteria: Heart rate <55 beats/min, SBP consistently <100 mm Hg, severe first-degree or advanced heart block, and wheezing or significant COPD.

Treatment: Immediate β-blockade group received metoprolol 5 mg intravenously for three doses (given within 2 hours of rt-PA) then 50–100 mg twice daily. The deferred β-blockade group received metoprolol 50 mg twice daily on day 6 followed by 100 mg twice daily. All patients received aspirin, heparin (intravenously for 5 days, then subcutaneously every 12 hours), and lidocaine (1.0–1.5 mg/kg then 2.0–4.0 mg/min for 24 hours).

Results: No significant differences in mortality or LVEF were observed at discharge, but the subgroup of low-risk patients receiving β-blockade had a lower rate of death and nonfatal reinfarction (5.4% vs. 13. 7%; $p = 0.01$), as well as less recurrent chest pain (18.8% vs. 24.1%; $p < 0.02$).

55. **Gottlieb SS**, et al. Cooperative Cardiovascular Project. Effect of beta-blockade on mortality among high-risk and low-risk patients after MI. *N Engl J Med* 1998;339:489–497.

    Design: Retrospective, observational study. Primary efficacy end point was 2-year mortality rate.

    Purpose: To compare the mortality rates of patients in high- and low-risk subgroups who were treated with β-blockers with rates among those not receiving these agents.

    Population: 201,752 patients from the Cooperative Cardiovascular Project data base (most discharges occurred between February 1994 and July 1995) with a principal diagnosis of acute MI. Approximately two thirds of patients had relative contraindications to β-blocker administration [per ACC/American Heart Association (AHA) guidelines]. Only 8,464 patients were not followed for 24 months.

    Treatment: 34.3% of patients received β-blockers (based on discharge prescription data).

    Results: Patients with the following characteristics received β-blockers less frequently: very elderly, blacks, low ejection fraction, heart failure, COPD, elevated creatinine, or type 1 diabetes mellitus. However, mortality was lower in all of these subgroups of patients who were treated with β-blockers. Overall, 2-year mortality was 40% lower among patients without complications. Mortality also was 40% lower with β-blockers in patients with a non–Q-wave MI or COPD, whereas slightly smaller reductions (28%–35%) were seen in those with an ejection fraction <20%, blacks, age >80 years, creatinine > 1.4 mg/dL, and diabetes. However, absolute mortality reduction in these latter groups was similar to or greater than that among patients with no risk factors.

    Comments: Inadequate information was provided about the severity of conditions. All patients with a specific risk factor were grouped together (e.g. mild, moderate, and severe heart failure). The accompanying editorial stresses the need for randomized trials before ACC/AHA guidelines on contraindications to β-blockade after MI are revised.

56. **Hjalmarson A**, et al. Effect on mortality of metoprolol in acute MI. *Lancet* 1981;2:823–827.

    A total of 1,395 patients with chest pain lasting ≥30 minutes and ECG changes were randomized at an average of 11 hours from onset of symptoms to 15 mg intravenously then 100 mg twice daily or placebo. MI was confirmed in 69.6% of patients. The metoprolol group had a 36% lower 90-day mortality rate (5.7% vs. 8.9%; $p < 0.03$).

57. **Ryden L**, et al. A double-blind trial of metoprolol in acute MI. Effects on ventricular arrhythmias. *N Engl J Med* 1983;308:614–618.

    A total of 1,395 patients with suspected MI were given metoprolol 15 mg intravenously, 50 mg every 6 hours for 2 days, then 100 mg twice daily for 3 months. Antiarrhythmic drugs were given only for ventricular fibrillation and sustained ventricular tachycardia. Only 58% of patients had a definite MI. The metoprolol group had less ventricular fibrillation (0.9% vs. 2.4%; $p < 0.05$) and less lidocaine use ($p < 0.01$).

58. **Soumerai SB**, et al. Adverse outcomes of underuse of β-blockers in elderly survivors of acute MI. *JAMA* 1997;227:115–121 (editorial pp. 155–156).

This large retrospective cohort study was composed of 5,332 patients; 1987–1992 Medicare and drug claims data were utilized. Only 21% received treatment (no change in frequency from 1987 to 1991). A threefold greater likelihood of being started on a calcium-channel blockers was observed. Underuse of β-blockers was predicted by use of calcium-channel blockers and increasing age. Overall, β-blocker use was associated with an adjusted 43% better survival, an effect seen in all age groups.

59. **Vantrimpoint P**, et al. Additive beneficial effects of beta-blockers to angiotensin converting enzyme inhibitors in the SAVE study. *J Am Coll Cardiol* 1997;29:229–236.

This retrospective analysis of SAVE data showed that β-blocker use was associated with a 30% lower rate of adjusted risk of cardiovascular mortality ($p = 0.002$), 21% less severe CHF ($p = 0.02$), and a nonsignificant 11% lower rate of recurrent MI. Importantly, these lower rates were independent of captopril use.

60. **Basu S**, et al. Beneficial effects of intravenous and oral carvedilol treatment in acute MI. *Circulation* 1997;96:183–191.

This small study showed the benefits of carvedilol, an agent with both and β- and α-adrenergic features. A total of 151 consecutive patients were randomized to carvedilol (2.5 mg intravenously over 15 minutes, 6.25 mg orally 4 hours later, then 6.25 mg twice daily for 2 days and 12.5–25 mg twice daily for 6 months). ETT, ambulatory monitoring, and echocardiography were performed before discharge and at 3 and 6 months postdischarge. The carvedilol group had an impressive 45% reduction in cardiac events (death, MI, heart failure, unstable angina, revascularization, cerebrovascular accident, ventricular arrhythmia; 24% vs. 44%, $p < 0.02$). In particular, 45% less death and MI ($p = 0.12$) was observed. There were no significant differences in predischarge ejection fraction, although the carvedilol-treated patients did have a better predischarge stroke volume and attenuated remodeling in the subgroup with an ejection fraction of <45%.

Thrombolytic Therapy

Review Articles, Meta-Analyses, and Miscellaneous

61. **White HD**. Thrombolytic therapy for patients with MI presenting after six hours. *Lancet* 1992;340:221–222.

This analysis of trials with late thrombolytic administration showed a significant 12% reduction in 35-day mortality with treatment at 7–12 hours. A nonsignificant 6% reduction was seen with treatment at 13–24 hours.

62. Fibrinolytic Therapy Trialists (**FTT**) Collaborative Group. Indications for fibrinolytic therapy in suspected acute MI: collaborative overview of early mortality and major morbidity results from all randomised trials of >1000 patients. *Lancet* 1994;343:311–322.

This analysis focused on nine studies (GISSI-1, ISAM, AIMS, ISIS-2 and ISIS-3, ASSET, USIM, EMERAS, and LATE) with >1,000 patients (58,600 total). During days 0 and 1, the use of thrombolytics was associated with a higher mortality rate, especially in the elderly and those treated >12 hours after symptom onset. However, much greater benefit was seen on days 2–35. Thrombolytic-treated patients with ST-segment elevation or bundle branch block had a 3% lower mortality rate when treated from 0 to 6 hours versus 2% lower at 7–12 hours and only 1% lower (p = NS) at 13–18 hours.

63. **Boersma E**, et al. Early thrombolytic therapy in acute MI: reappraisal of the golden hour. *Lancet* 1996;348:771–775.

This analysis focused on 22 randomized trials enrolling ≥100 patients (total 50,246 patients). Substantial mortality benefit (6.5% absolute reduction) was seen when a thrombolytic was given within 1 hour of onset of symptoms (vs. 2.6% at 1–2 hours, 2.6% at 2–3 hours, and 2.9% at 3–6 hours). Comparing those treated within 2 hours with those treated after 2 hours, the proportional mortality reduction was –44% versus –20% (p = 0.001). These data fit a nonlinear regression equation (i.e., most benefit early). In contrast, a similar prior analysis by the FTT Collaborative Group (*see Lancet* 1994;343:311) had generated a linear model (1.6 additional lives per 1,000 treated patients for each hour of delay). However, their analysis included data from 4,250 patients who had unstable angina (USIM trial) and minimal or no ST elevation (ISIS-3).

64. **Krumholz HM**, et al. Thrombolytic therapy for eligible elderly patients with MI. *JAMA* 1997;277:1683–1688 (editorial pp. 1723–1724).

This retrospective, multicenter cohort study was composed of 753 of 3,093 MI patients ≥65 years of age with ST elevation ≥1 mm, new left bundle branch block, and no thrombolytic contraindications. Only 44% were administered a thrombolytic agent. Predictors of no thrombolysis were advanced age, no chest pain, presenting >6 hours after onset of symptoms, left bundle branch block, ST elevation <6 mm, presence of Q waves, ST elevation in only two leads, and altered mental status. Reasons for no thrombolysis were cited in the chart in only 19% of cases (top two reasons were delay and age). Of note, a 75% thrombolysis rate was observed if the patient had chest pain and presented within 6 hours. The accompanying editorial points out that this issue is being addressed because thrombolysis rates have recently risen proportionally faster in the elderly.

65. **White HD,** Van de Werf FJJ. Thrombolysis for acute MI. *Circulation* 1998;97:1632–1646.

This excellent review article discusses the importance of early treatment and achieving infarct artery patency, eligibility criteria and contraindications, specific patient subgroups (e.g., anterior and inferior location, cardiogenic shock, ST-segment depression), prehospital and late treatment, cost-effectiveness issues, newer agents (reteplase, lanoteplase, TNK-tPA, saruplase, staphylokinase), and future treatment strategies.

65a. **Zeymer U**, et al. for the **ALKK** Study Group. Influence of time to treatment on early infarct-related artery patency after different thrombolytic regimens. *Am Heart J* 1999;137:34–38 (editorial pp. 1–3).

This retrospective analysis focused on six angiographic trials of patients receiving six different thrombolytic regimens. Comparing patency rates of patients treated within 3 hours with those treated after 3 hours to 6 hours, there was no difference in TIMI grade 3 flow rates after front-loaded alteplase (72.5% vs. 76.3%) and reteplase (63.6% vs. 63.2%). In contrast, TIMI grade 3 patency decreased with later treatment in those receiving streptokinase [36.8% (≤3 hours) vs. 27.6%; $p = 0.09$], APSAC (59.5% vs. 34.8%; $p = 0.004$), and urokinase (62.3% vs. 41.7%; $p = 0.03$). The accompanying editorial points out that other studies also have shown that the efficacy of non–fibrin-specific thrombolytic agents decreases with increasing time to treatment.

Thrombolytic Comparative Studies

66. **TIMI-1**. The Thrombolysis in MI (TIMI) Trial. Phase I findings. *N Engl J Med* 1985;312:932–936.
   Design: Prospective, randomized, double-blind, placebo-controlled, multicenter study. Primary end point was infarct-related artery patency at 90 minutes.
   Purpose: To evaluate the efficacy of intravenously administered thrombolytic therapy and to compare the effects of tPA and streptokinase.
   Population: 316 patients <76 years of age presenting ≤7 hours from onset of symptoms with chest pain lasting ≥30 minutes and ST-segment elevation in at least two ECG leads.
   Exclusion Criteria: Uncontrolled hypertension, cardiogenic shock, recent cerebrovascular events, active hemorrhage or hemorrhagic diathesis, prior streptokinase treatment, prior coronary bypass surgery, and prolonged CPR.
   Treatment: Streptokinase 1.5 million U over 60 minutes and a 3-hour infusion of tPA placebo, or a 3 hour infusion of plasminogen activator [80 mg (40 mg in first hour, then 20 mg for 2 hours)] and a 1-hour infusion of streptokinase placebo.
   Results: 290 patients received treatment; 26 had a <50% reduction in the diameter of the IRA not treated. Among the 214 patients with total baseline occlusion, tPA achieved better reperfusion at 90 minutes: 60% versus 35% (TIMI grade 2 or 3 flow; $p < 0.001$). No significant differences in rates of bleeding events were observed.

67. Gruppo Italiano per lo Studio della Streptochinasi nell'Infarto Miocardico (**GISSI-2**). GISSI-2: a factorial randomised trial of alteplase vs. streptokinase and heparin vs. no heparin among 12,490 patients with acute MI. *Lancet* 1990;336:65–71.
   Design: Prospective, randomized, open, parallel-group, 2 × 2 factorial, multicenter study. Primary end point was death, clinical heart failure, and ejection fraction ≤35%.
   Purpose: To compare the efficacy of intravenous streptokinase and tPA for the treatment of suspected acute ST-elevation MI and to study the effects of heparin on the incidence of recurrent ischemia.
   Population: 12,490 patients presenting within 6 hours of onset of symptoms with chest pain and ≥1 mm ST elevation in any limb lead or ≥2 mm in any precordial lead.
   Exclusion Criteria: Recent treatment with streptokinase (≤6 months), SBP ≥200 mm Hg or DBP ≥110 mm Hg, cerebrovascular accident within prior 6 months, and recent or current bleeding.
   Treatment: (a) streptokinase 1.5 million U over 30–60 minutes and heparin 12,500 U subcutaneously twice daily (starting 12 hours after initiation of the thrombolytic and continued through hospital discharge); (b) tPA 10-mg bolus, then 50 mg

over 1 hour, then 40 mg over 2 hours and heparin 12,500 U subcutaneously twice daily; (c) streptokinase 1.5 million U over 30–60 minutes without heparin; or (d) tPA 10 mg bolus, then 50 mg over 1 hour, then 40 mg over 2 hours without heparin.
Results: No significant difference was observed in combined end points between streptokinase and tPA [22.5% vs. 23.1% (mortality 8.6% vs. 9.0%)]. No difference was observed in the rates of recurrent infarction, postinfarction angina, stroke, or bleeding. And no differences were observed between heparin and no heparin, except for increased bleeding with heparin (1.0% vs. 0.6%, relative risk 1.64, 95% CI 1.09–2.45).
Comments: The International Study Group recruited an additional 8,401 patients (*see Lancet* 1990;336:71). Among these 20,891 patients, there was no difference in in-hospital mortality rates (tPA 8.9%, streptokinase 8.5%), but tPA was associated with a significantly higher stroke rate (1.33% vs. 0.94%).

68. **ISIS-3** Collaborative Group. A randomised comparison of streptokinase versus tissue plasminogen activator versus anistreplase and of aspirin and heparin versus aspirin alone among 41,299 cases of suspected acute MI. *Lancet* 1992;339:753–770.
Design: Prospective, randomized, double-blind (thrombolytic agents) and open-label (heparin), 3 × 2 factorial, multicenter study. Primary end point was 35-day mortality rate.
Purpose: To compare the effects on mortality of tPA, streptokinase, and APSAC and to compare aspirin alone with aspirin plus subcutaneously administered heparin.
Population: 41,299 patients with suspected MI presenting within 24 hours of onset of symptoms (no ECG criteria).
Exclusion Criteria (suggested): Recent severe trauma, stroke, gastrointestinal bleeding or ulcer, and streptokinase allergy.
Treatment: (a) Streptokinase 1.5 million U over 60 minutes; (b) rt-PA 0.6 million U/kg over 4 hours (0.04 million U/kg as a bolus, 0.36 million U/kg over 1 hour, then 0.067 million U/kg/h for 3 hours); or (c) APSAC 30 U over 3 minutes. All patients received aspirin (162.5 mg daily), and half of the patients also received heparin 12,500 U twice daily subcutaneously for 7 days (started 4 hours after initiation of thrombolytic therapy).
Results: No differences in 35-day mortality rate were seen between the three thrombolytic groups: streptokinase, 10.6%; tPA, 10.3%; APSAC, 10.5%. The streptokinase group did have fewer strokes (1.04% vs. 1.39% for tPA; *p* < 0.01), whereas tPA was associated with fewer reinfarctions [2.9% vs. 3.5% (streptokinase)]. There was a trend toward a lower mortality difference with heparin while it was being administered [7-day mortality rate 7.4% vs. 7.9% (aspirin alone); *p* = 0.06], but this disappeared at 35-day and 6-month follow-ups. Heparin was associated with an excess of major noncerebral and cerebral hemorrhages (1.0% vs. 0.8%, *p* < 0.01; 0.56% vs. 0.40%, *p* < 0.05), but there was no difference in the total stroke rate (1.28% vs. 1.18%).
Comments: No difference in mortality seen with tPA and streptokinase, but questions remained because of the suboptimal heparin regimen (i.e., delayed and subcutaneous).

69. **GUSTO I**: The Global Utilization of Streptokinase and tPA for Occluded Coronary Arteries Study (GUSTO) Investigators. An international randomized trial comparing four thrombolytic

strategies for acute MI. *N Engl J Med* 1993;329:673–682 (editorial pp. 723–724).

Design: Prospective, randomized, open label, multicenter study. Primary end point was 30-day all-cause mortality rate.

Purpose: To compare the effects of four thrombolytic regimens utilizing streptokinase and/or tPA.

Population: 41,021 patients presenting <6 hours from onset of symptoms with chest pain lasting >20 minutes and ST elevation ≥1 mm in at least two limb leads or ≥2 mm in at least two precordial leads.

Exclusion Criteria: Prior stroke, active bleeding, prior treatment with streptokinase or anistreptlase, and recent trauma or major surgery; relative contraindication was SBP ≥180 unresponsive to therapy.

Treatment: (#1) streptokinase 1.5 million U over 60 minutes with subcutaneous heparin 12,500 U twice daily; (#2) streptokinase 1.5 million U over 60 minutes and intravenous heparin (5,000-U bolus then 1,000 U/h); (#3) accelerated tPA [15-mg bolus, then 0.75 mg/kg (maximum 50 mg) over 30 minutes, then 0.5 mg/kg (maximum 35 mg) over 60 minutes] with intravenous heparin (5, 000-U bolus then 1,000 U/h); or (#4) tPA 1.0 mg/kg over 60 minutes (10% given as a bolus; maximum dose 90 mg) and streptokinase 1 million U over 60 minutes with intravenous heparin (5,000-U bolus then 1,000 U/h).

Results: Accelerated tPA with intravenous heparin (regimen #3) was associated with the lowest 30-day mortality rate: 6.3% (vs. 7.2%, 7.4%, and 7. 0% for regimens #1, #2, and #4), which corresponds to a 14% reduction compared with the streptokinase-only regimens ($p = 0.001$). Despite an increased intracranial hemorrhage risk seen with tPA (0.72% vs. 0.49%, 0.54%, and 94%), tPA still was associated with a significant reduction in the combined end point of death or disabling stroke (6.9% vs. 7.8% in streptokinase-only groups; $p = 0.006$). tPA appeared to confer more of a benefit in patients with anterior MI (8.6% vs. 10.5% mortality). A mortality benefit similar to that of tPA overall was seen in patients >75 years of age (1.3% vs. 1.1%), although limited numbers prevented the subgroup analysis from having the power to achieve statistical significance.

Comments: The mortality rate was only 4.3% in patients treated within 2 hours versus 5.5% at 2–4 hours and 8.9% at 4–6 hours. Thus, time to therapy is also an important factor. A secondary analysis showed age to be a powerful mortality predictor: 3% if <65 years old versus 9.5%, 19.6%, and 30.3% if 65–74, 75–85, and >85 years of age, respectively (*see Circulation* 1996;94:1826). One-year follow-up showed a persistent benefit of tPA with an increase in mortality of only 1.4% from 30 days to 1 year (*see Circulation* 1996;94:1233). Another secondary analysis showed the optimal PTT range to be 50–70 seconds (lowest 30-day mortality, stroke and bleeding rates) with a clustering of reinfarctions in the first 10 hours after discontinuation of heparin (*see Circulation* 1996; 93:870). Finally, a cost-effectiveness analysis (*see N Engl J Med* 1995;332:1418) showed that tPA costs $32,678 per year of life saved.

70. The GUSTO Angiographic Investigators. The effects of tissue plasminogen activator, streptokinase, or both on coronary artery

patency, ventricular function and survival after acute MI. *N Engl J Med* 1993;329:1615–1622 (editorial pp. 1650–1652).
Design: prospective, randomized, open label, multicenter study. Primary end point was TIMI grade flow at 90 minutes.
Purpose: To compare the patency rates and the effect on left ventricular function of tPA and streptokinase.
Population: 2,431 patients presenting <6 hours from onset of symptoms with chest pain lasting >20 minutes and ST elevation ≥1 mm in at least two limb leads or ≥2 mm in at least two precordial leads.
Exclusion Criteria: See GUSTO I trial summary.
Treatment: Four thrombolytic regimens (see GUSTO I trial summary). Patients were then randomized to cardiac catheterization at 90 minutes, 180 minutes, 24 hours, or 5–7 days. The 90 minute group underwent repeat catheterization at 5–7 days.
Results: Highest patency (TIMI grade 2 or 3 flow) at 90 minutes was seen with tPA and intravenous heparin: 81% versus 54% with streptokinase and subcutaneous heparin, 60% with streptokinase and intravenous heparin, and 73% with combination therapy ($p < 0.001$ for tPA vs. streptokinase groups). Normal flow (TIMI grade 3) was seen in 54% of the tPA patients versus 29%, 32%, and 38% in the other three groups. Surprisingly, the differences between the tPA and streptokinase groups disappeared at 180 minutes. The reocclusion rate was low and similar in all four groups (4.9%–6.4%). Left ventricular function paralleled patency at 90 minutes, with the tPA group having better regional wall motion. Mortality was also strongly correlated with 90-minute patency: a low 4.4% with TIMI grade 3 flow versus 8.9% with grade 1 flow ($p = 0.009$).
Comments: Results support the open artery theory asserting that early reperfusion of the IRA results in improved outcome (see accompanying editorial). A subsequent analysis of the 559 patients who underwent catheterization twice (at 90 minutes and 5–7 days) showed that early patency results were not predictive of reocclusion (*see J Am Coll Cardiol* 1994;24:1439). Another analysis showed that the mortality benefit of achieving 90-minute TIMI grade 3 flow was amplified beyond the initial 30 days: unadjusted mortality hazard ratio (TIMI grade 3 vs. ≤2) from 30 days to 688 days was only 0.39 (vs. 0.57 at 30 days) (*see Circulation* 1998;97:1549).

71. **Cannon CP**, et al. **TIMI-4**. Comparison of front-loaded recombinant tissue plasminogen activator, anistreplase and combination thrombolytic therapy for acute MI. *J Am Coll Cardiol* 1994; 24:1602–1610.
Design: Prospective, randomized, double-blind, multicenter study. Primary end points comprised an in-hospital composite consisting of death, severe CHF or cardiogenic shock, low ejection fraction, reinfarction, TIMI grade flow <2 at 90 minutes or 18 to 36 hours, reocclusion (on sestamibi imaging), major spontaneous hemorrhage, and severe anaphylaxis.
Purpose: To compare the efficacy and side effects of anistreplase, front-loaded rt-PA, and the combination of these agents.
Population: 382 patients <80 years of age presenting within 6 hours of onset of symptoms with ischemic pain lasting ≥30 minutes and ≥1 mm of ST elevation in at least two contiguous leads or new left bundle branch block.

Exclusion Criteria: Prior left bundle branch block, oral anticoagulation, recent (<2 weeks) tPA administration, or prior anistreptlase or streptokinase administration.

Treatment: Front-loaded rt-PA [15-mg bolus, then 0.75 mg/kg (maximum 50 mg) over 30 minutes, then 0.50 mg/kg (maximum 35 mg) over 30 minutes]; or anistreptlase 30-U bolus over 2–5 minutes; or rt-PA [15-mg bolus then 0.75 mg/kg (maximum 50 mg) over 30 minutes] and anistreptlase 20-U bolus. All patients received intravenous heparin and aspirin.

Results: rt-PA group had higher patency (TIMI grade 2 or 3 flow) at 60 minutes: 78% vs. 59% for two other groups ($p = 0.02$). Similar results were observed at 90 minutes [TIMI grade 3 flow in 60%, 43% (anistreptlase only), and 44% (combination)]. No significant differences were seen in the composite primary end points: rt-PA, 41.3%; anistreptlase, 49%; combination, 53.6%. However, the 6-week mortality rate was lowest in the rt-PA group: 2.2% vs. 8.8% with anistreptlase ($p = 0.02$) and 7.2% with combination therapy ($p = 0.06$). The rt-PA group had less major hemorrhage: 10.9% vs. 21.8% and 21.6%.

Comments: This was an angiography trial, so the availability and use of revascularization procedures may have affected the clinical results. This double-blind trial showed similar benefits of tPA as open-label GUSTO I.

72. **Smalling RW**, et al. **RAPID**. More rapid, complete and stable coronary thrombolysis with bolus administration of reteplase compared with alteplase infusion in acute MI. *Circulation* 1995;91:2725–2732.

Design: Prospective, randomized, open-label, parallel-group, multicenter study. Primary end point was TIMI grade 2 or 3 flow at 90 minutes.

Purpose: To compare bolus administration of reteplase with a standard infusion of alteplase.

Population: 606 patients 18–75 years of age presenting within 6 hours of onset of symptoms with chest pain lasting ≥30 minutes and ST elevation ≥1 mm in inferior or lateral leads or ≥2 mm in precordial leads.

Exclusion Criteria: Left bundle branch block, prior coronary artery bypass surgery, prior Q-wave MI in same anatomic region, recent (≤2 weeks) coronary angioplasty, prior cerebrovascular accident, and SBP >180 mm Hg or DBP >110 mm Hg.

Treatment: (a) Reteplase 15 million U single bolus; (b) reteplase 10 million U bolus then 5 million U bolus 30 minutes later; (c) reteplase 10 million U bolus then 10 million U bolus 30 minutes later; or (d) alteplase, given as a 6-to 10-mg bolus followed by an infusion over the first hour to a total dose of 60 mg, then 20 mg/h for 2 hours.

Results: Reteplase group receiving two 10 million U boluses had better TIMI grade 3 flow than the alteplase group at 90 minutes (63% vs. 49%) and at 5–14 days (88% vs. 71%). This group also had a better ejection fraction prior to hospital discharge (53% vs% 49%; $p = 0.034$). The incidence of bleeding complications was similar in all four treatment groups.

Comments: The results of this study demonstrate the efficacy of bolus reteplase administration, but the lack of a front-loaded alteplase regimen (used in RAPID II) was a major limitation of this trial.

73. International Joint Efficacy Comparison of Thrombolytics (**INJECT**). Randomized, double-blind comparison of reteplase double-bolus administration with streptokinase in acute MI: trial to investigate equivalence. *Lancet* 1995;346:329–336.

Design: Prospective, randomized, double-blind, double-dummy, multicenter study. Primary end point was 35-day mortality rate.

Purpose: To determine whether the effect of reteplase on 35-day mortality is at least equivalent to that of streptokinase.

Population: 6,010 patients presenting within 12 hours of onset of symptoms with chest pain lasting ≥30 minutes and ST elevation ≥1 mm in at least two of three inferior leads or leads I and aVL, ≥2 mm in at least two contiguous precordial leads, or new left bundle branch block.

Exclusion Criteria: Any prior cerebrovascular event, increased bleeding risk (e.g., recent major surgery, prolonged CPR, oral anticoagulants, SBP >200 mm Hg), and streptokinase or anistreptlase in prior 12 months.

Treatment: Streptokinase 1.5 million U over 60 minutes or reteplase 10 million U bolus and repeated 30 minutes later. All patients received heparin for 24 hours.

Results: 35-day mortality rates were similar: 9.0% (reteplase) and 9.5% (streptokinase). Results show that reteplase is at least as effective as streptokinase. Reinfarction and bleeding rates also were similar (5.0% vs. 5.4%; 0.7% vs. 1.0%), whereas the reteplase group had less atrial fibrillation (7.2% vs. 8.8%; $p < 0.05$), cardiogenic shock (4.7% vs. 6.0%; $p < 0.05$), heart failure (23.6% vs. 26.3%; $p < 0.05$), and hypotension (15.5% vs. 17.6%; $p < 0.05$).

Comments: No angiographic substudy has been conducted to confirm the high TIMI grade 3 patency achieved in the phase II study. The accompanying editorial suggests a probable lower TIMI grade 3 flow rate, especially because delay to treatment was longer in INJECT than in GUSTO.

74. **Bode C**, et al. for the **RAPID II** Investigators. Randomized comparison of coronary thrombolysis achieved with double-bolus reteplase (recombinant plasminogen activator) and front-loaded, accelerated alteplase (recombinant tissue plasminogen activator) in patients with acute MI. *Circulation* 1996;94:891–898.

Design: Prospective, randomized, open-label, parallel-group, multicenter study.

Purpose: To compare the bolus-administered thrombolytic reteplase with an accelerated infusion of alteplase on infarct-related patency and major events.

Population: 324 patients 18–75 years of age presenting within 12 hours (from onset of symptoms to planned administration of treatment) with chest pain lasting ≥30 minutes and ST elevation ≥1 mm in at least two of three inferior leads or lateral leads or ≥2 mm in at least two contiguous leads, or left bundle branch block.

Exclusion Criteria: Prior coronary artery bypass surgery, recent (<2 weeks) PTCA, prior MI in same anatomic region, prior stroke or known intracranial structural abnormalities, severe hypertension (>180/110 mm Hg) not rapidly responding to treatment, oral anticoagulation, and other increased bleeding risks.

Treatment: Reteplase 10 million U over 2–3 minutes then 10 million U repeated 30 minutes later, or front-loaded alteplase. All patients got aspirin and intravenous heparin.

Results: Reteplase group had better TIMI grade 3 flow at 90 minutes (60% vs. 45%; $p = 0.01$) and 51% fewer coronary interventions (13.6% vs. 26.5%; $p < 0.01$); a >50% statistically nonsignificant mortality reduction (4.1 vs. 8.4%) also was observed, as were similar rates of transfusion, hemorrhage, and stroke.

75. **GUSTO III** Investigators. A comparison of reteplase with alteplase for acute MI. *N Engl J Med* 1997;337:1118–1123 (editorial pp. 1159–1161).
Design: Prospective, randomized (2:1), open-label, parallel-group, multicenter study. Primary end point was 30-day mortality rate.
Purpose: To determine if reteplase is superior to alteplase in reducing mortality in acute MI.
Population: 15,059 patients presenting with ≥30 minutes of continuous symptoms and within 6 hours of their onset and ≥1 mm ST elevation in at least two limb leads or ≥2 mm in precordial leads or bundle branch block.
Exclusion Criteria: Active bleeding, history of stroke, recent major surgery, SBP ≥200 mm Hg or DBP ≥110 mm Hg, and requirement for oral anticoagulation.
Treatment: Reteplase given as two 10 million U boluses 30 minutes apart or an accelerated infusion of alteplase [15-mg bolus, then 0.75 mg/kg (maximum 50 mg) over 30 minutes, then 0.50 mg/kg (maximum 35 mg) over 60 minutes].
Results: Reteplase and alteplase groups had similar 30-day mortality rates: 7.47% vs. 7.24% ($p = 0.54$; 95% CI for absolute difference in mortality rates was −1.1% to 0.66%). Stroke rate and combined end points of death or nonfatal, disabling stroke were both similar (1.64% vs. 1.79%; 7.89% vs. 7.91%).
Comments: Although this trial was designed as a superiority trial, the accompanying editorial points out that these results do not demonstrate equivalence according to the extremely strict COBALT trial criterion. Nonetheless, clinical equivalence of reteplase was observed in this large trial.

76. **InTIME-II.** Preliminary results presented at the 48th ACC Scientific Session in New Orleans, LA, March 1999.
This prospective, randomized, multicenter, double-blind, double-dummy trial was composed of 15,078 patients who presented within 6 hours of pain and were randomized in 2:1 fashion to lanoteplase 120 IU/kg (single intravenous bolus) or tPA. The 30-day mortality rate between the two groups was statistically similar (and also met the FDA requirement for equivalence): 6.6% in the tPA group and 6.77% in the lanoteplase group. The incidence of intracranial hemorrhage was significantly higher in the nPA group (1.13% vs. 0.62; $p = 0.003$), whereas there was a trend toward a lower incidence of several secondary end points, including death plus MI, recurrent MI, urgent revascularization, and severe heart failure.

77. Assessment of the Safety and Efficacy of a New Thrombolytic: TNK-tPA (**ASSENT-2**). Single-bolus tenecteplase compared with front-loaded alteplase in acute MI: the ASSENT-2 double-blind randomized trial. *Lancet* 1999;354:716–722 (editorial pp. 695–697).
Design: Prospective, randomized, open-label, multicenter study. Primary end point was all-cause mortality at 30 days.
Purpose: To assess the efficacy and safety of tenecteplase (TNK-tPA) compared with alteplase (tPA).
Population: 16,949 patients presenting within 6 hours of symptom onset with ST segment elevations of ≥1 mm in ≥2 limb leads

or $\geq$2 mm in $\geq$2 contiguous precordial leads; or new left bundle branch block.

Treatment: TNK-tPA administered over 5 to 10 seconds (30 mg if <60 kg, 35 mg if 60–60.9 kg, 40 mg if 70–79.9 mg, 45 mg if 80–89.9 kg, 50 mg if $\geq$90 kg) or accelerated infusion of tPA over 90 minutes ($\leq$100 mg).

Results: All-cause mortality rate at 30 days was nearly identical in the two groups: 6.18% (TNK-tPA) and 6.15% (tPA). Intracranial hemorrhage rates were also similar (0.43% [TNK-tPA], 0.44% [tPA], but fewer non-cerebral bleeding complications (26.4% vs 29.0%, p = 0.0003) and less need for blood transfusion (4.3% vs 5.5%, p = 0.0002) were observed with TNK-tPA. Subgroup analysis showed that the mortality rate among patients treated over 4 hours after the onset of symptoms was significantly lower with TNK-tPA (7.1% vs 9.2%, p = 0.018). This finding may be due to the increased fibrin specificity of TNK-tPA.

78. **Anderson JL**, et al. Second Thrombolytic Trial of Eminase in Acute MI (**TEAM-2**). Multicenter patency trial of intravenous anistreplase compared with streptokinase in acute MI. *Circulation* 1991;83:126–140.

This randomized, double-blind trial was composed of 370 patients $\leq$75 years of age presenting within 4 hours of suspected MI. They were treated with anistreplase 30 U over 2–5 minutes or streptokinase 1.5 million U over 60 minutes. Angiography was performed at 90–240 minutes and again at 18–48 hours. Similar early patency [72% vs. 73% (TIMI grade 2 or 3 flow)] and mortality rates (5.9% vs. 7.1%) were observed. However, the anistreplase group did have a higher TIMI grade 3 flow rate (83% vs. 72%; p = 0.03) and less residual stenosis (mean diameter 74% vs. 77%; p = 0.02).

79. **Neuhaus K-L**, et al. rt-PA-APSAC Patency Study (**TAPS**). Improved thrombolysis in acute MI with front-loaded administration of alteplase. Results of the rt-PA-APSAC Patency Study. *J Am Coll Cardiol* 1992;19:885–891.

This randomized trial enrolled 421 patients to APSAC or frontloaded rt-PA (15-mg bolus, 50 mg over 30 minutes, 35 mg over 60 minutes). Higher 90-minute patency (TIMI grade 2 or 3 flow) was achieved with rt-PA (84% vs. 70%; p = 0.0007), as were fewer in-hospital deaths (2.4% vs. 8.1%; p < 0.01). Similar reinfarction rates [3.8% (rt-PA) vs. 4.8%] were observed despite the rt-PA group having more frequent early occlusion (10.3% vs. 2.5%).

80. **Anderson JL**, et al. **TEAM-3**. Anistreptlase vs. alteplase in acute MI: comparative effects on left ventricular function, morbidity and one-day coronary patency. *J Am Coll Cardiol* 1992;20:753–766.

This study randomized 325 patients presenting within 4 hours of symptom onset to anistreptlase 30 U over 2–5 minutes or rt-PA 100 mg over 3 hours. All patients were given aspirin (160 mg/day) and intravenous heparin. The rt-PA group had a higher ejection fraction prior to discharge (51.3% vs. 54.2%; p < 0.05) and at 1 month (54.8% vs. 50.2%; p < 0.01). Similar rates of coronary artery patency were assessed at 1 day (anistreplase 89%, alteplase 86%). No statistically significant difference in mortality was observed (6.2% vs. 7.9%), but the study was not powered to detect one.

81. **Zarich SW**, et al. Pro-urokinase and t-PA Enhancement of Thrombolysis (**PATENT**). Sequential combination thrombolytic

therapy for acute MI: results of PATENT trial. *J Am Coll Cardiol* 1995;26:374–379.

In this open label study, 1,011 patients were given a 5- to 10-mg bolus of rt-PA then a 90-minute infusion of prourokinase (40 mg/h). Reasoning behind combination was that rt-PA initiates fibrinolysis, overcoming relative resistance of intact fibrin to prourokinase [urokinase monotherapy achieved TIMI 3 flow in 52% in one study (*see J Am Coll Cardiol* 1995;24:1242)]. All patients received aspirin and intravenous heparin. TIMI grade 3 flow at 90 minutes was an impressive 60%, with only one in-hospital death.

82. **Vanderschueren S**, et al. A randomized trial of recombinant staphylokinase vs. alteplase for coronary artery patency in acute MI. *Circulation* 1995;92:2044–2049 (editorial pp. 2026–2028).

In this open trial, 100 patients presenting within 6 hours were randomized to accelerated or weight-adjusted rt-PA over 90 minutes or staphylokinase 10–20 mg over 30 minutes. In animal models, staphylokinase had been more potent at lysing platelet-rich thrombi. Similar TIMI grade 3 flow rates at 90 minutes were observed: staphylokinase, 62% (10 mg, 50%; 20 mg, 74%); rtPA, 58%. However, staphylokinase patients had increased residual fibrinogen at 90 minutes (118% vs. 68%). This fibrin specificity leads to a decreased systemic lytic state. As a result, the intravenous heparin bolus was increased to 10,000 U early in the study.

83. **O'Connor CM**, et al. for the Duke University Clinical Cardiology Group Study (**DUCCS**) II Investigators. A randomized factorial trial of reperfusion strategies and aspirin dosing in acute MI. *Am J Cardiol* 1996;77:791–797.

The trial was terminated early after GUSTO I reported that 162 patients had been randomized to front-loaded tPA and intravenous heparin or anistreptlase without heparin. The tPA group had 19% fewer end points [recurrent ischemia or heart failure, reinfarction, cardiogenic shock, stroke, and death (25.4% vs. 31.3%; $p = 0.32$)]. Patency rates were similar (on predischarge angiography), whereas the tPA group had fewer in-hospital interventions (5.3% vs. 11.5%). In an ECG substudy, the tPA group had greater frequency of >50% ST-segment resolution.

84. **Tebbe U**, et al. for the Comparative Trial of Saruplase versus Streptokinase (**COMPASS**) Investigators. Randomized, double-blind study comparing saruplase with streptokinase therapy in acute MI: the COMPASS equivalence trial. *J Am Coll Cardiol* 1998;31:487–493.

This equivalence trial demonstrated the safety and efficacy of the new agent saruplase. A total of 3,089 patients presenting within 6 hours of onset of symptoms were randomized to streptokinase (1.5 million U over 60 minutes) or saruplase (20-mg bolus then 60 mg over 60 minutes). All patients received heparin infusions for 24 hours starting 30 minutes after the end of thrombolytic therapy, whereas only the saruplase patients received a 5,000-U bolus (prior to start of saruplase). Mortality rates at 30 days were 5.7% for the saruplase group and 6.7% for the streptokinase group (odds ratio 0.84; $p < 0.01$ for equivalence). Overall stroke rates and reinfarction rates were similar, whereas the saruplase patients had less hypotension and cardiogenic shock.

85. **Den Heijer P**, et al. Intravenous nPA for Treatment of Infarcting Myocardium Early (**InTIME I**) Investigators. Evaluation of a

weight-adjusted single-bolus plasminogen activator in patients with MI. A double-blind, randomized angiographic trial of lanoteplase vs. alteplase. *Circulation* 1998;98:2117–2125.

This prospective, multicenter, double-placebo study of 602 patients presenting ≤6 hours after onset of symptoms were randomized to a single bolus of lanoteplase 15,000, 30,000, 60,000 or 120,000 U/kg bolus or accelerated alteplase. Lanoteplase demonstrated a dose response in TIMI grade 3 flow at 60 and 90 minutes (23.6% to 47.1% and 26.1% vs. 57.1%). Patency rate at 90 minutes was significantly better with lanoteplase 120,000 U/kg versus alteplase (83% vs. 71.4%). However, alteplase only achieved a 90-minute TIMI grade 3 flow rate of 37.4% (vs. 54% in GUSTO I).

86. **Cannon CP**, et al. for the **TIMI-10B** Investigators. TNK-tissue plasminogen activator compared with front-loaded alteplase in acute MI. *Circulation* 1998;98:2805–2814.

This prospective, randomized, multicenter trial was composed of 886 acute ST-elevation MI patients presenting within 12 hours of onset of symptoms. Patients received TNK-tPA 30 mg or 50 mg or front-loaded tPA. All patients underwent immediate angiography. The 50-mg dose of TNK-tPA was discontinued early due to an increased rate of intracranial hemorrhage and was replaced by a 40-mg dose, and heparin doses were decreased. TNK-tPA 40 mg and tPA produced similar rates of TIMI grade 3 flow at 90 minutes (62.8% vs. 62.7%, p = NS; TNK-tPA 30 mg, 54.3%, p = 0.035). TNK-tPA doses of 0.5 mg/kg resulted in higher TIMI grade 3 flow and lower median corrected TIMI frame counts (i.e., faster flow) than lower doses. Lower rates of major bleeding and intracranial hemorrhage were observed after the heparin doses were lowered and titration of heparin was begun at 6 hours.

Single Agent Studies

87. **GISSI-1**. Effectiveness of intravenous thrombolytic treatment in acute MI. *Lancet* 1986;327:397–401.

Design: Prospective, randomized, open, parallel-group, multicenter study. Primary end point was 21-day mortality rate.

Purpose: To evaluate the safety and efficacy of intravenous streptokinase in acute MI and to determine if any effect is dependent on the interval between onset of pain and treatment.

Population: 11,806 patients presenting within 12 hours of onset of symptoms with chest pain and ST elevation or depression ≥1 mm in any limb or ≥2 mm in any precordial lead.

Exclusion Criteria: Recent or current bleeding, recent (<2 months) stroke, surgery or trauma in prior 10 days, SBP ≥200 mm Hg, DBP ≥110 mm Hg, and prior treatment with streptokinase. Relative contraindications were severe renal or hepatic failure, pregnancy, and left ventricular thrombi.

Treatment: Streptokinase 1.5 million U over 60 minutes.

Results: Streptokinase-treated patients had a 21-day mortality rate that was 18% lower than controls (10.7% vs. 13.0%; p = 0.0002). The largest mortality advantage [23% (p = 0.0005)] was associated with administration to those presenting within 3 hours of onset of symptoms (relative risk 0.74 vs. 1.19 for 9–12 hours). At 1 year, the mortality benefit persisted (17.2% vs. 19.0%; p = 0.0008).

Comments: 10-year follow-up showed that the mortality benefit was still significant, with 19 lives saved/1,000 patients (p = 0.02) (*see Circulation* 1998;98:2659).

88. **ISIS-2** Collaborative Group. Randomised trial of intravenous streptokinase, oral, both, or neither among 17,187 cases of suspected acute MI. *Lancet* 1988;332:349–360.
    Design: Prospective, randomized, double-blind, placebo-controlled, multicenter study. Primary end point was vascular mortality.
    Purpose: To assess the separate and combined effects on mortality of intravenous streptokinase and oral aspirin in patients with suspected acute MI.
    Population: 17,187 patients with suspected MI presenting within 24 hours (median 5 hours) of onset of symptoms.
    Exclusion Criteria: Any history of stroke, gastrointestinal hemorrhage, or ulcer. Possible contraindications included recent trauma, severe persistent hypertension (not defined), allergy to streptokinase or aspirin, and low risk of cardiac death.
    Treatment: Streptokinase 1.5 million U over 60 minutes and/or aspirin 162.5 mg daily; or placebo.
    Results: Streptokinase and aspirin-alone groups had 25% and 23% lower 5-week vascular mortality rates, respectively [9.2% vs. 12.0% (placebo), $p < 0.00001$; 9.4% vs. 11.8%, $p < 0.00001$). The streptokinase and aspirin group had an even larger 42% mortality reduction (8% vs. 13.2%). Combination therapy was also effective in patients with left bundle branch block (mortality 14% vs. 27.7%). Streptokinase was associated with hypotension in 10% and more bleeds requiring transfusion (0.5% vs. 0.2%), but fewer strokes (0.6% vs. 0.8%). Aspirin reduced nonfatal reinfarction and stroke rates (1.0% vs. 2.0%; 0.3% vs. 0.6%).

89. Intravenous Streptokinase in Acute MI (**ISAM**) Study Group. A prospective trial of intravenous streptokinase in acute MI: mortality, morbidity and infarct size at 21 days. *N Engl J Med* 1986; 314:1465–1471.
    Design: Prospective, randomized, double-blind, placebo-controlled, multicenter study. Primary end point was 21-day mortality rate.
    Purpose: To assess the effects of intravenous streptokinase on 21-day mortality and to compare results in those treated within 3 hours with those treated at 3–6 hours.
    Population: 1,741 patients ≤75 years of age presenting within 6 hours of onset of symptoms.
    Exclusion Criteria: History of stroke, oral anticoagulation, hemorrhagic diathesis, streptokinase treatment in prior 9 months, SBP ≥200 mm Hg or DBP ≥120 mm Hg, and trauma or surgery in previous 10 days.
    Treatment: Streptokinase 1.5 million U over 60 minutes, or placebo. All patients received heparin for 72–96 hours and coumadin for 3 weeks.
    Results: Streptokinase group had nonsignificant reduction in 21-day mortality (6.3% vs. 7.1%), significantly higher LVEF (56.8% vs. 53.9%) and an earlier CK-MB peak (13.9 vs. 19.2 hours). Among those treated within 3 hours, the mortality rates were lower [5.2% (streptokinase) vs. 6.5%; $p = NS$].
    Comments: A subsequent publication (*see Eur Heart J* 1990; 11:885–896) reported that anterior MI patients treated with streptokinase had higher ejection fractions (50% vs. 42%; $p = 0.013$), especially those treated within 3 hours ($p = 0.004$). These

differences persisted through 3-year follow-up (*see J Am Coll Cardiol* 1991;18:1610).

90. **Wilcox RG**, et al. Anglo-Scandinavian Study of Early Thrombolysis (**ASSET**). Trial of tissue plasminogen activator for mortality reduction in acute MI. *Lancet* 1988;332:525–530.
    Design: Prospective, randomized, double-blind, placebo-controlled, multicenter study. Primary end point was mortality at 1 month.
    Purpose: To evaluate the effects of tPA on mortality after acute MI.
    Population: 5,013 patients 18–75 years of age with suspected acute MI who were treated within 5 hours of onset of symptoms.
    Exclusion Criteria:
    Treatment: tPA 10 mg bolus followed by 50 mg over 1 hour then 20 mg/h for 2 hours (100 mg total), or placebo.
    Results: tPA group had a 26% lower 1-month mortality rate: 7.2% vs. 9.8% (26% relative risk reduction [95% confidence interval, 11% to 39%]). This benefit persisted at 6 months: 10.4% vs. 13.1%. Among patients with proven MI, the mortality difference was more impressive: 12.6% vs. 17.1%. tPA group did have more bleeding and more frequent bradycardia (27 vs. 5 patients).

91. **Topol EJ**, et al. and the Thrombolysis and Angioplasty in MI (**TAMI-6**) Study Group. A randomized trial of late reperfusion therapy for acute MI. *Circulation* 1992;85:2090–2099.
    Design: Prospective, randomized, double-blind, placebo-controlled, multicenter study. Primary end point was infarct vessel patency at 6–24 hours.
    Purpose: To evaluate whether thrombolysis is effective when administered after 6 hours from onset of symptoms and whether PTCA is beneficial when performed in those with persistent occlusion of the IRA.
    Population: 197 patients ≤75 years of age presenting 6–24 hours after onset of symptoms with ≥1 mm ST elevation in at least contiguous leads.
    Exclusion Criteria: History of stroke, recent surgery or trauma, hemorrhagic diathesis, prior Q-wave MI in the distribution of IRA, and BP >180/110 mm Hg. PTCA exclusion criteria (second randomization) were left main stenosis >50%, severe diffuse disease, and small or unidentifiable IRA.
    Treatment: tPA over 2 hours [1 mg/kg over first 60 minutes (10% as bolus; maximum 80 mg) then 20 mg over 2nd hour], or placebo. Angiography was performed within 24 hours; 71 patients had persistent IRA occlusion and met eligibility criteria for randomization to PTCA or no PTCA.
    Results: Better early patency was achieved with tPA [65% vs. 27% (placebo)] but similar rates were observed for late (6-month) patency (both 59%), in-hospital mortality, and LVEF. At 6 months, the tPA group had no increase in left ventricular end-diastolic volume (vs. ~25% increase in the placebo group). PTCA patients had an 81% initial recanalization rate and improved ventricular function at 1 month, but there was also no advantage evident at late follow-up (of note, no PTCA group had a 38% spontaneous recanalization rate).

92. The European MI Project (**EMIP**) Group. Prehospital thrombolytic therapy in patients with suspected MI. *N Engl J Med* 1993;329:383–389.

Design: Prospective, randomized, double-blind, crossover, multicenter study. Primary end point was overall 30-day mortality rate.
Purpose: To evaluate the safety and efficacy of prehospital thrombolytic administration compared with in-hospital thrombolysis.
Population: 5,469 patients presenting within 6 hours of symptom onset with ≤1 mm ST elevation in at least two limb leads or ≥2 mm in at least two precordial leads.
Exclusion Criteria: Oral anticoagulation, hemorrhagic diathesis, recent (≤6 months) stroke, surgery or major trauma, SBP >200 mm Hg or DBP >120 mm Hg, and PTCA in prior 2 weeks.
Treatment: Anistreplase 30 U prior to hospitalization followed by placebo in hospital or placebo followed by anistreplase.
Results: Trial was terminated early due to failure to reach target of 10,000 patients in a 2-year period. Patients in the prehospital group received anistreplase 55 minutes earlier on average than those in hospital group. Prehospital anistreplase was associated with a nonsignificant 13% overall mortality reduction (9.7% vs. 11.1%; $p = 0.08$) and a significant 16% cardiac mortality reduction (8.3% vs. 9.8%; $p = 0.049$). More adverse events [ventricular fibrillation ($p = 0.02$), shock ($p < 0.001$), symptomatic hypotension ($p < 0.001$), bradycardia ($p = 0.001$)] occurred in the prehospital group prior to hospitalization, but this was offset by a higher incidence during the hospital period in the hospital group.

93. **Weaver WD**, et al. MI Triage and Intervention (**MITI**). Prehospital versus hospital-initiated thrombolytic therapy. *JAMA* 1993;270:1211–1216.
Design: Prospective, randomized, open, parallel-group study. Primary end point was a composite score that combined death, stroke, major bleeding, and infarct size.
Purpose: To compare prehospital and hospital initiation of thrombolytic therapy in patients with chest pain and ST-segment elevation.
Population: 360 patients ≤75 years of age presenting within 6 hours of onset of symptoms with ST elevation.
Exclusion Criteria: History of stroke, recent bleeding or surgery, SBP <180 mm Hg or DBP >120 mm Hg.
Treatment: Prehospital or hospital administration of alteplase (100 mg over 3 hours) plus aspirin (325 mg).
Results: Despite earlier time to treatment in the prehospital initiated group (77 vs. 110 minutes), no significant differences were seen in primary composite end point score (p = 0.64), mortality rate (5.7 % vs. 8.1%; $p = 0.49$), ejection fraction, or infarct size. A secondary analysis showed that when treatment was initiated at <70 minutes, prehospital therapy was associated with a lower mortality rate (1.2% vs. 8.7%) and better ejection fraction (53% vs. 49%; $p = 0.03$). However, at 2-year follow-up (*see Am J Cardiol* 1996;78:497), the mortality benefit in this subgroup was no longer statistically significant [2% (<70 minutes) vs. 12%; $p = 0.12$].
Comments: Lack of statistical benefit with prehospital treatment could have been due to the unanticipated reduction of 40 minutes in hospital treatment times and sample size.

94. Late Assessment of Thrombolytic Efficacy (**LATE**) Study Group. Late Assessment of Thrombolytic Efficacy study with alteplase 6–24 hours after onset of MI. *Lancet* 1993;342:759–766.

Design: Prospective, randomized, double-blind, placebo-controlled, multicenter study. Primary end point was 35-day mortality rate.

Purpose: To compare administration of alteplase with placebo in acute MI patients presenting at 6–24 hours.

Population: 5,711 patients presenting 6–24 hours after onset of symptoms with ≥1 mm ST elevation in at least two limb leads, ≥2 mm ST elevation in at least two precordial leads, ST depression ≥2 mm in at least two leads, pathologic Q waves, or abnormal T-wave inversion in at least two leads thought to represent a non–Q-wave infarct.

Exclusion Criteria: Cardiogenic shock, major surgery or trauma in the past month, SBP >200 mm Hg or DBP >110 mm Hg, recent (≤6 months) stroke, and transient ischemic attack.

Treatment: Alteplase 100 mg over 3 hours (10-mg intravenous bolus, 50 mg over 1 hour, 20 mg/h for 2 hours); or placebo.

Results: Intention-to-treat analysis showed a nonsignificant 14% 35-day mortality reduction in the alteplase group (8.9% vs. 10.3%). However, prespecified survival analysis according to treatment within 12 hours showed that the alteplase group had a 25.6% mortality reduction (8.9% vs. 11.9%; $p = 0.023$). Treatment for 12–24 hours was associated with a nonsignificant 5% mortality reduction (8.7% vs. 9.2%). Alteplase was not associated with a higher cardiac rupture rate, but rather earlier occurrence of rupture (within 24 hours, post thrombolysis).

95. **Rawles J**, et al. on behalf of the Grampian Region Early Anistreptlase Trial (**GREAT**) Group. Halving of mortality at one year by domociliary thrombolysis in the GREAT. *J Am Coll Cardiol* 1994;23:1–5.

Design: Prospective, randomized, double-blind, parallel-group, multicenter study.

Purpose: To evaluate the feasibility, safety, and efficacy of home-administered thrombolysis by general practitioners compared with hospital thrombolysis.

Population: 311 patients with suspected MI seen by their general practitioners within 4 hours of symptom onset (ECG recordings required but not reported).

Exclusion Criteria: Thrombolytic therapy in past 6 months, surgery or major trauma in prior 10 days, hemorrhagic diathesis or significant bleeding in past 6 months, current anticoagulation, recent cerebrovascular accident (≤2 months), and BP >200/120 mm Hg.

Treatment: Anistreptlase 30 U at home or in hospital.

Results: Home-administered anistreptlase was given over 2 hours sooner, at a median 101 versus 240 minutes. The home-treated group had a 52% lower 1-year mortality rate (10.4% vs. 21.6%; $p = 0.007$).

Comments: Subsequent analysis showed the highest mortality rate in those randomized earliest. However, among patients at 2 hours, a 2.1% higher 30-day mortality per hour delay to thrombolytic therapy and a 6.9% higher 30-month mortality per hour delay were observed (*see BMJ* 1996;312:212).

96. The Continuous Infusion versus Double-Bolus Administration of Alteplase (**COBALT**) Investigators. A comparison of continuous infusion of alteplase with double-bolus administration for acute MI. *N Engl J Med* 1997;337:1124–1130 (editorial pp. 1159–1161).

Design: Prospective, randomized, open, multicenter study. Primary end point was 30-day mortality rate.

Purpose: To compare an accelerated infusion of alteplase over 90 minutes with a two-bolus regimen in patients with acute MI.

Population: 7,169 patients presenting within 6 hours of symptom onset with ≥1 mm ST elevation in at least two limb leads and/or ≥2 mm in at least two contiguous precordial leads.

Exclusion Criteria: Active bleeding, history of stroke or CNS structural abnormalities, major surgery or trauma in previous 6 months, pregnancy, and SBP ≥180 mm Hg or DBP ≥110 mm Hg despite treatment.

Treatment: Front-loaded alteplase [15-mg bolus then 0.75 mg/kg over 30 minutes (maximum 50 mg) and 0.50 mg/kg over final 60 minutes (maximum 35 mg)] or bolus regimen [50 mg over 1–3 minutes followed by 50 mg 30 minutes later (or 40 mg if <60 kg)]. Adjunctive therapy included aspirin and intravenous heparin (goal aPTT 60–85 seconds).

Results: Double-bolus group had a 0.44% higher 30-day mortality rate (7.98% vs. 7.53%). The upper boundary of the 95% CI was +1.48%, which exceeded the prespecified upper limit of 0.40% to indicate equivalence. The double-bolus group also had statistically nonsignificant higher rates of stroke and hemorrhage stroke (1.92% vs. 1.53%, $p = 0.24$; 1.12% vs. 0.81%).

Comments: The accompanying editorial points out that the definition of equivalence used was very strict because a sample size of 50,000 patients is required to rule out with 80% power an excess mortality of 0.4% when the true mortality rates are identical and in the 7.5% range.

97. **Ross AM**, et al. Plasminogen Activator-Angioplasty Compatibility Trial (**PACT**). Presented at the 47th Scientific Sessions of the ACC, Atlanta, GA, March 1998.

In this trial, 606 patients with acute MI presenting within 6 hours of onset of symptoms were randomized to precatheterization thrombolysis (tPA 50-mg bolus) or placebo. If TIMI grade 3 flow was present, a second bolus of tPA 50 mg was given. If TIMI grade 0–2 flow was present, angioplasty was performed. Initial angiography showed that the tPA group had better TIMI grade 3 flow (32.8% vs. 14.8%). After angioplasty, TIMI flow grade was similar between the two groups, indicating that tPA administration did not adversely impact procedural outcomes. There were no significant differences in bleeding rates, suggesting that immediate angioplasty could be performed safely after reduced-dose tPA. There was also no significant difference between the groups in predischarge ejection fraction (primary end point).

98. **Kennedy JW**, et al. Western Washington randomized trial of intracoronary streptokinase in acute MI. *N Engl J Med* 1985; 312:1073–1078.

This early trial used intracoronary streptokinase (4,000 U/min started at average 4.5 hours; average dose 286,000 U). Streptokinase was beneficial in patients in which reperfusion occurred (1-year mortality rate 2.5% vs. 17%).

99. **White HD**, et al. Effect of intravenous streptokinase on left ventricular function and early survival after acute MI. *N Engl J Med* 1987;317:850–855.

This randomized, double-blind trial was composed of 219 patients with first MIs presenting within 4 hours of onset of symptoms and treated with 1.5 million U over 30 minutes or placebo. All patients were given intravenous heparin for 48 hours, aspirin, and dipyridamole. At 3 weeks, the streptokinase group had increased LVEF (primary end point): 59% vs. 53%; $p < 0.005$. The streptokinase group also had a significantly lower mortality rate (2.5% vs. 12.9%; $p = 0.012$).

100. **Meinertz T**, et al. The German Multicenter Trial of anisoylated plasminogen streptokinase activator complex versus heparin for acute MI. *Am J Cardiol* 1988;62:347–351.

A total of 313 patients presenting within 4 hours of onset of suspected MI were randomized to intravenous heparin or APSAC (30-U bolus). APSAC patients had less cardiogenic shock at 24 hours and a 56% lower 28-day mortality rate (5.6% vs. 12.6%; $p = 0.03$).

101. APSAC Intervention Mortality Study (**AIMS**). Long-term effects of intravenous anistreplase in acute MI: final report of AIMS study. *Lancet* 1990;335:427–431.

This randomized, double-blind trial was composed of 1,258 patients presenting within 6 hours of onset of suspected MI. The trial was terminated early (target size 2,000 patients) due to 47% lower 30-day mortality in patients receiving anistreplase. This benefit persisted at 1 year: 11% vs. 18% ($p = 0.0007$).

102. **Carney RJ**, et al. Randomized angiographic trial of recombinant tissue-type plasminogen activator (alteplase) in MI. *J Am Coll Cardiol* 1992;20:17–23.

This study demonstrated that the commonly used accelerated tPA regimen safely achieves more rapid reperfusion. A total of 281 patients were randomized in open fashion to a standard regimen (initial 10-mg bolus, then 50 mg over 1 hour, then 20 mg/h for 2 hours) or an accelerated regimen (15-mg bolus, 50 mg over 30 minutes, then 35 mg over 60 minutes). The accelerated tPA group had better patency at 60 minutes (76% vs. 63%; $p = 0.03$) but not at 90 minutes (81% vs. 77%; $p = 0.21$). Similar rates of recurrent ischemia, reinfarction, stroke, and bleeding were observed.

103. **Steg PG**, et al. for the Prospective Evaluation of Reperfusion Markers (**PERM**) Study Group. Efficacy of streptokinase, but not tissue-type plasminogen activator, in achieving 90-minute patency after thrombolysis for acute MI decreases with time to treatment. *J Am Coll Cardiol* 1998;31:776–779 (editorial pp. 781–782).

This retrospective analysis focused on 481 patients treated within 6 hours of symptom onset; all underwent angiography at 90 minutes. Streptokinase but not tPA was found to be less effective when administered after 3 hours, regardless of whether TIMI flow grades 2 and 3 were pooled [86.9% (<3 hours) vs. 54.9%; $p = 0.0001$] or grade 3 flow was considered alone (81.7% vs. 53.6%; $p = 0.0001$). Of note, these data confirm an observation noted in the TIMI-1 study and may be a phenomenon specific to nonfibrinspecific agents because the same effect has been reported with anistreplase and urokinase.

Percutaneous Transluminal Coronary Revascularization

Angioplasty With or Without Thrombolytics

104. **Weaver, WD**, et al. Comparison of primary coronary angioplasty and intravenous thrombolytic therapy for acute MI: a quantitative review. *JAMA* 1997;278:2093–2098.

Data analysis from 10 randomized trials with a total of 2,606 patients. Mortality at 30 days or less was significantly lower in patients treated with primary PTCA compared with thrombolysis (4.4% vs 6.5%; odds ratio 0.66 [95% CI 0.46–0.94], p = 0.02). Primary PTCA was also associated with lower rates of reinfarction (7.2% vs 11.9%, or 0.58 [95% CI 0.44–0.75], p <0.001). Authors point out that the primary angioplasty results were primarily achieved in specialized, high volume centers.

105. **Bates DW**, et al. Coronary angiography and angioplasty after acute MI. *Ann Intern Med* 1997;126:539–550.

This extensive review focused on the English-language literature from 1970 to June 1995. Interesting data include the high yearly cost (~$1 billion) of catheterizations after MI, significant variability (30%–81%) in use of angiography after MI, and high correlation ($r = 0.91$) between catheterization and subsequent revascularization (clinical cascade). The review systemically examines the data for use of angiography and angioplasty at various time points and situations after MI and in patients with complications of MI. An excellent overview is provided of major current controversies such as primary angioplasty versus thrombolysis and indications for angiography after MI.

106. **Gibson CM**. Primary angioplasty compared with thrombolysis: new issues in the era of glycoprotein IIb/IIIa inhibition and intracoronary stenting. *Ann Intern Med* 1999;130:841–847.

This review discusses data from trials comparing conventional balloon angioplasty with thrombolysis and more recent studies involving intracoronary stenting and the use of glycoprotein IIb/IIIa inhibitors in conjunction with angioplasty and reduced-dose thrombolysis.

Primary Angioplasty

107. **Eckman MH**, et al. Direct angioplasty for acute MI. *Ann Intern Med* 1992;117:667–676.

This review of the English-language literature from 1983 to October 1991 focuses on studies involving angioplasty without prior thrombolysis (23 articles with a total of 4,368 patients). The average hospital mortality rate was 8.3%, but was much higher (44.2%) in those with cardiogenic shock. Nonrandomized trial data suggest a mortality benefit of PTCA over thrombolysis in those with cardiogenic shock.

108. **Grines CL**, et al. Primary Angioplasty in MI (**PAMI**). A comparison of immediate angioplasty with thrombolytic therapy for acute MI. *N Engl J Med* 1993;328:673–679 (editorial pp. 726–728).

Design: Prospective, randomized, open, multicenter study. End points included in-hospital death, reinfarction, and intracranial bleeding and ejection fraction at 6 weeks.

Purpose: To compare immediate PTCA with thrombolytic therapy in acute MI.

Population: 395 patients presenting within 12 hours of ischemic pain with ≥1 mm ST elevation in at least two contiguous ECG leads.

Exclusion Criteria: Complete left bundle branch block, cardiogenic shock, and increased bleeding risk.

Treatment: tPA 100 mg intravenously (or 1.25 mg/kg if patient weighed <65 kg) over 3 hours; or immediate PTCA. All patients received intravenous heparin for 3–5 days.

Results: A 97% PTCA success rate was observed. The PTCA group had a 60% lower in-hospital mortality rate (2.6% vs. 6.5%; $p = 0.06$) and a significant 58% reduction in in-hospital death or reinfarction (5.1% vs. 12.0%; $p = 0.02$). The PTCA group also had less intracranial bleeding (0% vs. 2.0%; $p = 0.05$). No difference was seen between groups in ejection fraction at 6 weeks (both at rest and during exercise). The benefits of primary angioplasty were maintained at 2-year follow-up: lower incidence of death or MI (14.9% vs. 23%; $p = 0.034$), less recurrent ischemia (36.4% vs. 48%; $p = 0.026$), lower reintervention rates (27.2% vs. 46.5%; $p < 0.0001$), and lower rehospitalization rates (58.5% vs. 69.0%; $p = 0.035$) (*see Circulation* 1999;33:640).

Comments: An impressively short randomization to balloon time was observed (average 60 minutes vs. 42 minutes for door to thrombolysis). At 6 months, the PTCA benefit persisted: death or reinfarction in 8.2% vs. 17.0% ($p = 0.02$). The accompanying editorial asserts that high-risk patients are most likely to gain the most benefit from immediate PTCA (e.g., >75 years of age, anterior MI, cardiogenic shock). The editorial also points out that PTCA was available in only 18% of hospitals (even fewer with emergency and/or CABG capability).

109. **Every NR**, et al. for the MI Triage and Intervention (**MITI**) Investigators. A comparison of thrombolytic therapy with primary coronary angioplasty for acute MI. *N Engl J Med* 1996; 335:1253–1260 (editorials pp. 1311–1317).

Design: Retrospective cohort analysis of MITI Registry (19 Seattle area hospitals, 10 with primary angioplasty capability).

Purpose: To compare outcomes in acute MI patients receiving thrombolytic therapy and primary angioplasty.

Population: 3,145 MITI patients (thrombolytic group, n = 2,095; PTCA group, n = 1,050) treated between 1988 and 1994.

Exclusion Criteria: Lack of ECG data and angioplasty ≥6 hours after admission.

Treatment: Thrombolysis with alteplase (65%), streptokinase (32%), or urokinase (3%; 8% were treated prior to hospitalization); or coronary angiography within 6 hours of admission followed by angioplasty if indicated.

Results: No significant differences were observed between thrombolysis and PTCA in in-hospital [5.6% (thrombolytic) vs. 5.5%] or 3-year mortality rates. At 3-year follow-up, the thrombolysis group had 30% less coronary angiography, 15% fewer coronary angioplasties, and 13% lower costs. Of note, thrombolysis patients were treated faster (1 vs. 1.7 hours after arrival) and sooner after chest pain than the PAMI thrombolysis group (198 vs. 230 minutes). Low-volume PTCA hospitals did provide later treatment (2.3 vs. 1.5 hours) and had higher in-hospital mortality rates (8.1% vs. 4.5%).

Comments: Compared with PAMI, there was lower procedural success (89% vs. 98%) and less aggressive heparinization. The accompanying pro-thrombolytic editorial asserts that PTCA is not widely available and prompt use is infrequent and that PAMI showed benefit of PTCA only in the elderly. The accompanying pro-PTCA editorial points out that PTCA achieves higher TIMI grade 3 flow (93%–97% vs. 54% with front-loaded tPA) and better long-term patency (87%–91% vs. 50%), is associated with fewer strokes (0.3% vs. 2.5%) and no intracranial hemorrhage (0% vs. 1.4%), reocclusion is more treatable (e.g., more heparin and/or stenting), and can be performed when thrombolysis is contraindicated. A meta-analysis (including GUSTO IIb data) showed lower mortality rates with PTCA (4.5% vs. 7.1%; $p < 0.01$).

110. **GUSTO IIb** Angioplasty Substudy. The Global Use of Strategies to Open Occluded Arteries in Acute Coronary Syndromes Angioplasty Substudy Investigators. *N Engl J Med* 1997;336: 1621–1628.

Design: Prospective, randomized, open, multicenter substudy (57 sites; all performed 200 angioplasties/yr, with one operator doing 50/yr). Thirty-day primary end point was death, MI, and stroke.

Purpose: To compare thrombolytic therapy with primary angioplasty in patients with acute ST-elevation MI.

Population: 1,138 patients presenting within 12 hours of ST-elevation MI.

Exclusion Criteria: Same as main GUSTO IIb trial (see Chapter 3, ref. 34).

Treatment: Accelerated tPA [15-mg intravenous bolus, 0.75 mg/kg over 30 minutes (maximum 50 mg), 0.50 mg/kg over 60 minutes (maximum 35 mg)] or primary angioplasty (average door to balloon time 1.9 hours).

Results: PTCA group had one-third lower rate of death, MI, and stroke (odds ratio 0.67; 9.6% vs. 13.7%, $p = 0.033$). Most of the observed benefit occurred from days 5 to 10. By 6 months, the difference was no longer significant (14% vs. 16%). Breakdown by end point (at 30 days): death, 5.7% vs. 7% ($p = 0.37$); MI, 4.5% vs. 6.5% ($p = 0.13$); stroke, 0.2% vs. 0.9% ($p = 0.11$). Of note, PTCA was not associated with any extra benefit in high-risk groups. Also, PTCA achieved TIMI grade 3 flow in a surprisingly low 73% of cases (technical success rate 93%), which was associated with a 1.6% mortality rate (vs. 21.4%, 14.3%, 19.9% for TIMI flow grades 0–2).

111. **Brener SJ**, et al. on behalf of the Reopro and Primary PTCA Organization and Randomized Trial (**RAPPORT**) Investigators. Randomized, placebo-controlled trial of primary glycoprotein IIb/IIIa blockade with primary angioplasty for acute MI. *Circulation* 1998;98:734–741.

Design: Prospective, randomized, double-blind, placebo-controlled, multicenter study. Primary end point was death, MI, and any TVR at six months.

Purpose: To evaluate whether platelet IIb/IIIa receptor blockade with abciximab reduces ischemic events in acute MI patients undergoing primary angioplasty.

Population: 483 patients presenting within 12 hours of onset of symptoms with ischemic chest pain lasting >20 minutes accompanied by significant ST elevation in at least two contiguous leads or new left bundle branch block.

Exclusion Criteria: Severe thrombocytopenia, ongoing internal bleeding or recent major surgery, previous stroke, severe uncontrolled hypertension, PTCA of IRA in prior 3 months, cardiogenic shock, and prior abciximab or thrombolytic therapy.

Treatment: Abciximab 0.25 mg/kg bolus then 0.125 µg/kg/min (maximum 10 µg/min) for 12 hours. All patients received aspirin and heparin 100 U/kg bolus before PTCA (with further boluses as needed to keep activated clotting time >300 seconds). Stenting was discouraged but was allowed for residual dissection with >50% restenosis and for abrupt or threatened closure.

Results: No difference was observed between the two groups in incidence of 6-month primary end point (28.1% vs. 28.2%). However, the abciximab group had less death, MI, and urgent TVR at 7 days (3.3% vs. 9.9%; p = 0.003), 30 days (5.8% vs. 11.2%; p = 0.03), and 6 months (11.6% vs. 17.8%; p = 0.05). The abciximab group had 42% less bailout stenting (11.9% vs. 20.4%; p = 0.008). Abciximab was associated with increased major bleeding (defined as a hematocrit decrease of >5%; 16.6% vs. 9.5%, p = 0.02), mostly at the arterial access site. On treatment analysis showed that abciximab was associated with decreased death and MI at 7 days (1.4% vs. 4.7%; p = 0.047) with a trend at 6 months (6.9% vs. 12%; p = 0.07).

Comments: Low-risk population (30-day mortality rates ~2%) may have attenuated the impact of abciximab. Increased bleeding with abciximab was likely due to the double-blind design because the investigators were unwilling to discontinue heparin immediately after the procedure(s) for early sheath removal.

112. **O'Neill W**, et al. A prospective randomized clinical trial of intracoronary streptokinase versus coronary angioplasty for acute MI. *N Engl J Med* 1986;314:812–818.

In this first randomized trial of angioplasty vs. thrombolysis (albeit intracoronary), only 56 patients were enrolled, all <75 years of age and with symptoms <12 hours. No differences were seen in the recanalization rate (83% vs. 85%), but the angioplasty group had decreased residual stenosis (43% vs. 83%) and significant ejection fraction improvement (+8% vs. +1%; p < 0.001). However, only 44 of 56 had undergone the requisite serial ventriculographic studies.

113. **Ribeiro EE**, et al. Randomized trial of direct coronary angioplasty versus intravenous streptokinase in acute MI. *J Am Coll Cardiol* 1993;22:376–380.

This randomized trial was composed of 100 patients presenting within 6 hours. Patients received streptokinase 1.2 million U over 1 hour or immediate PTCA. The PTCA group had a longer time to treatment (238 vs. 179 minutes). No significant differences in mortality rate (6% vs. 2%), 48-hour infarct artery patency (74% vs. 80%), or ejection fraction (59% vs. 57%) were observed.

114. **Zijlstra F**, et al. A comparison of immediate angioplasty with intravenous streptokinase in acute MI. *N Engl J Med* 1993; 328:680–684.

In this small randomized trial of 142 patients presenting within 6 hours of onset of pain, patients were randomized to balloon angioplasty or streptokinase 1.5 million U over 60 minutes. The angioplasty group had a lower reinfarction rate (0% vs. 12.5%) and higher ejection fraction by discharge (51% vs. 45%; p = 0.004).

115. **Gibbons RJ**, et al. Immediate angioplasty compared with the administration of a thrombolytic agent followed by conservative treatment for MI. *N Engl J Med* 1993;328:685–691.

In this small randomized trial of 108 patients presenting within 12 hours of chest pain, the PTCA group did not have better myocardial salvage (by technetium 99 scan). Nor were any differences in ejection fraction or mortality rate observed. However, PTCA patients did have a shorter stay (7.7 vs. 10.6 days; $p = 0.01$) and less rehospitalization (in first 6 months, 4% vs. 18%).

116. **Tiefenbrunn AJ**, et al. Clinical experience with primary percutaneous transluminal coronary angioplasty compared with alteplase (recombinant tissue-type plasminogen activator) in patients with acute MI. A report from the Second National Registry of MI (**NRMI-2**). *J Am Coll Cardiol* 1998;31:1240–1245.

This analysis showed that the outcomes of PTCA and rt-PA are comparable in thrombolysis-eligible patients not in cardiogenic shock. Data were from 4,939 nontransfer primary PTCA patients treated within 12 hours of symptom onset and 24,705 rt-PA–treated patients. Longer delay to treatment was seen in the PTCA group: 111 minutes (door to balloon) versus 42 minutes ($p < 0.0001$). Cardiogenic shock patients did better with PTCA: in-hospital mortality rate 32% versus 52% ($p < 0.0001$). A similar mortality rate was observed among thrombolytic-eligible patients not in cardiogenic shock [5.4% (rt-PA) vs. 5.2%]. A higher stroke rate was observed in the thrombolytic group (1.6% vs. 0.7%; $p < 0.0001$), but no difference in combined incidence death and nonfatal stroke (6.2% vs. 5.6%). There were also no significant differences in reinfarction rates (2.9% vs. 2.5%).

117. **Danchin N**, et al. Treatment of acute myocardial infarction by primary coronary angioplasty or intravenous thrombolysis in the "real world." *Circulation* 1999;99:2639–2644.

This analysis of the nationwide prospective registry focused on all patients admitted for acute MI to French ICUs in November 1995. Primary angioplasty patients (n = 152) had a higher incidence of a history of prior cerebrovascular accident than thrombolysis patients (n = 569; 10% vs. 2%, $p < 0.01$). Other baseline characteristics were similar between the two groups. There was no significant difference in 1-year survival between groups [85.0% (angioplasty) vs. 89.5%; $p = 0.18$]. Multivariate predictors of 1-year mortality were older age, anterior location of infarction, female sex, and history of heart failure.

PTCA after Thrombolysis

118. **Topol EJ**, et al. and the Thrombolysis and Angioplasty in MI (**TAMI**) Study Group. A randomized trial of immediate versus delayed elective angioplasty after intravenous tissue plasminogen activator in acute MI. *N Engl J Med* 1987;317:581–588 (editorial pp. 624–626).

Design: Prospective, randomized, multicenter study. Primary end point was infarct-related vessel patency and global left ventricular function.

Purpose: To compare immediate with delayed elective angioplasty in patients undergoing thrombolysis for acute MI.

Population: 386 patients met initial criteria (≤75 years of age, within 6 hours of onset of symptoms, and ≥1 mm ST elevation in at least two contiguous leads); 197 patients had appropriate catheterization findings (i.e., lesions amenable to angioplasty) and were randomized to immediate or delayed angioplasty.

Exclusion Criteria: Pain <20 minutes or relieved by nitroglycerin, increased bleeding risk, prior CABG, and cardiogenic shock. Contraindications related to angiographic findings included >50% left main stenosis, severe/diffuse disease, and infarct-related vessel unidentifiable.

Treatment: Predominantly single-chain tPA 150 mg intravenously over 6–8 hours followed by angiography with either immediate angioplasty or deferred angioplasty (latter performed at 7–10 days and if indicated). The immediate group also had angiography at 7–10 days to assess for reocclusion and left ventricular function.

Results: Immediate PTCA success rate was 86%. Similar reocclusion rates were observed [11% (immediate) vs. 13%]. Neither group had an improvement in global left ventricular function. In the delayed group, 14% did not require angioplasty (residual stenosis <50%), but there was a higher crossover rate to emergency angioplasty (16% vs. 5%). Immediate angioplasty had its own risks: Seven of nine patients with abrupt closure required emergency CABG surgery.

119. **Rogers WJ**, et al. for the **TIMI-IIA** Investigators. Comparison of immediate invasive, delayed invasive and conservative strategies after tissue-type plasminogen activator. *Circulation* 1990; 81;1457–1476.

    Design: Prospective, randomized, open, multicenter study. Primary end point was predischarge LVEF.

    Purpose: To compare immediate versus delayed (at 18–48 hours) PTCA or CABG versus conservative treatment in acute MI patients treated with tPA.

    Population: 586 patients ≤75 years of age presenting within 4 hours of chest pain and with ≥1 mm ST elevation in at least two contiguous ECG leads.

    Exclusion Criteria: PTCA in preceding 6 months, prior CABG or prosthetic valve surgery, history of cerebrovascular disease or uncontrolled hypertension, increased bleeding risk, recent trauma, and prolonged CPR.

    Treatment: All patients received tPA [first 195 patients, 150 mg over 6 hours; next 391 patients, 100 mg over 6 hours (6-mg intravenous bolus, 54 mg over 1st hour, 20 mg in 2nd hour, 5 mg/h for 4 hours)]; 195 underwent immediate invasive treatment, 194 delayed invasive treatment, and 197 conservative treatment [angiography ± angioplasty allowed with ischemic symptoms (spontaneous or provoked with testing)]. All patients received heparin for 5 days.

    Results: All groups had similar predischarge LVEF (average 49.3%) and IRA patency (TIMI grade 2 or 3 flow; mean 83.7%). The immediate invasive group had a significantly higher CABG rate [7.7% vs. 2.1% (delayed invasive) vs. 2.5% (conservative); $p < 0.01$], and more transfusions were required among non-CABG patients (13.8% vs. 3.1% vs. 2.0%). Similar 1-year mortality rates were observed despite higher PTCA rates in immediate and delayed invasive groups (76% vs. 64% vs. 24%)

120. **Califf RM**, et al. for the TAMI Study Group. Evaluation of combination thrombolytic therapy and timing of cardiac catheterization in acute MI. *Circulation* 1991;83:1543–1556.

Design: Prospective, randomized, open, parallel-group, factorial (3×2), multicenter study. Primary end point was global left ventricular ejection fraction (LVEF).

Purpose: To evaluate combination thrombolytic therapy by comparison with monotherapy and to compare an aggressive with a deferred angiography strategy.

Population: 575 patients ≤75 years of age presenting within 6 hours of symptoms and with >1 mm ST elevation in at least two contiguous ECG leads.

Exclusion Criteria: Prior CABG, prior Q-wave MI in same distribution, cardiogenic shock, and contraindications to thrombolysis.

Treatment: Urokinase (1.5 million U intravenous bolus then 1.5 million U over 60 minutes), rt-PA [100 mg over 3 hours (6-mg intravenous bolus, 60 mg over 1 hour, 20 mg/h for 2 hours)], or combination therapy [urokinase 1.5 million U over 1 hour and rt-PA 1 mg/kg over 1 hour (10% as intravenous bolus, maximum dose 90 mg)]. Aggressive strategy consisted of immediate angiography while deferred strategy involved angiography prior to discharge (days 5–10).

Results: Global LVEF was well preserved and nearly identical at predischarge angiography (54%), regardless of thrombolytic or catheterization strategy. Combination thrombolysis did result in higher 90-minute patency: TIMI grade 2 or 3 flow in 76% [tPA 71% (p = NS), urokinase 62% (p = 0.049)]. Less reocclusion [2% vs. 12% (p = 0.04) and 7% (p = NS)] and recurrent ischemia (25% vs. 31% vs. 35%) were observed. An aggressive strategy yielded better results with fewer adverse outcomes: death, stroke, reinfarction, heart failure, or recurrent ischemia in 55% vs. 67% (p = 0.004), as well as a trend toward a higher predischarge patency rate (94% vs. 90%; p = 0.065).

121. Should We Intervene Following Thrombolysis (**SWIFT**) Trial Study Group. SWIFT trial of delayed elective intervention v conservative treatment after thrombolysis with anistreplase in acute MI. *BMJ* 1991;302:555–560.

    In this prospective, multicenter (n = 21) trial of 800 patients <70 years of age, patients randomized to early angiography and appropriate intervention (PTCA 43%, CABG 15%) or conservative care [PTCA 2.5%, CABG 1.7% (initial admission)]. All patients were treated with anistreplase 30 U over 5 minutes. No differences in 1-year mortality (5.8% vs. 5%) and reinfarction rates (15% vs. 13%) were observed. Intervention group did have longer stay (11 days vs. 10 days).

122. **Madsen JK**, et al. Danish Trial in Acute MI (**DANAMI**). Danish multicenter randomized study of invasive vs. conservative treatment in patients with inducible ischemia after thrombolysis in acute MI (DANAMI). *Circulation* 1997;748–755 (editorial pp. 713–715).

    Design: Prospective, randomized, open, multicenter study. Median follow-up period was 2.4 years. Primary end point was death, acute MI, and admission with unstable angina.

    Purpose: To compare an invasive strategy of PTCA or CABG with a conservative strategy in patients with inducible ischemia after thrombolysis for MI.

    Population: 1,008 patients <70 years of age with a first MI and inducible ischemia [spontaneous ischemia ≤36 hours after admission or positive bicycle exercise tolerance test result (≥ 0.1 mm ST depression, ≥ 0.2 mm ST elevation)].

Exclusion Criteria: Prior MI, PTCA, or CABG; incomplete thrombolysis; BP decrease during exercise; significant noncoronary disease; ECG abnormalities precluding ST-segment evaluation during exercise (e.g., left bundle branch block).

Treatment: Invasive therapy group received angiography within 2 weeks, PTCA and CABG if significant disease ($\geq 50\%$ stenosis). In the conservative arm, angiography was allowed if severe angina developed (e.g., Canadian Cardiovascular Society class 3 or 4).

Results: In the invasive group, PTCA was performed in 52.9% and CABG in 29.2% (at 2–10 weeks). In the conservative group, at 2 months, only 1.6% had undergone revascularization (at 1 year, 15%). At follow-up, no significant mortality difference was observed [3.6% (invasive) vs. 4.4%], but the invasive group had 47% fewer MIs (5.6% vs. 10.5%; $p = 0.0038$) and fewer unstable angina admissions (17.9% vs. 29.5%; $p < 0.00001$). Overall, the invasive group had 36% fewer primary end points (death, MI, and unstable angina) at 2 years (23.5% vs. 36.6%; $p < 0.0001$).

Comments: Data support the use of angiography if stress test positive. The accompanying editorial points out that few U.S. cardiologists follow the ACC/AHA guidelines that recommend stress testing prior to invasive testing. They propose performing angiography for medium or large MIs, and revascularization if evidence of an incomplete infarct (e.g., lower than expected CK peak, ECG evolution, preserved wall motion of infarct zone) is present, and stress testing first those with only small MIs (e.g., leads II, III, aVF only).

123. **Simoons ML**, et al. European Cooperative Study Group (**ECSG-4**). Thrombolysis with tissue plasminogen activator in acute MI: no additional benefit from immediate percutaneous coronary angioplasty. *Lancet* 1988;331:197–202.

This randomized trial was composed of 367 patients. Treatment was tPA 100 mg intravenously over 3 hours then invasive (angiography and PTCA) or noninvasive strategy. The noninvasive group had a lower mortality rate (3% vs. 7%), recurrent ischemia within 24 hours (3% vs. 17%), and bleeding complications. The invasive group had a high rate of periprocedural reocclusion (transient 16%, sustained 7%).

Rescue PTCA

124. **Abbottsmith CW**, et al. Fate of patients with acute MI with patency of the infarct-related vessel achieved with successful thrombolysis versus rescue angioplasty. *J Am Coll Cardiol* 1990; 16:770–778.

This retrospective analysis focused on 776 TAMI patients with a patent IRA; 607 received only thrombolysis and 169 had rescue angioplasty. The rescue success rate was 88%. However, at 7–10 days, the thrombolysis group had less reocclusion [11% vs. 21% (successful rescue), $p < 0.001$] and better ejection fractions (52.3% vs. 48.1%; $p < 0.01$), whereas the in-hospital mortality rates were similar (4.6% vs. 5.9%). Failed rescue angioplasty was associated with a high mortality rate [39.1% vs. 5.9% (successful rescue)].

125. **Ellis SG**, et al. Present status of rescue coronary angioplasty: current polarization of opinion and randomized trials. *J Am Coll Cardiol* 1992;19:681–686.

     This overview of 12 trials (only one randomized) included a total of 560 patients. The average success rate of rescue PTCA was 80%. Reocclusion occurred in 18%. The overall mortality rate 10.6%, but it was much higher (up to 39%) in those who failed rescue.

126. **Ellis SG**, et al. **RESCUE**. Randomized comparison of rescue angioplasty with conservative management of patients with early failure of thrombolysis for acute anterior MI. *Circulation* 1994;90:2280–2284.

     Design: Prospective, randomized, multicenter study. Primary end point was LVEF at 25–35 days.

     Purpose: To assess the clinical benefit of rescue angioplasty in a relatively high-risk population.

     Population: 151 patients 21–79 years of age presenting with ST elevation ≥2 mm in at least two precordial leads.

     Exclusion Criteria: Cardiogenic shock, prior MI, and left main stenosis ≥50%.

     Treatment: Thrombolysis followed by PTCA or aspirin, heparin, and vasodilators.

     Results: Rescue PTCA was successful in 92%. The rescue PTCA group had less death and severe heart failure (6% vs. 17%; $p = 0.05$) and better exercise (but not rest) ejection fractions (43% vs. 38%; $p = 0.04$).

127. **Gibson CM**, et al. Rescue angioplasty in the thrombolysis in MI (**TIMI**) 4 trial. *Am J Cardiol* 1997;80:21–26.

     This retrospective analysis focused on 402 TIMI-4 patients with either successful rescue angioplasty (PTCA) or successful thrombolysis. The successful PTCA group had better 90-minute TIMI grade 3 flow (87% vs. 65%; $p = 0.002$) and a lower TIMI frame count (27 vs. 39; $p < 0.001$). The successful versus failed rescue PTCA group had fewer in-hospital adverse end points, consisting of death, MI, severe CHF/shock, ejection fraction ≤40% (29% vs. 83%; $p = 0.01$). The rescue PTCA (all) versus other groups had similar event rates (both with adverse outcomes in 35%).

128. **Ross AM**, et al. Rescue angioplasty after failed thrombolysis: technical and clinical outcomes in a large thrombolysis trial. *J Am Coll Cardiol* 1998;31:1511–1517.

     This retrospective analysis focused on GUSTO-I angiographic substudy data. Rescue PTCA was performed in 198 patients; the artery was successfully opened in 88.4%, with 68% achieving TIMI grade 3 flow. Successful rescue PTCA resulted in better left ventricular function and 30-day mortality than failed rescue, comparable with outcomes in those with closed infarct arteries managed conservatively (266 patients), but less favorable than those with successful thrombolysis (1,058 patients). Failed rescue was associated with high 30.4% mortality (multivariate analysis predictor, severe heart failure).

Cardiogenic Shock

129. **Hochman JS**, et al. Should We Emergently Revascularize Occluded Coronaries for Cardiogenic Shock (**SHOCK**) Investigators. Early revascularization in acute MI complicated by car-

diogenic shock. *N Engl J Med* 1999;341:625–634 (editorial pp. 686–688).

This prospective, randomized, multicenter trial was composed of 302 patients with ST-elevation MI (or new left bundle branch block), pulmonary capillary wedge pressure ≥15 mm Hg, cardiac index ≤2.2, SBP >90 mm Hg for 30 minutes before inotropes/ vasopressors or IABP initiated, and heart rate 60 beats/min. Patients underwent emergent revascularization within 6 hours (PTCA or CABG) or medical management [thrombolysis recommended (given in 64%), delayed revascularization allowed at 54 hours]. The emergency revascularization (ERV) group had a 97% angiography rate and 87% revascularization rate [PTCA 49% (at average 0.9 hours), CABG 38% (average 2.7 hours)]. Among initial medical stabilization (IMS) patients, 4% had revascularization performed before 54 hours and 22% underwent late revascularization. There was no significant difference in 30-day all-cause mortality (primary end point) between the two groups (ERV 46.7% vs. IMS 56.0%; $p = 0.11$); however, at 6 months there was a significant mortality benefit associated with early revascularization strategy (50.3% vs 63.1%, p = 0.027). In the subgroup of patients ≤75 years of age, ERV was significantly better than IMS (at 30 days, 41% vs. 57%, $p < 0.01$; 6 months, 48% vs. 69%, $p < 0.01$). Of note, the PTCA success rate was 76%, and the mortality rate was 100% if PTCA did not achieve TIMI grade 2 or 3 flow.

Stenting

130. **Stone GW**, et al. for the **PAMI Stent Pilot** Trial Investigators. Prospective, multicenter study of the safety and feasibility of primary stenting in acute MI: in-hospital and 30-day results of the PAMI Stent Pilot Trial. *J Am Coll Cardiol* 1998;31:23–30.

Design: Prospective, multicenter, open study. Follow-up period was 30 days.

Purpose: To evaluate the feasibility of routine primary stenting strategy acute MI and its impact on recurrent ischemia, reinfarction, and late restenosis.

Population: 312 consecutive patients treated with PTCA for acute MI.

Exclusion Criteria: Cardiogenic shock; absolute contraindications to heparin, aspirin, or ticlopidine; thrombolytic therapy for index MI; previous bypass surgery; and vein graft occlusion.

Treatment: Primary PTCA followed by stenting of all eligible lesions (3–4 mm, lesion length no more than two stents, absence of giant thrombus burden, major side branch jeopardy, excessive tortuosity or calcification). All patients received aspirin, ticlopidine 250–500 mg, and heparin 5,000- to 10,000-U bolus in the emergency room.

Results: Stenting was attempted in 77%, with a 98% success rate. TIMI grade 3 flow was restored in 96%. The stented group had low rates of in-hospital death (0.8%), reinfarction (1.7%), and recurrent ischemia (1.3%). At 30-day follow-up, only one additional event (TVR) was observed.

Comments: Preliminary STENT PAMI results were presented at the 71st AHA Scientific Session (Dallas, TX, November 1998): 900 patients were randomized to balloon angioplasty or heparin-coated Palmaz-Schatz stenting. acute procedural success rates were >99% in both groups. Postprocedural TIMI grade 3 flow rates were 89% and 92% in the angioplasty and stent groups, respectively. At 6 months, the stent group had a larger mean luminal diameter and lower restenosis rate (20.3% vs. 30.5%). The stent group showed a trend toward fewer primary composite end point events at 30 days (death, MI, disabling stroke, ischemia-driven TVR; 4.2% vs. 5.4%) and a significant reduction at 6 months (12.4% vs. 20.1%). The stent group also had significantly lower 6-month rates of total TVR (12.8% vs. 21.4%); bleeding rates were similar.

131. **Antoniucci D**, et al. Florence Randomized Elective Stenting in Acute Coronary Occlusions (**FRESCO**). A clinical trial comparing primary stenting of the infarct-related artery with optimal primary angioplasty for acute MI. *J Am Coll Cardiol* 1998;31: 1234–1239.

Design: Prospective, randomized, multicenter study. Primary end point was death, reinfarction, and repeat TVR due to recurrent ischemia at 6 months.

Purpose: To compare primary stenting of the IRA with optimal PTCA for clinical and angiographic outcomes in acute MI.

Population: 150 patients presenting within 6 hours of onset of symptoms with ST-elevation MI and who underwent successful primary PTCA.

Exclusion Criteria: No PTCA was attempted if stenosis was <70% or the IRA could not be identified. No randomization to PTCA alone or stenting was performed if reference diameter was <2.5 mm. Patients could have no anatomical contraindications to stenting (e.g., tortuosity, thrombus).

Treatment: Primary PTCA or primary PTCA followed by stenting. All patients received intravenous heparin for 3 days and were routinely treated with aspirin (325 mg daily) and ticlopidine (500 mg/day for 2 weeks).

Results: Stenting success rate was 100%. At 6 months, the incidence of primary end point was only 9% in the stent group versus 28% in the PTCA group ($p = 0.003$). Repeat angiography was performed at 6 months, and the incidence of restenosis or reocclusion was 17% in the stent group and 43% in the PTCA group ($p = 0.001$).

132. **Suryapranata H**, et al. Randomized comparison of coronary stenting with balloon angioplasty in selected patients with acute MI. *Circulation* 1998;97:2502–2505 (editorial pp. 2483–2485).

Design: Prospective, randomized, single-center study. Clinical end points were death, recurrent MI, bypass surgery, and repeat angioplasty of infarct-related vessel.

Purpose: To compare routine primary stenting with balloon angioplasty in acute MI.

Population: 227 acute MI patients presenting within 6 hours of symptom onset or after 6–24 hours if there was evidence of ongoing ischemia.

Exclusion Criteria: Cardiogenic shock, prior bypass surgery or angioplasty, and prior MI. Angiographic criteria included unprotected left main disease, severe disease necessitating urgent bypass surgery, significant side branch jeopardy, excessive tortuosity, extensive thrombus, or inability to cross lesion with guidewire.

Treatment: Primary stenting (Palmaz-Schatz) or angioplasty (with bailout stenting only if prolonged inflation unsuccessful).

All patients received aspirin (80 mg/day). Initial patients received warfarin for 3 months, but patients enrolled after January 1996 received ticlopidine 250 mg/day for 2 weeks.

Results: Overall 6-month mortality rate was only 2%. The stent group had fewer reinfarctions (1% vs. 7%; $p = 0.036$) and less need for subsequent target vessel revascularization (4% vs. 17%; $p = 0.0016$). The stent group also had better cardiac event-free survival rate (95% vs. 80%; $p = 0.012$). Of note, the stent group had a larger reference vessel.

Comments: Generalizability of results were limited by small sample, single-center design, and highly experienced operators. A significant proportion of patients were excluded (50% vs. only 23% in PAMI Stent Pilot Trial).

133. **Rodriguez A**, et al. Gianturco-Roubin in AMI (**GRAMI**). In-hospital and late results of coronary stents versus conventional balloon angioplasty in acute MI (GRAMI trial). *Am J Cardiol* 1998; 81:1286–1291.

This small randomized trial showed the superiority of stent base intervention in the acute MI setting. A total of 104 patients were assigned to balloon angioplasty followed by elective stenting (group 1) or angioplasty alone (group 2; 15 of 52 would require bailout stenting). Procedural success rates were 98% and 94.2%, respectively ($p = \text{NS}$). Group 1 patients had significantly fewer adverse in-hospital events (death, nonelective bypass surgery, recurrent ischemia, reinfarction; 3.8% vs. 19.2%, $p = 0.03$). Group 1 patients also had a higher incidence of TIMI grade 3 flow at pre-discharge angiography (95% vs. 83%; $p < 0.03$) and better event-free survival at 1-year follow-up (83% vs. 65%; $p = 0.002$).

ACE Inhibitors With or Without Nitrates

General Reviews and Meta-Analyses

134. **Ball SG**, et al. ACE inhibitors after MI: indications and timing. *J Am Coll Cardiol* 1995;25(suppl):42–46.

This review article emphasizes the significant benefit of ACE inhibition in patients with left ventricular dysfunction. Early initiation and total length of therapy (e.g., 4–6 weeks vs. longer or indefinite) are also discussed.

135. ACE Inhibitor MI Collaborative Group. Indications for ACE inhibitors in the early treatment of acute MI. Systematic overview of individual data from 100,000 patients in randomized trials. *Circulation* 1998;97: 2202–2212 (editorial pp. 2192–2194).

This meta-analysis was composed of four randomized trials (CONSENSUS II, GISSI-3, ISIS-4, and CCS-1) 98,496 total patients, in which ACE inhibitors were started within 36 hours of acute MI. ACE inhibition was associated with a 7% reduction in 30-day mortality (7.1% vs. 7.6%; $p < 0.004$). Most of the benefit was observed within the first week of treatment. The greatest mortality benefit was seen in high-risk groups (e.g., anterior MI, Killip class 2 to 3, heart rate 100 beats/min at entry). ACE inhibition also was associated with a reduction in nonfatal cardiac failure (14.6% vs. 15.2%; $p = 0.01$) but led to more frequent hypotension (17.6% vs. 9.3%; $p < 0.01$) and renal dysfunction (1.3% vs. 0.6%; $p < 0.01$).

136. **Domanski MJ**, et al. Effect of angiotensin converting enzyme inhibition on sudden cardiac death in patients following acute MI. *J Am Coll Cardiol* 1999;33:598–604.

The results of this meta-analysis of 15 trials with 15,134 patients suggest that part of the benefit of ACE inhibition in acute MI is related to a reduction in risk of sudden cardiac death. The majority of deaths (87%) were cardiovascular, of which 38.2% were deemed sudden cardiac deaths. Overall, ACE inhibitor therapy was associated with significant reductions in overall mortality [odds ratio 0.83 (95% CI 0.71–0.97)], cardiovascular death [odds ratio 0.82 (95% CI 0.69–0.97)], and sudden cardiac death [odds ratio 0.80 (95% CI 0.70–0.92)].

Studies

137. **Pfeffer MA**, et al. on behalf of the Survival and Ventricular Enlargement (**SAVE**) Investigators. Effect of captopril on mortality and morbidity in patients with left ventricular dysfunction after MI. *N Engl J Med* 1992;327:669–677.
Design: Prospective, randomized, double-blind, placebo-controlled, multicenter study. Mean follow-up period was 42 months. Primary end point was all-cause mortality.
Purpose: To determine the effect of captopril on mortality and morbidity when started 3–16 days after MI in patients with left ventricular dysfunction.
Population: 2,231 patients 21–80 years of age with an ejection fraction ≤40% but no overt heart failure.
Exclusion Criteria: Requirement or contraindication to ACE inhibition, creatinine >2.5 mg/dL, unstable post-MI course.
Treatment: Captopril initiated 3–16 days after MI and titrated from 12.5 mg three times daily to 25 mg three times daily by hospital discharge (and later 50 mg three times daily if tolerated); or placebo.
Results: Captopril group had the following risk reductions: 19% lower all-cause mortality (20% vs. 25%; $p = 0.019$), 21% lower cardiovascular mortality ($p = 0.014$), 25% fewer recurrent MIs (11. 9% vs. 15.2%; $p = 0.015$), and 22% less severe heart failure requiring hospitalization ($p = 0.019$). No difference was observed in deterioration of 9 percentage points in ejection fraction as measured by repeat radionuclide ventriculography at mean 36 months (13% vs. 16%; $p = 0.17$).
Comments: Later analysis showed that the reduction in recurrent MI was independent of ejection fraction and that mortality after a recurrent MI was 32% lower in the captopril group ($p = 0.029$). Captopril patients underwent fewer revascularization procedures ($p = 0.01$), but there was no reduction in unstable angina admissions. Overall, captopril was associated with a 14% reduction in composite ischemic index of recurrent MI, revascularization, and unstable angina ($p = 0.047$) (*see Circulation* 1994; 90:1731).
138. **Swedeberg K**, et al. on behalf of the Cooperative New Scandinavian Enalapril Survival Study (**CONSENSUS II**) Group. Effects of early administration of enalapril on mortality in patients with acute MI. *N Engl J Med* 1992;327:678–684.
Design: Prospective, randomized, double-blind, placebo-controlled, multicenter study. Average follow-up period was 188 days. Primary end point was all-cause mortality rate.
Purpose: To evaluate the effect on mortality of early intravenous administration of enalapril in acute MI patients.

Population: 6,090 patients within 24 hours of symptom onset and 1 of the following: ST elevation in at least two contiguous leads, new Q waves, or elevated serum enzymes.
Exclusion Criteria: Blood pressure <105/65 mm Hg, history of adverse reaction to or requirement for ACE inhibition, severe valvular stenosis, and vasopressor requirement.
Treatment: Intravenous enalaprilat 1 mg over 2 hours (stopped if BP fell below 90/60 mm Hg). Oral enalapril was begun at 6 hours (initial dose 2.5 mg and increased up to 20 mg/day); or placebo.
Results: Trial was terminated early by the safety committee. There was no significant mortality difference observed at 180 days: 10.2% (placebo) vs. 11.0% (enalapril). Enalapril was associated with more frequent hypotension (BP <90/50 mm Hg): 12% vs. 3% ($p < 0.001$).

139. Acute Infarction Ramipril Efficacy (**AIRE**) Study Investigators. Effect of ramipril on mortality and morbidity of survivors of AMI with clinical evidence of heart failure. *Lancet* 1993;342:821–828.
Design: Prospective, randomized, double-blind, parallel-group, placebo-controlled, multicenter study. Average follow-up period was 15 months. Primary end point was all-cause mortality.
Purpose: To evaluate if ramipril started 3–10 days after MI reduces mortality in patients whose course is complicated by heart failure.
Population: 2,006 patients with a definite acute MI and clinical evidence of heart failure at any point after MI.
Exclusion Criteria: Heart failure due to valvular disease, unstable angina, contraindications to ACE inhibition, and severe and resistant heart failure.
Treatment: Ramipril 2.5 mg twice daily for 2 days then 5 mg twice daily if tolerated.
Results: All-cause mortality was significantly lower in the ramipril group: 27% risk reduction (17% vs. 23%; $p = 0.002$). Ramipril patients also a had 30% lower risk of sudden death ($p = 0.011$) and a 19% risk reduction in combined end points consisting of death, severe heart failure, MI, and stroke ($p = 0.008$). No significant difference was observed in reinfarction or stroke rates.

140. **GISSI-3**. GISSI-3: effects of lisinopril and transdermal glyceryl trinitrate singly and together on 6-week mortality and ventricular function after acute MI. *Lancet* 1994;343:1115–1122.
Design: Prospective, randomized, open-label, 2×2 factorial, multicenter study. Primary outcomes were 6-week all-cause mortality and combination of death, heart failure at 5 days after MI, and ejection fraction $\leq 35\%$ or $\geq 45\%$ myocardial segments with abnormal motion.
Purpose: To evaluate the effect of lisinopril and nitrates, alone and in combination, on all-cause mortality and left ventricular function after acute MI.
Population: 18,895 patients (lisinopril, n = 4,713; nitrates, n = 4,731; both, n = 4,722; controls, n = 4,729) presenting within 24 hours of chest pain onset and with ≥ 1 mm ST elevation or depression in at least one limb lead or ≥ 2 mm in at least one precordial lead.
Exclusion Criteria: Severe heart failure, SBP <100 mm Hg, serum creatinine >177 μM, and severe comorbidity.
Treatment: (a) Lisinopril 5 mg in first 24 hours then 10 mg once daily for 6 weeks or open control; (b) glyceryl nitrate 5 μg/min

intravenously and increased by 5–20 μg/min or until SBP was lowered by 10%. At 24 hours, transdermal GTN was started (10 mg/day, 14 hours each day) for 6 weeks. If not tolerated, isosorbide mononitrate (50 mg once daily) or open control. Overall, 72% of patients received a thrombolytic agent, 31% were on a β-blocker and 84% on aspirin.

Results: Overall, 6-week mortality rate was only 6.7%. Lisinopril was associated with significant mortality reduction (6.3% vs. 7.1%, odds ratio 0.88; $p = 0.03$) with survival curves beginning to diverge on the first day. Reduction also was seen in combined primary outcome (15.6% vs. 17.0%, odds ratio 0.90; $p = 0.009$). No difference between lisinopril and controls was observed in recurrent infarction, postinfarct angina, cardiogenic shock, and stroke. No difference in mortality was observed between patients with and without glyceryl nitrate (18.4% vs. 18.9%; $p = 0.39$). Of note, 13.3% of controls received nonstudy ACE inhibitors, and 57.1% received nonstudy nitrates.

Comments: At 6 months, the lisinopril group had fewer deaths and left ventricular dysfunction (18.1% vs. 19.3%; $p = 0.03$) (*see J Am Coll Cardiol* 1996;27:337). A retrospective analysis showed that lisinopril was more beneficial in diabetic patients (6-week mortality 8.7% vs. 12.4%, odds ratio 0.68) than in nondiabetic patients ($p < 0.025$) (*see Circulation* 1997;26:4245).

141. **Ambrosioni E**, et al. for the Survival of MI Long-term Evaluation (**SMILE**) Study Investigators. The effect of the angiotensin-converting-enzyme inhibitor zofenopril on mortality and morbidity after anterior MI. *N Engl J Med* 1995;332:80–85 (editorial pp. 110–118).

Design: Prospective, randomized, double-blind, placebo-controlled, multicenter study. Follow-up period was 1 year. Primary end point was death or severe heart failure (at least three of the following: S3, bilateral pulmonary rales, radiologic evidence, and peripheral edema).

Purpose: To determine if short-term ACE inhibition after MI reduces mortality and severe heart failure.

Population: 1,556 patients (out of 20,261 cardiac care unit patients) at <24 hours from symptom onset and not administered thrombolytic therapy.

Exclusion Criteria: Cardiogenic shock, SBP <100 mm Hg, creatinine >2.5 mg/dL, and history of CHF or ACE inhibitor use.

Treatment: Zofenopril 7.5–30 mg twice daily or placebo.

Results: At 6 weeks, the zofenopril group had a significant 34% reduction in the incidence of death and severe heart failure (7.1% vs. 10.6%; $p = 0.018$). There was a significant 46% reduction in severe heart failure and a statistically nonsignificant 25% reduction in death (7.1% vs. 10. 6%; $p = 0.19$). At 1 year, the zofenopril group had 29% lower mortality (10.0% vs. 14.1%; $p = 0.011$).

Comments: This was a highly selected patient population. The accompanying editorial points out that ACE inhibitors in broader MI groups have a reduced but still significant effect of five lives saved per 1,000 (vs. 40–70 for high-risk patients). It is unclear if patients gained left ventricular function benefit from long-term therapy.

142. **ISIS-4** Collaborative Group. ISIS-4: a randomised factorial assessing early oral captopril, oral mononitrate and intravenous

magnesium sulfate in 58,050 patients with suspected acute MI. *Lancet* 1995;345:669–685.

Design: Prospective, randomized, double-blind, partially placebo-controlled (including captopril arm), multicenter study. Primary end point was 5-week mortality rate.

Purpose: To assess the effects of early initiation of captopril, oral nitrate, and intravenous magnesium on mortality and morbidity in acute MI patients.

Population: 58,050 patients with suspected acute MI (confirmed in 92%) presenting within 24 hours (median 8 hours) of symptom onset.

Exclusion Criteria (recommended): Cardiogenic shock, persistent severe hypotension, severe fluid depletion, and negligibly low risk of cardiac death.

Treatment: Captopril arm received 6.25 mg, 12.5 mg 2 hours later, 25 mg at 10–12 hours, then 50 mg twice daily for 28 days; or placebo. The imdur arm received 30 mg, 30 mg 10–12 hours later, 60 mg once daily for 28 days); 70% received thrombolytic therapy and 94% antiplatelet therapy.

Results: Captopril was associated with a 7% reduction in mortality: 7.19% vs. 7.69% ($p^2 = 0.02$). The benefit doubled in high-risk groups (prior MI, CHF, anterior ST elevation). More hypotension was seen with captopril, but no increased deaths were seen among patients with low BP (90–100 mm Hg). Imdur administration did not have a significant effect on mortality (7.34% vs. 7.54%).

143. Chinese Cardiac Study (**CCS-1**). Oral captopril versus placebo among 13,634 patients with suspected acute MI: interim report from the Chinese Cardiac Study (CCS-1). *Lancet* 1995;345:686–67.

Design: Prospective, randomized, placebo-controlled, multicenter study. Primary end point was 4-week all-cause mortality.

Purpose: To assess the effect of ACE inhibition in a broad group of MI patients.

Population: 13,634 patients with or without ST elevation presenting within 36 hours of symptom onset.

Exclusion Criteria: Persistent hypotension (SBP <90 mm Hg), chronic use of large doses of diuretics, and contraindications to ACE inhibitors.

Treatment: Captopril 6.25 mg initial dose, 12.5 mg 2 hours later, then 12.5 mg three times daily; or placebo.

Results: Captopril group had a nonsignificant mortality reduction at 4 weeks: 9.05% vs. 9.59% ($p = 0.03$). Captopril was associated with a significant excess of hypotension, but there was no adverse effect on early mortality.

Comments: The additive results of CCS-1, ISIS-4, CONSENSUS-II, GISSI-3, and 11 smaller trials show a clear benefit of ACE inhibitors: 6.5% odds reduction (7.27% vs. 7.73%; total of 100,963 patients).

144. **Kober L**, et al. for the Trandolapril Cardiac Evaluation (**TRACE**) Study Group. A clinical trial of the angiotensin-converting-enzyme inhibitor trandolapril in patients with left ventricular dysfunction after MI. *N Engl J Med* 1995;333:1670–1676.

Design: Prospective, randomized, double-blind, placebo-controlled, multicenter study. Follow-up period was 24–50 months. Primary end point was all-cause mortality rate.

Purpose: To evaluate the effect of long-term ACE inhibition with trandolapril on mortality in acute MI complicated by left ventricular dysfunction.

Population: 1,749 of 2,606 eligible patients with an ejection fraction ≤35% and an acute MI 3–7 days prior to enrollment.

Exclusion Criteria: Contraindications to or need for ACE inhibition, severe diabetes, hyponatremia (<125 m*M*), unstable angina requiring immediate intervention, and severe comorbidity.

Treatment: Trandolapril 1 mg/day and titrated up to 4 mg/day; or placebo.

Results: Trandolapril group with a 22% reduction in the relative risk of death (34.7% vs. 42.3%; *p* = 0.001), as well as significantly fewer cardiovascular and sudden cardiac deaths (relative risks 0.75 vs. 0.76) and less frequent progression to severe heart failure (relative risk 0.71). There was a nonsignificant reduction in recurrent MI (relative risk 0.86; *p* = 0.29).

Comments: Subsequent analysis revealed that the benefit of trandolapril increased with increasing age: placebo group with 14% excess of mortality in those ≤55 years of age versus 28% in those ≥75 years of age (*see Am J Cardiol* 1996;78:158). Of note, TRACE showed a benefit of ACE inhibition whether clinical signs of heart failure were present or not.

145. **Pfeffer MA**, et al. for the Healing and Early Afterload Reducing Therapy (**HEART**) Trial Investigators. Early versus delayed angiotensin-converting-enzyme inhibition therapy in acute MI. *Circulation* 1997;95:2643–2651.

    Design: Prospective, randomized, double-blind, placebo-controlled, multicenter study. Follow-up period was 90 days.

    Purpose: To compare the safety and efficacy of immediate versus delayed ACE inhibition on echocardiographic evidence of ventricular dilatation in patients with anterior MI.

    Population: 352 patients presenting within 24 hours of symptom onset.

    Exclusion Criteria: Contraindications or need for ACE inhibitor, creatinine 2.5 mg/dL, cardiogenic shock, SBP <100 mm Hg, and persistent ischemia.

    Treatment: Three groups: (#1) early (days 1–14) placebo, then full-dose ramipril (10 mg/day); (#2) early and late low-dose ramipril (0.625 mg); and (#3) early and late full-dose ramipril.

    Results: Trial was terminated early (600 patients planned) based on GISSI-3 and ISIS-4 results showing benefit of early initiation of ACE inhibition. Early full-dose ramipril (group 3) showed the largest increase in ejection fraction at 90 days [+4.9 vs. 3.9 (low dose) vs. 2.4 (delayed full dose); *p* trend < 0.05). No significant differences were observed in left ventricular diastolic area. Groups had similar event rates and incidence of low BP (≤90 mm Hg).

146. Placebo-controlled, Randomized, ACE Inhibitor, Comparative Trial in Cardiac Infarction and Left Ventricular Function (**PRACTICAL**). Comparison of enalapril versus captopril on left ventricular function and survival three months after acute MI. *Am J Cardiol* 1994;73:1180–1186.

    A total of 225 patients were enrolled within 24 hours and randomized to enalapril 5 mg three times daily, captopril 25 mg three times daily, or placebo. ACE inhibition was associated with a significantly increased ejection fraction (from 45% to 47%; $p = 0.005$) and less ventricular dilatation [left ventricular end-diastolic volume, from 168 to 172 mL vs. from 175 to 189 mL ($p = 0.051$); left ventricular end-systolic volume, from 94 to 94 mL vs. from 99 to 108 mL ($p = 0.026$)].

Nitrates

General Reviews

147. **Yusuf S**, et al. Effect of intravenous nitrates on mortality in acute MI: an overview of the randomized trials. *Lancet* 1988;1: 1088–1092.

    Analysis of data from seven small intravenous nitroglycerin trials enrolling 851 patients found that use of intravenous nitroglycerin was associated with a significant 41% mortality reduction (12. 0% vs. 20.5%; $p < 0.001$). Analysis of three trials studying intravenous nitroprusside found that its use was associated with a nonsignificant mortality reduction (14.3% vs. 17.8%).

Studies

148. **Jugdutt BI**, et al. Intravenous nitroglycerin therapy to limit myocardial infarct size, expansion and complications: effect of timing, dosage, and infarct location. *Circulation* 1988;78:906–919.

    This small randomized study showed that mortality benefit was associated with intravenous nitroglycerin. A total of 310 patients were randomized to intravenous nitroglycerin (infusion titrated to lower mean blood pressure 10% if normotensive, 30% if hypertensive) or control. The intravenous nitroglycerin group had a smaller CK infarct size ($p < 0.0001$), less cardiogenic shock (5% vs. 15%; $p < 0.005$), and decreased left ventricular thrombi (5% vs. 22%; $p < 0.0005$). At 10-day follow-up, a 22% higher ejection fraction, 40% less left ventricular asynergy, 41% lower Killip class, and no difference in expansion index (vs. +31%) were observed. Importantly, the nitroglycerin group had lower 30-day and 1-year mortality rates (14% vs. 26%, $p < 0.005$; 21% vs. 31%, $p < 0.05$). Subgroup analysis showed that this benefit was limited to those with anterior infarcts.

149. **ISIS-4** Collaborative Group. ISIS-4: a randomised factorial assessing early oral captopril, oral mononitrate and intravenous magnesium sulfate in 58,050 pts with suspected acute MI. *Lancet* 1995;345:669–685.

    This megatrial that enrolled 58,050 patients with suspected acute MI admitted within 24 hours of symptom onset included a randomization to oral mononitrate (30 mg, 30 mg 10–12 hours later, then 60 mg/day for 28 days), or placebo. In the nitrate arm, there was a nonsignificant reduction in 35-day mortality (7.34% vs. 7.54%). Of note, nearly half the placebo group received intravenous nitrate therapy, which could have diluted the results. The reader is referred to reference 143 for a full summary.

150. **Cohn JN**, et al. Effect of short-time infusion of sodium nitroprusside on mortality rate in acute MI complications by left ventricular failure. *N Engl J Med* 1982;306:1129–1135.

    This prospective, double-blind, placebo-controlled trial was composed of 812 men with left ventricular filling pressures ≥ 12 mmHg randomized to nitroprusside (10–200 µg/min) or placebo for 48 hours. The goal of therapy was to reduce left ventricular filling pressures by 40%. Overall, no differences were seen in 13-week mortality [19% vs. 17% (placebo)]. However, nitroprusside appeared beneficial if given late (>9 hours; 13-week mortality rates 14.4% vs. 22.3%, $p = 0.04$) and harmful if given early (24.2% vs. 12.7%; $p = 0.025$).

151. **Flaherty JT**, et al. A randomized prospective trial of intravenous nitroglycerin in patients with acute MI. *Circulation* 1983;68: 576–588.

In this prospective, blinded study, 104 patients were randomized to nitroglycerin (initially 5 µg/min, goal SBP decrease of 10%) or placebo for 48 hours. Early nitroglycerin [started within 10 hours of symptoms (post hoc definition)] was associated with less cardiac death, new CHF, and infarct extension at 10 days [15% vs. 39% (other three groups); $p = 0.003$]. Also, more early treated patients had an ejection fraction improvement of 10% at 7–14 days [35% vs. 6% (late nitroglycerin) vs. 11% and 0%; $p = 0.004$]. No significant differences were observed in 3-month mortality (15% vs. 25%) or peak CK or infarct size.

152. **Mahmarian JJ**, et al. Transdermal nitroglycerin patch therapy improves left ventricular function and prevents remodeling after acute MI. *Circulation* 1998;97:2017–2024.

This prospective, randomized, double-blind, placebo-controlled trial showed a benefit of low-dose nitroglycerin patch therapy in a subgroup of patients with depressed left ventricular function. All 291 patients had baseline radionuclide angiography then were randomized to 0.4, 0.8, or 1.6 mg/h, or placebo patch. Radionuclide angiography was repeated at 6 months and 6.5 days after the patch was discontinued. The low-dose group (0.4 mg/h) had a lower end-systolic volume index (primary end point), as well as lower end-diastolic volume index (-11.4 and -11.6 mL/m^2, respectively; $p < 0.03$). This beneficial effect was observed primarily in patients with baseline ejection fraction $\leq$40% (-31 and -33 mL/m^2; both $p < 0.05$). After patch withdrawal, end-systolic volume index significantly increased, but not to pretreatment values. A larger study needs to assess whether these remodeling effects translate into fewer major cardiac events.

Calcium-Channel Blockers

153. **Wilcox RG**, et al. Trial of Early Nifedipine in Acute MI (**TRENT**). Trial of early nifedipine in acute MI: the TRENT study. *BMJ* 1986;293:1204–1208.

Design: Prospective, randomized, double-blind, placebo-controlled, multicenter study. Primary end point was all-cause mortality rate.

Purpose: To evaluate the effects of early nifedipine on mortality in acute MI patients.

Population: 4,491 patients $\leq$70 years of age presenting within 24 hours of onset of chest pain.

Exclusion Criteria: SBP <100 mm Hg or DBP <50 mm Hg, heart rate >120 beats/min, and current treatment with calcium-channel blocker.

Treatment: Nifedipine 10 mg four times daily or placebo.

Results: 64% had confirmed MI. Nifedipine was associated with a nonsignificant 7% increase in mortality at 1 month (6.7% vs. 6.3%).

154. The Multicenter Diltiazem Post-Infarction Trial (**MDPIT**) Research Group. The effect of diltiazem on mortality and reinfarction after MI. *N Engl J Med* 1988;319:385–392.
Design: Prospective, randomized, double-blind, placebo-controlled, multicenter study. Mean follow-up period was 25 months. Primary end point was total mortality, cardiac death, and nonfatal MI.
Purpose: To evaluate the effects of long-term diltiazem on mortality on reinfarction rates after documented MI.
Population: 2,466 patients 25–75 years of age with a documented MI (enzyme confirmation required).
Exclusion Criteria: Cardiogenic shock, pulmonary hypertension with right ventricular failure, second- or third-degree heart block, heart rate <50 beats/min, and requirement for calcium antagonist.
Treatment: Diltiazem 60 mg twice or four times daily, or placebo.
Results: No difference was observed in total mortality between the diltiazem and placebo groups (166 and 167 patients, respectively). However, among patients without pulmonary congestion (1,909 patients), diltiazem was associated with fewer cardiac events (hazard ratio 0.77, 95% CI 0.61–0.98), whereas diltiazem-treated patients with pulmonary congestion had more cardiac events (hazard ratio 1.41, 95% CI 1.01–1.96).

155. The Danish Study Group on Verapamil in MI (**DAVIT II**). Effect of verapamil on mortality and major events after acute MI (DAVIT II). *Am J Cardiol* 1990;66:779–785.
Design: Prospective, randomized, double-blind, placebo-controlled, multicenter study. Average follow-up period was 16 months. Primary end point was death and reinfarction.
Purpose: To evaluate the effect on total mortality and major cardiac events of verapamil started in the second week after MI.
Population: 1,975 patients <75 years of age enrolled 7–15 days after proven MI.
Exclusion Criteria: SBP <90 mm Hg, second- or third-degree heart block at 3 days, heart failure not stabilizing on furosemide ≤160 mg/day, treatment with β-blockers or calcium antagonists due to angina pectoris, arrhythmias, hypertension, postoperative infarction, and significant valvular or congenital heart disease.
Treatment: Verapamil 120 mg three times daily (once or twice daily dosing allowed in cases of adverse drug reactions), or placebo.
Results: Verapamil group had 17% fewer major events (18.0% vs. 21. 6%; *p* = 0.03) and 20% lower mortality (11.1% vs. 13.8%; *p* = 0.11). A significant mortality reduction was seen in patients without CHF (7.7% vs. 11.8%; *p* = 0.02), whereas no benefit was seen in those without CHF (17.9% vs. 17.5%).

156. **Goldbourt U**, et al. Secondary Prevention Reinfarction Israel Nifedipine Trial (**SPRINT 2**). Early administration of nifedipine in suspected acute MI. *Arch Intern Med* 1993;153:345–353.
Design: Prospective, randomized, double-blind, placebo-controlled study. Primary end point was 6-month all-cause mortality rate.
Purpose: To evaluate the effect on mortality of nifedipine started early after acute MI in high-risk patients.
Population: 1,006 patients 50–79 years of age meeting at least one of the following criteria: prior MI, angina in preceding month,

hypertension, New York Heart Association (NYHA) class II or higher, anterior MI, and lactate dehydrogenase three times the upper limit of normal.

Exclusion Criteria: Requirement for a calcium antagonist, titration to 60 mg/day not tolerated, SBP <90 mm Hg, prior heart surgery, and complete left bundle branch block or Wolff-Parkinson-White syndrome.

Treatment: Nifedipine 20 mg three times daily (6-day titration period), or placebo.

Results: Trial was terminated early. The nifedipine group had a 20% higher 6-month mortality rate (18.7% vs. 15.6%; 95% CI 0.94–1.84). The majority of the mortality difference was due to excessive mortality during the first 6 days (7.8% vs. 5.5%; CI 0.86–3.0). No differences were observed in reinfarction rates (5.1% vs. 4.2%) or in outcomes based on CHF status.

157. **Rengo F**, et al. Calcium Antagonist Reinfarction Italian Study (**CRIS**). A controlled trial of verapamil in patients after acute MI: results of the CRIS. *Am J Cardiol* 1996;77:365–369 (editorial pp. 421–422).

Design: Prospective, randomized, double-blind, placebo-controlled study. Mean follow-up period was 2 years. Primary end point was all-cause mortality rate.

Purpose: To evaluate the effects of verapamil on mortality and major cardiac end points in acute MI patients.

Population: 1,073 patients 30–75 years of age who survived 5 days after an acute MI.

Exclusion Criteria: NYHA class III/IV heart failure, heart rate <50 beats/min, SBP <90 mm Hg or >190 mm Hg, DBP >110 mm Hg, and chronic therapy with calcium antagonists or β-blockers.

Treatment: Verapamil 120 mg orally every 8 hours or placebo started 7–21 days (mean 13.8 days) after admission.

Results: No differences were observed between the verapamil and placebo groups in all-cause mortality (30 and 29 deaths, respectively). The verapamil group did have 20% fewer reinfarctions and 20% less angina.

Comments: Consistent with the CRIS data, the accompanying editorial reports that pooled data from nine trials shows that verapamil is associated with a favorable effect on reinfarction (odds ratio 0.81; 95% CI 0.67–0.98) but no overall mortality benefit (odds ratio 0.93; 95% CI 0.78–1.10).

158. Incomplete Infarction Trial of European Research Collaborators Evaluating Progressing Post-Thrombolysis (**INTERCEPT**). Preliminary results presented at the 71st AHA Scientific Session in Dallas, TX, November 1999.

A total of 874 patients at 63 European sites who received thrombolytic therapy for acute MI were randomized at 36–96 hours to long-acting diltiazem 300 mg once daily or placebo for 6 months. All patients received aspirin. At 6 months, the diltiazem group had a nonsignificant 23% relative reduction in death, MI, and refractory ischemia (22.6% vs. 29.5%). The diltiazem group did have a significant reduction in the incidence of repeat revascularization (7% vs. 12%) and a strong trend toward fewer episodes of refractory ischemia (17.2% vs. 23.2%).

159. The Danish Study Group on Verapamil in MI (**DAVIT I**). Verapamil in acute MI. *Eur Heart J* 1984;5:516–528.

This randomized trial was composed of 3,498 patients <75 years of age with suspected MI. Patients received verapamil 0.1 mg/kg intravenously followed by 120 mg orally three times daily; or matched placebo. Treatment continued for 6 months in the 1,436 patients (41%) with confirmed MI. Verapamil use was associated with a nonsignificant 9% mortality reduction at 6 months (12.8% vs. 13.9%, odds ratio 0.91; 95% CI 0.67–1.24).

160. **Behar S**, et al. **SPRINT**: a randomised intervention trial of nifedipine in patients with acute MI. *Eur Heart J* 1988;9: 354–364.

In this large randomized, placebo-controlled trial of low-dose nifedipine (30 mg once daily), patients were enrolled 7–21 days after MI and average follow-up was 10 months. No significant differences were seen in overall mortality or reinfarction rates (5.8% vs. 5.7%; 4.8% vs. 4.4%). SPRINT II was then designed to evaluate higher dose of nifedipine (157).

Magnesium

161. **Woods KL**, et al. Second Leicester Intravenous Magnesium Intervention Trial (**LIMIT-2**). Intravenous magnesium sulfate in suspected acute MI: results of LIMIT-2. *Lancet* 1992;339:1553–1558.
Design: Prospective, randomized, double-blind, placebo-controlled, single-center study. Primary end point was 28-day mortality rate.
Purpose: To evaluate the effect of intravenous magnesium on early mortality in acute MI.
Population: 2,316 patients with suspected acute MI (no ECG criteria specified) presenting within 24 hours of onset of symptoms.
Exclusion Criteria: Complete heart block, requirement for magnesium, serum creatinine >300 μM.
Treatment: Magnesium sulfate 8 mmol over 5 minutes followed by 65 mmol over 24 hours; or saline.
Results: Acute MI was confirmed in 65%. The magnesium group had a 24% lower 28-day mortality rate (7.8% vs. 10.3%; $p = 0.04$).
Comments: Long-term follow-up (mean 2.7 years) shows persistent significant mortality benefit (16%) associated with magnesium (*see Lancet* 1994;343:816).

162. **ISIS-4** Collaborative Group. ISIS-4: a randomised factorial assessing early oral captopril, oral mononitrate and intravenous magnesium sulfate in 58,050 patients with suspected acute MI. *Lancet* 1995;345:669–685.

This megatrial of 58,050 patients with suspected acute MI admitted within 24 hours of symptom onset included a randomization to intravenous magnesium sulfate (8-mmol bolus over 15 minutes and then 72 mmol over 24 hours) or no magnesium. The magnesium group had a nonsignificant 6% increase in mortality (7.64% vs. 7.24%) and a higher incidence of CHF (+12/1,000), hypotension (+11/1,000), and cardiogenic shock (+5/1,000). These data have generated much debate. Proponents of magnesium assert that magnesium was not systemically given prior to reperfusion therapy and that its benefits are not apparent because of its use in a low-risk population, whereas the ISIS-4 investigators point out that no benefit of magnesium was seen in any subgroup [e.g., those presenting within 6 hours, soon after thrombolytic therapy, with no thrombolytic therapy, in patients likely magnesium-depleted (elderly, diuretics), etc.].

163. **Horner SM**. Efficacy of intravenous magnesium in acute MI in reducing arrhythmias and mortality: meta-analysis of magnesium in acute MI. *Circulation* 1992;86:774–779.

    This analysis focused on eight randomized studies with 930 patients. Magnesium use was associated with 54% lower mortality, 49% less ventricular tachycardia and ventricular fibrillation, and 58% fewer cardiac arrests than placebo-treated patients.

164. **Shechter M**, et al. Magnesium treatment in acute MI when patients are not candidates for thrombolytic therapy. *Am J Cardiol* 1995;75:321–323.

    In this randomized, double-blind study of 194 patients ineligible for thrombolytic therapy, patients received 25 mmol (6 g) in the first 3 hours, 42 mmol over the next 21 hours, and 25 mmol over the last 24 hours, or placebo. The magnesium group had fewer arrhythmias (27% vs. 40%; $p = 0.04$), higher LVEF at 72 hours and 1–2 months (49% vs. 43%, 52% vs. 45%, both $p = 0.01$), and 79% lower in-hospital mortality rates (4% vs. 17%; $p < 0.01$).

165. **Seelig MS,** Elin RJ. Reexamination of magnesium infusions in MI. *Am J Cardiol* 1995;76:172–173.

    Several issues were discussed, including (a) time of initiation (prior to reperfusion theoretically better); (b) amount [>75 mmol may increase mortality via bradyarrhythmias (small studies, 50–65 mmol; LIMIT-2, 73 mmol; ISIS-4, variable)]; (c) length of post-MI infusion [short duration may cause tachyarrhythmias (as in smaller studies)]; and (d) use of thrombolytics (LIMIT-2, 35%; ISIS-4, 70%), with possible greater benefit in high-risk patients who are often thrombolytic ineligible.

166. **Antman EM**. Magnesium in acute MI: timing is critical. *Circulation* 1995;92:2368–2372.

    This editorial accompanies two experimental studies [Christensen CW, et al. (pp. 2617–2621), Herzog WR, et al (pp. 2622–2627)] that demonstrate that the timing of magnesium is important, best if given prior to reperfusion. Reperfusion models show that magnesium prevents calcium influx. Also, magnesium deficiency at the time of an infarct (due to dietary intake, advanced age, prior diuretic use, etc.) is associated with a larger infarct (data from 8 reports in four species). Possible mechanisms of action for benefit exist if given prior to reperfusion: (a) decreased vulnerability to oxygen free radicals; (b) decreased cytosolic calcium; (c) decreased myocardial oxygen demand via sinus slowing and decreased arterial pressure; (d) coronary vasodilatation and enhancement of collateral development; and (e) inhibition of platelet aggregation and prevention of coronary thrombosis.

167. **Antman EM**. Magnesium in acute MI: overview of available evidence. *Am Heart J* 1996;132:487–494.

    In-depth review of experimental and clinical data. LIMIT-2 and ISIS-4 designs and data are discussed most thoroughly. Magnesium appears beneficial if given prior to reperfusion in those at highest risk, such as the elderly and those ineligible for thrombolytic therapy.

Antiarrhythmics

168. **Burkart F**, et al. Basel Antiarrhythmic Study of Infarct Survival (**BASIS**). Effect of antiarrhythmic therapy on mortality in survivors of MI with asymptomatic complex ventricular arrhythmias: BASIS. *J Am Coll Cardiol* 1990;16:1711–1718.

Design: Prospective, randomized, three-center study. Follow-up period was 1 year.

Purpose: To compare individualized antiarrhythmic therapy with low-dose amiodarone and no therapy.

Population: 312 of 1,220 consecutively screened MI survivors <71 years of age with asymptomatic, complex ventricular arrhythmias (Lown class 3 or 4b) on 24-hour ECG prior to hospital discharge.

Exclusion Criteria: Death in hospital, symptomatic arrhythmias or cardiovascular surgery during hospitalization, and severe comorbidity.

Treatment: (a) Individualized: initially quinidine or mexiletine (if both failed, others tried: ajmaline, disopyramide, flecainide, propafenone, sotalol). (b) Amiodarone 1 g/day for 5 days then 200 mg/day for 1 year. (c) No therapy: drugs allowed if arrhythmias developed.

Results: Amiodarone group had a lower overall 1-year mortality rate compared with controls: 5.1% vs. 13.2% ($p < 0.05$); mortality for individually treated patients was 10% (p = NS vs. amiodarone).

Comments: Post hoc analysis showed that the benefit of amiodarone was restricted to those with an ejection fraction of 40% (1.5% vs. 8.9% 1 year mortality; $p < 0.03$) (*see Am J Cardiol* 1992;69:1399). Late follow-up showed persistent benefit of amiodarone (after discontinuation at 1 year) compared with placebo: at 7 years, 30% vs. 45% mortality (p = 0.03) (*see Circulation* 1993;87:309). An accompanying editorial points out that the data are consistent with a rebound effect of up to 31% (due to wide confidence intervals) and that further data are needed to assess whether amiodarone therapy beyond 1 year is of benefit (*see Circulation* 1993;87:637).

169. The Cardiac Arrhythmia Suppression Trial (**CAST**) Investigators. Preliminary report: effect of encainide and flecainide on mortality in a randomized trial of arrhythmia suppression after myocardial infarction. *N Engl J Med* 1989;321:406–412.

Design: Prospective, randomized, open-label (initial phase), double-blind (main phase), placebo-controlled, multicenter study. Follow-up period was 10 months.

Purpose: To evaluate whether suppression of asymptomatic or mildly asymptomatic ventricular arrhythmias after MI reduces death due to arrhythmia.

Population: 1,727 patients with MI in prior 6 days to 2 years, at least six ventricular premature contractions per hour on 24-hour Holter monitoring, ejection fraction ≤0.55 if ≤90 days after MI or ≤0.40 if >90 days after MI (if ejection fraction 30%, patients not eligible to receive flecainide), and suppressibility during open-label phase (at 4–10 days, 80% reduction of ventricular premature contractions and 90% reduction of unsustained runs of ventricular tachycardia).

Exclusion Criteria: Ventricular arrhythmias associated with severe symptoms; unsustained ventricular tachycardia with 15 beats at 120 beats/min; contraindications to drugs; and ECG abnormalities making rhythm interpretation difficult.

Treatment: Encainide 35 or 50 mg orally three times daily, flecainide 100 or 150 mg twice daily, or moricizine 200 or 250 mg three times daily.

Results: Encainide and flecainide arms were discontinued early. Encainide and flecainide patients had more arrhythmic deaths [4.5% vs. 1.2% (placebo); relative risk 3.6; 95% CI 1.7–8.5], as well as higher overall mortality (7.7% vs. 3.0%; relative risk 2.5; 95% CI 1.6–4.5).

Comments: The moricizine arm of the trial continued (170). Later analysis showed that those patients with easily suppressible arrhythmias (n = 1,778) had fewer arrhythmic deaths than the 1,173 patients with difficult to suppress arrhythmias (relative risk 0.59; p = 0.003). This likely explains the low placebo mortality rate (1.2%) (*see Circulation* 1995;91:79).

170. **CAST II** Investigators. Effect of the antiarrhythmic agent moricizine on survival after MI. *N Engl J Med* 1992;327:227–233.

Design: Prospective, randomized, open-label (titration phase), double-blind (main phase), placebo-controlled, multicenter study. Mean follow-up period was 18 months. Primary end point was death due to arrhythmia or cardiac arrest due to arrhythmia requiring resuscitation.

Purpose: To evaluate whether suppression of asymptomatic or mildly symptomatic ventricular arrhythmias after MI by moricizine reduces arrhythmia deaths.

Population: 1,325 patients in the initial 14-day phase, 1,155 patients in the long-term phase; inclusion criteria similar to CAST I (169).

Exclusion Criteria: Ventricular arrhythmias associated with severe symptoms; unsustained VT with 15 beats at 120 beats/min; contraindications to drugs; and ECG abnormalities making rhythm interpretation difficult.

Treatment: Moricizine 200 mg three times daily (initial trial), 200–300 mg three times daily (long-term trial), or placebo (both trials).

Results: In the initial 14-day trial, the moricizine group had higher mortality (2.3% vs. 0.3%, relative risk 5.6; 95% CI 1.7–19.1). In the long-term phase, the moricizine group had a nonsignificant excess of deaths (15% vs. 12%).

Comments: The trial was stopped early because of a <8% chance of observing a significant benefit if the trial were continued to completion.

171. **Waldo AL**, et al. for the Survival with Oral d-sotalol (**SWORD**) Investigators. Effect of d-sotalol on mortality in patients with left ventricular dysfunction after recent and remote MI. *Lancet* 1996;348:7–12.

Design: Prospective, randomized, double-blind, placebo-controlled, multicenter study. Mean follow-up period was 148 days. Primary end point was all-cause mortality rate.

Purpose: To determine if the NYHA class III antiarrhythmic agent d-sotalol can decrease all-cause mortality in high-risk MI survivors.

Population: 3,121 patients with ejection fraction ≤40% and recent MI (6–42 days) or symptomatic heart failure (class II or III) with remote (>42 days) MI.

Exclusion Criteria: Unstable angina, class IV heart failure, history of life-threatening arrhythmia, PTCA or CABG within the preceding 14 days, and creatinine clearance ≤50 mL/min.

Treatment: d-sotalol 200 mg orally twice daily or placebo.

Results: Trial was terminated early due to 65% higher overall mortality in the sotalol group: 5.0% vs. 3.1% ($p = 0.006$). Increased arrhythmic deaths (relative risk 1.77; $p = 0.008$) accounted for the excess mortality. The effect was greatest in those with ejection fraction ≤30% [relative risk 4.0 vs. 1.2; ejection fraction 31%–40%; $p = 0.007$).

172. **Julian DG**, et al. for the European MI Amiodarone Trial (**EMIAT**) Investigators. Randomised trial of effect of amiodarone on mortality in patients with left-ventricular dysfunction after recent MI: EMIAT. *Lancet* 1997;349:667–674 (editorial pp. 662–663).

Design: Prospective, randomized, double-blind, placebo-controlled, multicenter study. Mean follow-up period was 21 months. Primary end point was all-cause mortality rate.

Purpose: To evaluate the effect of amiodarone on mortality in post-MI patients with left ventricular dysfunction.

Population: 1,486 patients 18–75 years of age with MI in prior 5–21 days and ejection fraction ≤40% by multiple-gated nuclear angiography (~45% with ejection fraction ≤30%).

Exclusion Criteria: Amiodarone therapy in preceding 6 months, heart rate <50 beats/min, second-or third-degree atrioventricular block, significant hepatic or thyroid dysfunction, and need for antiarrhythmic(s) other than β-blockers or digoxin.

Treatment: Amiodarone 800 mg/day for 14 days, 400 mg/day for 14 weeks, and then 200 mg/day; or placebo.

Results: Among all patients, total mortality was 13.4% with no difference between amiodarone and placebo (relative risk 0.99). Also, no difference was observed in cardiac mortality (relative risk 0.94; $p = 0.67$). The amiodarone group did have fewer arrhythmic deaths (relative risk 0.35; $p = 0.04$).

Comments: Accompanying editorial points out that assignment of cause of death (e.g., arrhythmic) by committee is subjective and inexact.

173. **Cairns JA**, et al. for the Canadian Amiodarone MI Arrhythmia Trial (**CAMIAT**) Investigators. Randomised trial of outcome after MI in patients with frequent or repetitive ventricular premature depolarisations: CAMIAT. *Lancet* 1997;349:675–682 (editorial pp. 662–663).

Design: Prospective, randomized, double-blind, placebo-controlled, multicenter study. Median follow-up period was 1.8 years. Primary end point was resuscitated ventricular fibrillation or arrhythmic death.

Purpose: To determine the effect of amiodarone on overall mortality in post-MI patients with frequent or repetitive ventricular premature depolarizations.

Population: 1,202 patients with MI in prior 6–45 days, ejection fraction ≤40%, and 24-hour ECG monitoring showing 10 ventricular premature depolarizations per hour or one run of three beats of ventricular tachycardia at 100–120 beats/min.

Exclusion Criteria: Contraindications to amiodarone (prior intolerance, heart rate <50 beats/min, heart block (any degree), QT >480 msec, ventricular tachycardia at >120 beats/min.

Treatment: Amiodarone 10 mg/kg/day for 2 weeks, 300–400 mg/day for 3–5 months, 200–300 mg/day for 4 months, and 200 mg for 5–7 days/week for 16 months; or placebo.

Results: Amiodarone group with nearly 50% fewer arrhythmic deaths plus resuscitated ventricular fibrillation [3.3% vs. 6.0%; $p = 0.016$ (intention-to-treat analysis, $p = 0.029$)]. Total mortality was not different.

Comments: Primary analysis was not based on intention-to-treat analysis. The trial also had many dropouts (221 amiodarone and 152 placebo patients; >70% and >50%, respectively, stopped due to adverse effects).

174. **Ceremuzynski L**, et al. Effect of amiodarone on mortality after MI: a double-blind, placebo-controlled pilot study. *J Am Coll Cardiol* 1992;20:1056–1062.

A total of 613 MI patients not eligible to receive β-blockers were randomized to placebo or amiodarone 800 mg/day, then 400 mg six times per week. The amiodarone group had a 45% lower 1-year mortality rate (6.2% vs. 10.7%; $p = 0.048$). The amiodarone group also had fewer class 4 ventricular arrhythmias (7.5% vs. 19.7%). Mild pulmonary toxicity was seen in only one patient.

175. **Teo KK**, et al. Effects of prophylactic antiarrhythmic drug therapy in acute MI. *JAMA* 1993;270:1589–1595.

This analysis focused on 138 randomized trials with ~98,000 enrolled patients. Lower mortality was seen with β-blockers (26,973 patients; odds ratio 0.81; $p^2 = 0.00001$) and amiodarone (778 patients; odds ratio 0.71; [$p = 0.03$]). Higher mortality was seen with class I agents (11,712 patients; odds ratio 1.14; $p = 0.03$). A statistically nonsignificant impact of calcium-channel blockers was observed (10,154 patients; odds ratio 1.04; $p = 0.41$).

176. **Sadowski ZP**, et al. Multicenter randomized trial and a systematic overview of lidocaine in acute myocardial infarction. *Am Heart J* 1999;137:792–798 (editorial pp. 770–773).

A total of 903 patients presenting within 6 hours of symptom onset with ST elevation were randomized to lidocaine (four boluses of 50 mg each every 2 minutes, then 3 mg/min for 12 hours, then 2 mg/min for 36 hours) or no lidocaine. The lidocaine group had significantly less ventricular fibrillation (2.0% vs. 5.7%; $p = 0.004$) but tended toward increased mortality (9.7% vs. 7.0%; $p = 0.145$). A meta-analysis of these results and those from 20 other randomized studies with over 11,000 patients revealed nonsignificant trends toward reduced ventricular fibrillation (odds ratio 0.71; 95% CI 0.47–1.09) and increased mortality rates (odds ratio 1.12; 95% CI 0.91–1.36) with lidocaine. The accompanying editorial asserts that these results are consistent with current recommendations that lidocaine should not be given prophylactically in acute MI.

Intraaortic Balloon Pump

177. **Ohman EM**, et al. **IABP** Trial. Use of aortic counterpulsation to improve sustained coronary artery patency during acute MI. *Circulation* 1994;90:792–799.

Design: Prospective, randomized, multicenter study. Primary end point was angiographically detected reocclusion of IRA during initial hospitalization.

Purpose: To determine if 48 hours of aortic counterpulsation therapy after reperfusion established during emergent catheterization would reduce the rate of reocclusion of the IRA.

Population: 182 acute MI patients who underwent catheterization within 24 hours with successful restoration of IRA patency.

Exclusion Criteria: Cardiogenic shock, pulmonary edema requiring aortic counterpulsation, severe peripheral vascular disease, >75% restenosis in one or two major epicardial arteries and TIMI grade 2 or 3 flow achieved in IRA with thrombolytic therapy, and contraindication to heparin.

Treatment: IABP for 48 hours or standard care.

Results: Primary angioplasty was performed in 106 patients, rescue angioplasty in 51 patients, and other methods (e.g., intracoronary thrombolysis) in the remaining 25 patients. Both groups had a similar incidence of severe bleeding complications and transfusions. Catheterization performed at a median of 5 days demonstrated that the aortic counterpulsation group had a lower IRA reocclusion rate (8% vs. 21%) and nearly 50% fewer clinical events (death, stroke, reinfarction, emergency revascularization, and recurrent ischemia; 13% vs. 24%; $p < 0.04$).

178. **Stone GW**, et al. A prospective, randomized evaluation of prophylactic intraaortic balloon pump (IABP) counterpulsation in high risk patients with acute MI treated with primary angioplasty. *J Am Coll Cardiol* 1997;29:1459–1467.

Design: Prospective, randomized, multicenter study. Primary end points were death, MI, IRA occlusion, stroke, new heart failure, and sustained hypotension.

Purpose: To determine if acute MI patients stratified as high risk benefit from a routine IABP strategy after PTCA.

Population: 437 PAMI II patients classified as high risk (meeting at least one of the following criteria: age >70 years, three-vessel disease, ejection fraction ≤45%, saphenous vein graft occlusion, persistent malignant ventricular arrhythmia, or suboptimal angioplasty result).

Exclusion Criteria: Cardiogenic shock, bleeding diathesis, and thrombolytic therapy prior to catheterization.

Treatment: IABP for 36–48 hours or standard care.

Results: The two groups had similar outcomes [composite end point incidence 28.9% (IABP) vs. 29.2%]. The IABP group had fewer unscheduled repeat catheterizations (7.6% vs. 13.3%; $p = 0.05$), but had more strokes (2.4% vs. 0%; $p = 0.03$). Of note, the authors suggest that the IABP effect may not have been detected due to low control group mortality (3.1%) and IRA occlusion rate (5.5%).

179. **Ohman EM**, et al. The use of intraaortic balloon pumping as an adjunct to reperfusion therapy in acute MI. *Am Heart J* 1991; 121:895–901.

This retrospective analysis focused on 810 consecutive patients thrombolyzed within 6 hours of onset of symptoms. The balloon pump was inserted in 85 patients. This group had a higher frequency of three-vessel disease, left anterior descending artery disease, and other risk factors, as well as a high in-hospital mortality rate of 32%. Reocclusion occurred in only 2 of 85 patients (after discharge) and no reinfarctions occurred while the balloon was inserted.

180. **Kono T**, et al. Aortic counterpulsation may improve late patency of the occluded coronary artery in patients with early failure of thrombolytic therapy. *J Am Coll Cardiol* 1996;28:876–881.

A total of 45 patients with TIMI grade 0–2 flow at 60 minutes were randomized to IABP for 48 hours or conservative therapy. At 3 weeks, the IABP group had the higher TIMI grade 3 flow (74% vs. 32%; $p < 0.05$) and lower residual stenosis (42% vs. 68%; $p < 0.01$).

181. **Kovack PJ**, et al. Thrombolysis plus aortic counterpulsation: improved survival in patients who present to community hospitals with cardiogenic shock. *J Am Coll Cardiol* 1997;29:1454–1458.

This retrospective analysis focused on 27 of 46 thrombolyzed patients who had an IABP placed. The IABP group had more prior MIs, higher cardiac index (2.0 vs. 1.5), and better community hospital and 1-year survival rates (93% vs. 37%, $p < 0.001$; 67% vs. 32%, $p = 0.019$).

182. **Anderson RD**, et al. Use of intraaortic balloon bump counterpulsation in patients presenting with cardiogenic shock: observations from the GUSTO-I study. *J Am Coll Cardiol* 1997;30:708–715.

This analysis focused on 68 GUSTO I patients with cardiogenic shock who had an IABP placed (91% within 1 day). Early IABP use was associated with increased bleeding (moderate, 47% vs. 12%, $p = 0.0001$; severe, 10% vs. 5%, $p = 0.16$). IABP use also was associated with increased arrhythmias, procedures, and bypass surgery. However, these increases were due to longer time to death (2.8 days vs. 7.2 hours). However, in part a trend toward lower 30-day mortality was seen with IABP use [57% vs. 67%, adjusted $p = 0.11$ (if revascularization patients were excluded, 47% vs. 64%, $p = 0.07$)].

Other Treatments

183. **Malmberg K**, et al. Diabetic Insulin-Glucose Infusion in Acute MI (**DIGAMI**). Randomized trial of insulin-glucose infusion followed by subcutaneous insulin treatment in diabetic patients with acute MI: effects on mortality at 1 year. *J Am Coll Cardiol* 1995;26:57–65.

Design: Prospective, randomized, open, multicenter study. Primary end point was all-cause mortality.

Purpose: To evaluate whether rapid improvement of metabolic control in diabetic patients with an insulin-glucose infusion decreases early mortality and subsequent morbidity.

Population: 620 patients with suspected MI and blood glucose 11 mM on admission (with or without prior diagnosis of diabetes).

Exclusion Criteria: Severe comorbidity.

Treatment: Continuous intravenous insulin infusion for 24 hours (started at 5 U/h) or until normoglycemia was achieved (goal of 7–10 mM); then subcutaneous insulin for 3 months; or conventional therapy.

Results: At 24 hours, the insulin-treated patients had lower glucose (9.6 vs. 11.7 mM) and 29% lower mortality at 1 year (18.6% vs. 26.1%; p = 0.027). Mortality reduction was most marked (52%) in patients with a low cardiovascular risk profile or no previous insulin therapy. Only 10% stopped insulin due to hypoglycemia with no associated morbidity.

Comments: Intense insulin may restore impaired platelet function, decrease PAI-1 activity, and possibly improve metabolism of noninfarcted areas. Long-term follow-up (*see BMJ* 1997;314:1512) showed that lower mortality was maintained at a mean 3.4 years: 33% vs. 44% (relative risk 0.72; p = 0.011), with the largest benefit seen in patients with no prior insulin therapy (relative risk 0.49).

184. **Diaz R**, et al. on behalf of the Estudios Cardiologicos Latinoamerica (**ECLA**) Glucose-Insulin-Potassium Pilot Trial Collaborative Group. Metabolic modulation of acute MI. *Circulation* 1998;98:2227–2234 (editorial pp. 2223–2226).

Design: Prospective, randomized, open, multicenter study.

Purpose: To evaluate the feasibility of glucose-insulin-potassium (GIK) administration in contemporary practice and to assess its effect on clinical end points in patients with acute MI.

Population: 407 patients with suspected acute MI presenting within 24 hours of symptom onset.

Exclusion Criteria: Severe renal impairment or hyperkalemia.

Treatment: high dose GIK (25% glucose, 50 IU insulin/L and 80 mM KCl at 1.5 mL/kg/h for 24 hours), low-dose GIK (10% glucose, 20 IU insulin/L, and 40 mM KCl at 1.0 mL/kg/h for 24 hours), or control. GIK was started an average 10–11 hours after onset of symptoms.

Results: GIK-treated patients had nonsignificant reductions in several in-hospital events, including severe heart failure, cardiogenic shock, ventricular fibrillation, and reinfarction. Among the 252 patients (61.9%) treated with reperfusion strategies (thrombolysis, 95%; PTCA, 5%), GIK-treated patients had a significant 66% reduction in in-hospital mortality (5.2% vs. 15.2%; relative risk 0.34; p = 0.008). At 1-year follow-up, only the high-dose GIK patients undergoing reperfusion had a significant mortality benefit (relative risk 0.37, log rank test 0.046). The GIK group did have a higher frequency of phlebitis (severe in only 2%) and serum changes in plasma concentration of glucose or potassium

Comments: High-dose regimen achieves maximal suppression of free fatty acid levels (*see Am J Cardiol* 1975;36:929). A meta-analysis of 1932 patients showed no interaction between GIK and reperfusion. The accompanying editorial points out the unusually high control group mortality in this study and concurs with the authors that larger randomized trials are necessary before such therapy becomes standard practice.

185. **Iliceto S**, et al. on behalf of the L-Carnitine Ecocardiografia Digitalizzata Infarcto Miocardico (**CEDIM**) Investigators. Effects of L-

carnitine administration on left ventricular remodeling after acute MI: CEDIM trial. *J Am Coll Cardiol* 1995;26:380–387.

This randomized trial was composed of 472 patients with a first MI. They were randomized within 24 hours to intravenous infusion 9 g/d for 5 days, then 2 g orally three times daily for 1 year, or placebo. L-carnitine patients had a smaller increase in end-diastolic volume and end-systolic volume at 3, 6, and 12 months (of note, prior studies had have shown fewer adverse events with limitation of left ventricular dilatation (*see Circulation* 1994;89:68). No differences were seen in LVEF. After hospital discharge, the L-carnitine group had a nonsignificant reduction in death and CHF (6% vs. 9.6%).

186. **Fath-Ordoubadi F**, et al. Glucose-insulin-potassium therapy for treatment of acute MI. *Circulation* 1997;96:1156 (editorial pp. 1074–1077).

This analysis focused on nine well-designed randomized, placebo-controlled trials with 1,932 patients (all prethrombolytic era). GIK was associated with lower hospital mortality (16.1% vs. 21%, odds ratio 0.72; $p = 0.004$). A 48% reduction was seen in the four trials using high-dose GIK (to maximally suppress free fatty acid levels).

Specific Cases

Anterior MI

187. **Stone PH**, et al. Prognostic significance of location and type of MI: independent adverse outcome associated with anterior location. *J Am Coll Cardiol* 1988;11:453–463.

This retrospective analysis focused on 471 Multicenter Investigation of the Limitation of Infarct Size (MILIS) patients with a first MI showing anterior location associated with poor outcome. Anterior versus inferior patients: larger infarcts (higher CK-MB fraction; $p < 0.001$), approximately three times more heart failure (40.7% vs. 14.7%), more than four times more in-hospital deaths (11.9% vs. 2. 8%; $p < 0.001$), and higher cumulative cardiac mortality (27% vs. 11%; $p < 0.001$). Q wave vs. non–Q wave: worse in-hospital course [higher CK-MB, lower ejection fraction, more heart failure and deaths (9.3% vs. 4.1%; $p < 0.05$)], but no significant difference in long-term cardiac mortality (21% vs. 16%). After adjustment for infarct size, anterior patients still had higher mortality rates. If location and type were considered, anterior patients still had worse outcomes (whether Q wave or non–Q wave).

188. **Shalev Y**, et al. Does the electrocardiographic pattern of "anteroseptal" MI correlate with the anatomic location of myocardial injury? *Am J Cardiol* 1995;75:763–766.

Analysis of 80 patients who underwent echocardiography and angiography. Among patients with ST elevation in leads in V1 to V3, 48 of 52 (92%) had an anteroapical infarct and a normal septum. Lesions were located in the mid to distal left anterior descending artery in 85%. These data challenge the current ECG definition of anteroseptal MI (Q or QS >0.03 seconds in V1–V3, ±V4).

Inferior MI

189. **Nicod P**, et al. Long-term outcome in patients with inferior MI and complete atrioventricular block. *J Am Coll Cardiol* 1988; 12:589–594.

Retrospective analysis of 749 patients at four centers. The complete heart block group (12.8%) had a nearly four times higher in-hospital mortality rate (24.2% vs. 6.3%; $p < 0.001$). However, there was no difference seen in postdischarge 1 year mortality rates (10.1% vs. 6.4%; p = NS) or reinfarction (both 4%).

190. **Berger PB**, et al. Incidence and prognostic implications of heart block complicating inferior MI treated with thrombolytic therapy: results from TIMI II. *J Am Coll Cardiol* 1992;20:533–540.

This retrospective analysis focused on 1,786 patients. Complete heart block occurred in 12% (6.3% at presentation). The complete heart block group had a higher unadjusted 21-day mortality rate (7.1% vs. 2.7%; p = 0.007), but adjusted relative risk was not statistically significant. Mortality was nearly five times higher in those with complete heart block after thrombolysis (9.9% vs. 2.2%; $p < 0.001$). Increased deaths were attributable to more severe cardiac dysfunction.

191. **Behar S**, et al. Complete atrioventricular block complicating inferior acute wall MI: short and long-term prognosis. *Am Heart J* 1993;125:1622–1627.

This analysis focused on 2,273 SPRINT Registry patients with inferior Q-wave MIs. An 11% incidence of complete heart block was observed (women, 14%; 70 years of age, 15%). The complete heart block group had more than a threefold higher in-hospital mortality rate (37% vs. 11%, $p < 0.0001$; adjusted odds ratio 2.0; 95% CI 1.12–3.57). However, no difference in 5 year mortality was observed among hospital survivors (28% vs. 23%).

192. **Peterson ED**, et al. Prognostic significance of precordial ST segment depression during inferior MI in the thrombolytic era: results in 16,521 patients. *J Am Coll Cardiol* 1996;28: 305–312.

This post hoc GUSTO-I analysis focused on 6,422 patients without any precordial depression. The ST depression group had a 47% higher 30-day mortality rate (4.7% vs. 3.2%; at 1 year, 5% vs. 3.4%; $p < 0.001$). Magnitude of depression (sum of V1–6) added significant prognostic information after risk factor adjustment: 36% higher mortality per 0.5 mm.

193. **Bates ER**. Revisiting reperfusion therapy in inferior MI. *J Am Coll Cardiol* 1997;30:334–342.

This review article argues that thrombolytic therapy may not be helpful in low-risk patients (2%–4% mortality) or those with symptoms for >6 hours. High-risk patients include those with left precordial ST depression, complete atrioventricular block, and right precordial ST elevation. Review of data shows no advantage of angioplasty advantage over thrombolysis. However, the use of angioplasty is recommended in cardiogenic shock.

194. **Strasberg B**, et al. Left and right ventricular function in inferior acute MI and significance of advanced atrioventricular block. *Am J Cardiol* 1984;54:985–987.

This analysis focused on 139 patients with first inferior MI; 19% developed second-degree or complete heart block. The advanced block group had lower left and right ventricular ejection fractions (51% vs. 58%, $p < 0.01$; 32% vs. 39%, $p < 0.001$), higher left and right ventricular wall motion scores (5.6 vs. 3.1,

$p < 0.001$; 3.4 vs. 1.5, $p < 0.002$), and a trend toward higher mortality rates (15% vs. 6%).

195. **Matetzky S**, et al. Significance of ST segment elevations in posterior chest leads (V7 to V9) in patients with acute inferior MI: application for thrombolytic therapy. *J Am Coll Cardiol* 1998;31: 506–511.

   This analysis showed that ST elevation in V7 to V9 correlates with posterolateral involvement, and such patients benefit more from thrombolysis. Eighty-seven patients who had a first inferior MI and were treated with rt-PA were stratified according to the presence (46 patients) or absence (41 patients) of ST elevation in V7 to V9. The ST elevation group had a higher incidence of posterolateral wall motion abnormalities ($p < 0.001$) on radionuclide ventriculography, a larger infarct area (higher peak CK, $p < 0.02$), lower predischarge ejection fraction ($p < 0.008$), and higher incidence of death, reinfarction, or heart failure ($p < 0.05$). Patency of the IRA in the V7 to V9 elevation group resulted in an improved ejection fraction at discharge ($p < 0.012$), whereas ejection fraction in the nonelevation patients was unchanged, regardless of IRA patency.

Right Ventricular Infarction

196. **Mavric Z**, et al. Prognostic significance of complete atrioventricular block in patients with acute inferior MI with and without right ventricular involvement. *Am Heart J* 1990;119:823–828.

   This retrospective analysis focused on 243 patients with an acute inferior MI and complete heart block, 19% with a right ventricular infarction (≥1 mm ST elevation in V3R or V4R). Among complete heart block patients, right ventricular infarction was associated with a nearly fourfold higher mortality rate than inferior only patients (41% vs. 11%; $p < 0.05$). If no complete heart block was present, no mortality difference was observed between inferior MI and right ventricular infarction (14% vs. 11%; $p = $NS), and no increased mortality was associated with complete heart block if no right ventricular infarction was present..

197. **Zehender M**, et al. Right ventricular infarction as an independent predictor of prognosis after acute MI. *N Engl J Med* 1993; 328:981–988 (editorial pp. 1036–1038).

   This analysis of 200 consecutive patients showed that ST elevation in lead V4R was highly predictive of right ventricular infarction: sensitivity 88%, specificity 78%. ST elevation in V4R also was associated with higher mortality (31% vs. 19% overall) and more in-hospital complications (64% vs. 28%).

198. **Kinch JW**, Ryan TJ. Right ventricular infarction. *N Engl J Med* 1994;330:1211–1217.

   This excellent overview discusses the pathophysiology, diagnosis, complications, treatment, and prognosis of patients with right ventricular infarction.

199. **Zehender M**, et al. Eligibility for and benefit of thrombolytic therapy in inferior MI: focus on the prognostic importance of right ventricular infarction. *J Am Coll Cardiol* 1994;24:362–369.

   This prospective analysis focused on 200 patients with an inferior MI. Thrombolytic therapy (accelerated tPA regimen) was received by 36%; this group of patients had a lower mortality than patients ineligible for tPA (8% vs 25%, p <0.001). However, benefit of tPA was restricted to patients with right ventricular infarction (RVI) complicating acute inferior MI: 76% lower mortality (10% vs. 42%; $p < 0.005$) and fewer overall complications (34% vs. 54%; $p < 0.05$). In the absence of RVI, no difference was observed in mortality (7% vs 6%), whether or not patient received tPA.

200. **Bowers TR**, et al. Effect of reperfusion on biventricular function and survival after right ventricular infarction. *N Engl J Med* 1998;338:933–940 (editorial pp. 978–980).

This prospective study was composed of 53 inferior MI patients with echocardiographic evidence of right ventricular infarction (right ventricular free-wall dysfunction, dilatation, and depressed global performance). Complete reperfusion was achieved by balloon angioplasty in 77% of patients (i.e., normal flow in right coronary artery and its major right ventricular branches) and led to recovery of right ventricular function [mean score for free-wall motion 1.4 (at 3 days) vs. 3.0 (baseline); $p < 0.001$]. In contrast, unsuccessful reperfusion (no right ventricular branch flow) was associated with a lack of right ventricular recovery, as well as persistent hypotension and low cardiac output (83% vs. 12%; $p = 0.002$) and markedly higher mortality (58% vs. 2%; $p = 0.001$).

201. **Zeymer U**, et al. Effects of thrombolytic therapy in acute inferior MI with or without right ventricular involvement. *J Am Coll Cardiol* 1998;32:876–881.

This analysis of 522 inferior MI patients from the HIT-4 trial showed that right ventricular involvement is not an independent predictor of survival. Right ventricular involvement was associated with higher 30-day cardiac mortality rates (5.9% vs. 2.5%), but this was related to larger infarct size rather than to right ventricular infarction. Among large inferior MI patients (sum ST elevation >0.8 mV or precordial depression), a proximal right coronary artery lesion was seen in 52% with and 23% without right ventricular infarction. Among small MI patients, lesions were mostly distal in location, and cardiac mortality was <1% irrespective of the presence of right ventricular infarction.

202. **Bueno H**, et al. In-hospital outcome of elderly patients with acute inferior MI and right ventricular involvement. *Circulation* 1997;96:436–441.

This study highlighted the high mortality of right ventricular infarction in the elderly. This retrospective analysis focused on 198 consecutive patients ≥75 years of age with a first inferior MI, complicated by right ventricular infarction in 41% (ST elevation ≥0.1 mm in V3R or V4R and/or right ventricular free wall motion abnormalities or right ventricular dilatation). Right ventricular infarction was associated with a more than fourfold higher in-hospital mortality rate (47% vs. 10%; $p < 0.001$), mostly due to increased cardiogenic shock (32% vs. 5%). Increased complete heart block (33% vs. 9%) and rupture of the intraventricular septum (9% vs. 0%) also were observed. After risk factor adjustment (age, sex, diabetes, shock on admission, left ventricular function, atrioventricular block), the relative risk of mortality with right ventricular infarction was still 4.0 (95% CI 1.3–14.2).

203. **Shiraki H**, et al. Association between preinfarction angina and a lower risk of right ventricular infarction. *N Engl J Med* 1998; 338:941–947.

This retrospective analysis focused on 113 patients with a first MI due to occlusion of the right coronary artery. Absence of preinfarction angina (defined as chest pain <30 minutes ≤7 days before MI) was a strong predictor of right ventricular infarction (odds ratio 6.3; $p < 0.001$), complete atrioventricular block (odds ratio 3.6; $p = 0.01$), and combined hypotension and shock (odds ratio 12.4; $p < 0.001$). Angina in the preceding 24–72 hours was associated with a lower incidence of right ventricular infarction (odds ratio 0.2; $p = 0.02$) and hypotension/shock (odds ratio 0.1; $p = 0.02$).

Posterior MI

204. **Boden WE**, et al. Electrocardiographic evolution of posterior acute MI: importance of early precordial ST-segment depression. *Am J Cardiol* 1987;59:782–787.

   This analysis focused on 50 patients from the Diltiazem Reinfarction Study who had isolated precordial ST-segment elevation of ≥1 mm in at least two precordial leads (V1–V4). Serial ECGs showed that 46% developed evidence of posterior MI, defined as R-wave ≥0.04 seconds in lead V1 and R:S ≥1 in V2. The posterior group had a higher peak CK than the anterior group (1,051 vs. 663 IU; $p < 0.009$). All 23 posterior MI patients had horizontal ST depression and upright precordial T waves versus downsloping ST depression and T-wave inversion in 27 patients with an anterior non–Q-wave MI.

205. **Casas RE**, et al. Value of leads V7–V9 in diagnosing posterior wall acute MI and other causes of tall R waves in V1–V2. *Am J Cardiol* 1997;80:508–509.

   This retrospective analysis focused on 250 hospitalized patients with V7 to V9 leads obtained because of tall R in V1 and/or suspicion of posterior MI. A total of 110 patients (44%) had evidence of a new or old posterior MI; in 25%, they were the only leads diagnostic of MI.

Cocaine-associated MI

206. **Hollander JE**, et al. Prospective multicenter evaluation of cocaine-associated chest pain. *Acad Emerg Med* 1994;1:330–339.

   This prospective cohort study was composed of 246 patients with cocaine-associated chest pain. Pain began at a median 60 minutes after cocaine use and persisted for 120 minutes. Fourteen patients (5.7%) had a confirmed MI (elevated CK-MB). ECG showed a low sensitivity (35.7%) and high specificity (89.9%). No clinical differences were seen between those with and without MI.

207. **Hollander JE**. The management of cocaine-associated myocardial ischemia. *N Engl J Med* 1995;333:1267–1272.

   This review covers pathophysiology, initial evaluation, treatment, complications, diagnostic evaluation, long-term prognosis, and secondary prevention of cocaine-associated ischemia.

208. **Hollander JE**, et al. Predictors of coronary artery disease in patients with cocaine-associated MI. *Am J Med* 1997;102:158–163.

   This retrospective analysis focused on 70 patients from 29 centers. CAD was demonstrated in 49 patients (≥50% stenosis or positive stress test result). This group was older (42 vs. 31 years of age) and had more cardiac risk factors (2.3 vs. 1.5), hypertension (odds ratio 5.3), and bradyarrhythmias (odds ratio 8.0). A greater percentage also had inferior location ($p = 0.04$).

Non–Q-wave/Non-ST Elevation MI

See Chapter 3.

Assessment and Prognosis
General Review Articles

209. **Reeder GS,** Gibbons RJ. Acute MI: risk stratification in the thrombolytic era. *Mayo Clin Proc* 1995;70:87–94.

This thorough review of postthrombolytic therapy risk stratification focuses on noninvasive imaging, which is less predictive of late events in this patient population.

210. **Shaw LJ**, et al. A meta-analysis of pre-discharge risk stratification after acute MI with stress electrocardiography myocardial perfusion and ventricular function imaging. *Am J Cardiol* 1996;78:1327–1337.

This analysis of 54 studies (76% retrospective) with 19,874 patients shows the low positive predictive value of predischarge noninvasive testing.

211. **Peterson ED**, et al. ACP Guidelines. Guidelines for risk stratification after MI. *Ann Intern Med* 1997;126:556–560 (pt I), 561–582 (pt II).

Risk stratification was divided into three phases: acute evaluation, cardiac care unit phase, and hospital phase. During the initial evaluation, several baseline risk factors can be identified that are predictive of poor outcome: age, SBP, heart rate, heart failure on physical examination, infarct location, and history of prior MI. During the acute phase, patients with ST elevation or new left bundle branch block (25%–45%) should be identified and undergo reperfusion therapy (e.g., thrombolytic therapy, balloon angioplasty). During the cardiac care unit phase, patients given thrombolytic therapy should be monitored closely for evidence of reperfusion (resolution of pain and ST elevation); rescue angioplasty should be considered if reperfusion is not achieved. During the hospital phase, high-risk patients (e.g., CHF, recurrent ischemia, ventricular arrhythmias) should be considered for cardiac catheterization. Intermediate and low-risk patients should have a clinical evaluation of left ventricular function. The ~50%–60% of patients with a predicted ejection fraction of less than 40% or indeterminate clinical assessment should undergo testing to evaluate left ventricular function. If the ejection fraction is confirmed to be <40%, cardiac catheterization should be considered. Most patients with an ejection fraction of ≥40% should undergo noninvasive testing (e.g., ETT with or without pharmacologic stress imaging) prior to hospital discharge.

Electrocardiography, Arrhythmias, and Conduction System

212. **Volpi A**, et al. In-hospital prognosis of patients with acute MI complicated by primary ventricular fibrillation. *N Engl J Med* 1987;317:257–261.

This analysis focused on 11,112 GISSI patients. Primary ventricular fibrillation (defined as not due to shock or MI) occurred in 2.8% and was associated with a nearly twofold higher in-hospital mortality rate (10.8% vs. 5.9%, relative risk 1.94; 95% CI 1.35–2.78).

213. Multicenter Investigation of the Limitation of Infarct Size (**MILIS**). Prognosis after cardiac arrest due to ventricular tachycardia or ventricular fibrillation associated with acute MI. *Am J Cardiol* 1987;60:755–761.

This analysis focused on 849 MILIS study patients ≤75 years of age with a confirmed MI. Mean follow-up period was 32 months. Ventricular tachycardia and ventricular fibrillation patients had a fourfold higher in-hospital mortality rate (27% vs. 7%; $p < 0.001$). This difference was attributable to a sevenfold higher risk in patients with secondary causes of ventricular tachycardia and ventricular fibrillation (e.g., presence of heart failure, hypotension). A worse outcome was attained if the episode occurred after 72 hours (57% vs. 20%; $p < 0.05$). Of note, no cases of primary ventricular tachycardia and ventricular fibrillation occurred after 72 hours. No difference in mortality at follow-up was seen among hospital survivors.

214. **Berger PB**, et al. Incidence and significance of ventricular tachycardia and fibrillation in the absence of hypotension or heart failure in acute MI treated with recombinant tissue-type plasminogen activator: results from the Thrombolysis in Myocardial Infarction (TIMI) Phase II trial. *J Am Coll Cardiol* 1993;22: 1773–1779.

This analysis focused on 2,456 TIMI II patients without CHF or hypotension during the first 24 hours after study entry. Sustained ventricular tachycardia or ventricular fibrillation developed in 1.9% within 24 hours. Among patients undergoing angiography at 18 to 48 hours (per protocol), the ventricular tachycardia and ventricular fibrillation group had lower IRA patency (68% vs. 87%; $p = 0.01$). Mortality at 21 days was >10 times higher in the ventricular tachycardia and ventricular fibrillation patients (20.4% vs. 1.6%; $p < 0.001$). Survival from 21 days to 1 year was similar in both groups.

215. **Schroder R**, et al. Extent of early ST segment elevation resolution: a strong predictor of outcome in patients with acute MI and a sensitive measure to compare thrombolytic regimens. *J Am Coll Cardiol* 1995;26:1657–1664.

This prospective study was composed of 1,398 INJECT trial patients presenting within 6 hours of symptoms. ST-segment resolution at 3 hours was classified into three groups: complete (>70%), partial (30%–70%), and no (<30%) resolution. 35-day mortality rates in these groups were 2.5%, 4.3%, and 17.5% ($p < 0.0001$). Even after baseline characteristics were included, ST resolution was the most powerful predictor of 35-day mortality.

216. **Gill JB**, et al. Prognostic importance of myocardial ischemia detected by ambulatory monitoring early after acute MI. *N Engl J Med* 1996;334:65–70.

This study of 406 patients showed the independent prognostic value of ischemia on ambulatory ECG monitoring. Patients underwent 48 hours of monitoring at 5–7 days, and if possible, a predischarge submaximal stress test and ejection fraction assessment within 28 days. Ischemia on monitoring was seen in 23%; this group had a much higher 1-year mortality rate (16.6% vs. 3.9%; $p = 0.009$). The highest mortality rate occurred in patients without exercise tests and an ejection fraction <35% (16.4% and 18.2%). In a multiple regression analysis, ambulatory monitoring emerged as the only test that provided additional prognostic information (beyond that provided by clinical data), with a relative risk of 2.3 of death and nonfatal MI. The accompanying editorial points out that ACIP Pilot angiographic data showed most patients with ambulatory ischemia had complex coronary plaques as well as proximal lesions. It remains unclear if ambulatory ischemia is predictive of long-term outcomes, and its relationship to thallium scanning needs study.

217. **Mont L**, et al. Predisposing factors and prognostic value of sustained monomorphic ventricular tachycardia in early phase of acute MI. *J Am Coll Cardiol* 1996;28:1670–1676.

This retrospective analysis focused on 1,120 consecutive cardiac care unit patients. The incidence of monomorphic ventricular tachycardia was 1.9%. This group had larger infarcts (peak CK-MB 435 vs. 168 IU/L) and four times higher mortality (43% vs. 11%; $p < 0.001$). Ventricular tachycardia was an independent mortality predictor, whereas independent predictors of ventricular tachycardia were CK-MB (odds ratio 11.8), Killip class (odds ratio 4, 0), and bifascicular block (odds ratio 3.1).

218. **Jensen GVH**, et al. Does in-hospital ventricular fibrillation affect prognosis after MI? *Eur Heart J* 1997;18:919–924.

This retrospective analysis focused on the prospective registry of 4,259 patients at one center (during 1977–1988, thrombolytics, aspirin and β-blockers were not routinely used). In-hospital ventricular fibrillation occurred in 12.4%. Unadjusted in-hospital mortality was lower in primary ventricular fibrillation patients ($p < 0.0001$). In multivariate analysis, odds ratios for death on days 6–30 were 6.3 for primary ventricular fibrillation and 4.1 for ventricular fibrillation due to heart failure. If the patient survived 1 month, no prognostic value was observed (relative risk 1.11; $p = 0.26$). In logistic regression analysis, the prognostic importance of ventricular fibrillation was exhausted after 60 days.

219. **Crenshaw BS**, et al. Atrial fibrillation in the setting of acute MI: the GUSTO-I experience. *J Am Coll Cardiol* 1997;30:406–413.

Atrial fibrillation on admission ECG in 2.5%, rising to 7.9% after study enrollment. The group with early *and* late atrial fibrillation had more three-vessel disease, less TIMI grade 3 flow, more in-hospital strokes (3.1% vs. 1.3%; $p = 0.0001$), and more than twofold higher unadjusted 30-day *and* 1-year mortality rates (14.3% vs. 6.2%, $p = 0.0001$; 21.5% vs. 8.6%, $p < 0.0001$). In multivariate analysis, late atrial fibrillation predictors were age, peak CK, Killip class, and heart rate. Adjusted odds ratios of mortality were 1.1 for baseline atrial fibrillation (85% CI 0.88–1.3) and 1.4 for late atrial fibrillation (95% CI 1.3–1.5).

220. **Hathaway WR**, et al. Prognostic significance of the initial electrocardiogram in patients with acute MI. *JAMA* 1998;279:387–391.

This retrospective analysis focused on 34,166 GUSTO-I patients without paced or ventricular rhythms or left bundle branch block. In multivariate analysis, 30-day mortality predictors were found to be the sum of ST deviation (depression and elevation; odds ratio 1.53), heart rate (odds ratio 1.49), QRS duration (for anterior MIs, odds ratio 1.55), and ECG evidence of prior MI (for new inferior MI, odds ratio 2.47).

221. **Volpi A**, et al. Incidence and prognosis of early primary ventricular fibrillation in acute MI—results of the GISSI-2 database. *Am J Cardiol* 1998;82:265–271.

This retrospective analysis focused on 9,720 patients with a first MI. Early (≤4 hours) and late (>4 to 48 hours) late primary ventricular fibrillation occurred in 3.1% and 0.6%, respectively. Recurrence rates were 11% and 15%. Early primary ventricular fibrillation occurred more frequently if SBP < 120 mm Hg and in the presence of hypokalemia. In-hospital mortality was higher in patients with both early and late primary ventricular fibrillation [odds ratios 2.47 (95% CI 1.48–4.13) and 3.97 (95% CI 1.51–10.48)]. Mortality from hospital discharge to 6 months was similar for both primary ventricular fibrillation subgroups and controls.

222. **Go AS**, et al. Bundle-branch block and in-hospital mortality in acute MI. *Ann Intern Med* 1998;129:690–697.

This large retrospective cohort study of 297,832 patients from 1571 hospitals showed that the prevalences of right and left bundle branch block are similar (6.2% and 6.7%, respectively) and that right bundle branch block is a stronger independent predictor of in-hospital death [adjusted odds ratio 1.64 vs. 1.34 (left bundle branch block)].

223. **Cheema AN**, et al. Nonsustained ventricular tachycardia in the setting of acute MI. *Circulation* 1998;98:2030–2036.

This prospective database analysis showed that contrary to prevailing opinion, nonsustained ventricular tachycardia that occurs beyond several hours after acute MI is associated with adverse outcomes. Nonsustained ventricular tachycardia was identified in 118 patients within 72 hours of acute MI. The control group was matched for age, sex, type of MI, and thrombolytic therapy. The nonsustained ventricular tachycardia group had more frequent in-hospital ventricular fibrillation (9% vs. 0%; $p < 0.001$) but in-hospital mortality (10% vs. 4%) and follow-up mortality (10% vs. 17%) were not significantly different. However, a multivariate analysis showed that time from presentation to nonsustained ventricular tachycardia was the strongest mortality predictor (risk became significant at 13 hours and peaked at 24 hours; relative risk 7.5).

224. **Savonitto S**, et al. Prognostic value of the admission electrocardiogram in acute coronary syndromes. *JAMA* 1999;281:707–713 (editorial pp. 753–754).

This retrospective analysis focused on 12,142 GUSTO IIb patients. Presenting ECG characteristics included T-wave inversion in 22%, ST elevation in 28%, ST depression in 35%, and 15% with a combination of ST elevation and depression. The 30-day incidence of death or MI was 5.5% in patients with T-wave inversion, 9.4% in those with ST elevation, 10.5% in those with ST depression, and 12.4% in those with both ST elevation and depression. After adjusting for factors associated with increased death or MI at 30 days, compared to those with T-wave inversion only, patients with ST segment changes were at significantly increased risk (odds ratios 1.68, 1.62, and 2.27 for ST elevation, ST depression, and both, respectively). Admission CK levels were associated with increased risk of death (odds ratio 2.36) and death or MI (odds ratio 1.56). In a multivariate analysis, ECG category and CK levels at admission remained highly predictive of death and MI.

Exercise Testing

225. **Hamm LF**, et al. Safety and efficacy of exercise testing early after acute MI. *Am J Cardiol* 1989;63:1193–1197.

This analysis focused on 151,949 tests performed at 570 institutions; 42% were symptom-limited tests. Overall, only 41 fatal (0.03%) and 141 major cardiac complications (0.09%) were noted. Symptom-limited testing was associated with a similar mortality rate, but with 1.9 times more major cardiac complications.

226. **Chaitman BR**, et al. Impact of treatment strategy on predischarge exercise test in TIMI-II. *Am J Cardiol* 1993;71:131–138.

This analysis focused on 3,339 patients showing a fourfold higher 1-year mortality rate if no predischarge exercise test was done (7.7% vs. 1.8%; $p < 0.001$). No predictive value of ST depression or chest pain was observed: conservative, relative risk 0.6 (95% CI 0.1–2.9); invasive, relative risk 2.1 (95% CI 0.5–9.4). However, catheterization and revascularization are recommended if ETT is positive.

227. **Jain A**, et al. Comparison of symptom-limited and low level exercise tolerance tests early after MI. *J Am Coll Cardiol* 1993;22: 1816–1820.

This analysis focused on 150 consecutive patients [44 others were excluded (death, ischemia at rest or with minimal ambulation, complications, physician/patient preference)]. Bruce protocol was performed at 6.4 ± 3.1 days. Low-level test results were positive in only 23% versus 40% with symptom-limited tests ($p < 0.001$). At follow-up (15 ± 5 months), only five patients with a negative maximal test result versus 14 patients with a nondiagnostic symptom-limited test had cardiac events.

228. **Travin MI**, et al. Use of exercise technetium-99m sestamibi SPECT imaging to detect residual ischemia and for risk stratification after acute MI. *Am J Cardiol* 1995;75:665–669.

This study was composed of 134 patients tested within 14 days of acute MI. Ischemia was detected by SPECT in 11 of 13 (85%) patients who had subsequent cardiac events (mean follow-up 15 months), whereas chest pain only identified 23% and ECG 31%. If three sestamibi defects were detected, the event rate was 38%. Of note, among thrombolyzed patients (40%), extent of ischemia remained a strong correlate ($p = 0.008$) of events.

229. **Zaret BL**, et al. Value of radionuclide rest and exercise left ventricular in assessing survival of patients after thrombolytic therapy for acute MI: results of TIMI II Study. *J Am Coll Cardiol* 1995;26:73–79.

A total of 2,567 patients were studied at average 9 hours after onset of symptoms. Rest ejection fraction was strongly associated with 1 year mortality (overall 9.9%). The relative risk for ejection fraction of 30%–39% was 3.1; 40%–49%, 2.2; 50%–59%, 1.2. The differential between rest and exercise ejection fraction was not helpful.

230. **Villella A**, et al. Prognostic significance of maximal exercise testing after MI treated with thrombolytic agents: the GISSI-2 data base. *Lancet* 1995;346:523–529.

This post hoc analysis focused on 6,295 GISSI-2 patients tested an average of 28 days after acute MI. Interestingly, the same mortality rate (7.1%) was observed among those with a positive ETT result as those who did not undergo testing; lower rates were associated with nondiagnostic and negative tests (1.3% and 0.9%, respectively). Independent predictors of mortality were symptomatic ischemia and low work capacity (relative risks 2.1 and 1.8).

231. **Vanhees L**, et al. Comparison of maximum vs. submaximal exercise testing in providing prognostic information after acute MI and/or coronary artery bypass grafting. *Am J Cardiol* 1997;80: 257–262.

This retrospective analysis focused on 527 patients (MI, n = 297; bypass surgery, n = 119; both, n = 111) with a maximal test result at 12.9 ± 2.7 weeks after the event. After adjustments, peak oxygen uptake significantly related to all-cause and total mortality [hazard ratios 0.43 ($p < 0.05$) and 0.31 ($p < 0.01$)]. Five metabolic equivalents (METS) and anaerobic threshold were not predictive of mortality. In contrast, 7 METS (reached by 37%, encompasses 94% of events) was a strong predictor: hazard ratios 0.16 and 0.15 (both $p < 0.01$) and had excellent diagnostic accuracy (loss of specificity with a cutoff of 8 METS).

Echocardiography and Other Noninvasive Tests

232. **Sutton MSJ**, et al. Quantitative two-dimensional echocardiography measurements are major predictors of adverse cardiovascular events after acute MI. *Circulation* 1994;89:68–75.

A total of 521 SAVE trial patients had echocardiograms at 11.1 ± 3.2 days. At 1 year, left ventricular end-diastolic and left ventricular end-systolic areas were smaller in the captopril group ($p = 0.038, 0.015$). The captopril group had 35% fewer cardiovascular events. In these patients with cardiovascular events, a more than threefold increase in left ventricular cavity areas was observed.

233. **Picano E**, et al. Stress echocardiography results predict risk of reinfarction early after uncomplicated acute MI: large-scale multicenter study. *J Am Coll Cardiol* 1995;26:908–913.

A total of 1,080 patients underwent a dipyridamole echocardiography study at 10 ± 5 days. Follow-up period was 14 months. A positive test result (44%) was associated with a higher reinfarction rate (6.3% vs. 3.3%; $p < 0.01$).

234. **Sicari R**, et al. ECHO Dobutamine International Cooperative (**EDIC**) Study. Prognostic value of dobutamine-atropine stress echocardiography early after acute MI. *J Am Coll Cardiol* 1997; 29:254–260.

In this prospective, observational, multicenter trial, 778 patients with first MI were tested at an average of 12 days, with follow-up testing at 9 ± 7 months. Positive test results were attained in 56%. No difference in event rates (death, MI, unstable angina, angioplasty, bypass surgery) was observed regardless of positive or negative test results: 14% vs. 12% ($p = 0.3$). However, when only spontaneously occurring events were considered, myocardial viability was the best predictor (hazard ratio 2.0; $p < 0.002$). Wall motion stroke index is a very strong predictor of cardiac deaths only (hazard ratio 9.2; $p < 0.0001$).

235. **Migrino RQ**, et al. End-systolic volume index at 90 to 180 minutes into reperfusion therapy for acute MI is a strong predictor of early and late mortality. *Circulation* 1997;96:116–121.

A total of 1,300 patients underwent left ventriculography. End-systolic volume index of ≥40 mL/m^2 was independently associated with increased 30-day and 1-year mortality rates [adjusted odds ratios 3.4 (95% CI 2.0–5.9), 4.1 (95% CI 2.6–6.2); $p < 0.001$). Independent predictors of high end-systolic volume index ≥40 were

SBP <110 mm Hg, anterior MI, male, prior angina or MI, weight <70 kg, and heart rate ≥80 beats/min.

Flow and Vessel Patency

236. **Dewood MA**, et al. Prevalence of total coronary occlusion during the early hours of transmural MI. *N Engl J Med* 1980;303: 897–902.

    This classic angiography study demonstrated the central role of thrombotic occlusion in the pathogenesis of transmural MI. A total of 322 patients underwent catheterization at <24 hours. Total occlusion of the IRA was seen in 87% at <4 hours versus 65% at 12–24 hours.

237. **Califf RM**, et al. Failure of simple clinical measurements to predict perfusion status after intravenous thrombolysis. *Ann Intern Med* 1988;108:658–662.

    This retrospective analysis focused on 386 patients treated with tPA. Complete resolution of ST elevation prior to 90 minute angiography was associated with reperfusion in 96% and partial resolution in 84% of patients. However, ST resolution was only seen in 6% and 38%. Chest pain resolution was associated with reperfusion in 84% but was seen in only 29%. Overall, 56% of patients with no ST segment or symptom resolution had patent arteries. Of note, Holter monitoring and serum markers were not tested.

238. **Karagounis L**, et al. Does TIMI perfusion grade 2 represent a mostly patent artery or a mostly occluded artery? Enzymatic and electrocardiographic evidence from the TEAM-2 study (Trial of Eminase in Acute MI). *J Am Coll Cardiol* 1992;19:1–10.

    This analysis focused on 359 TEAM II patients treated with APSAC or streptokinase. Angiography was performed at 90–240 minutes. TIMI grade 3 flow was associated with earlier enzymatic peaks and better ECG indexes of MI than TIMI grade flows 0–2 ($p = 0.02$ to 0.0001). No differences were found between TIMI flow grades 0, 1, and 2.

239. **Gibson CM**, et al. Angiographic predictors of reocclusion after thrombolysis: results from TIMI-4. *J Am Coll Cardiol* 1995;25: 582–589.

    A total of 278 patients were randomized to APSAC, rt-PA, or combination therapy. Higher reocclusion (at 18–36 hours) was associated with TIMI grade 2 versus 3 flow (10% vs. 2%; $p = 0.003$), ulcerated lesions (10% vs. 3%; $p = 0.009$), and positive collateral vessels (18% vs. 5.6%; $p = 0.03$). Similar trends were seen for eccentric (7% vs. 2%; $p = 0.06$) and thrombotic lesions (8% vs. 3%; $p = 0.06$). Reocclusion also was associated with more severe mean stenosis at 90 minutes (78% vs. 74%; $p = 0.04$).

240. **Simes RJ**, et al. Link between the angiographic substudy and mortality outcomes in a large randomized trial of myocardial reperfusion: importance of early and complete infarct artery reperfusion. *Circulation* 1995;91:1923–1928 (editorial pp. 1905–1907).

    This GUSTO I substudy of 1,210 patients showed that TIMI grade 3 flow at 90 minutes was associated with decreased mortality. A model was developed that assumed any difference in treatment effects on 30-day mortality were mediated through differences in 90-minute infarct-related artery patency. The model showed a strong correlation ($r = 0.97$) between actual and predicted mortality rates. Thus, these data provide support for the idea that improved survival is due to achievement of early and complete reperfusion.

241. **Lamas GA**, et al. Effect of infarct artery patency on prognosis after acute MI. *Circulation* 1995;92:1101–1109.

This analysis focused on 946 SAVE patients. Catheterization (at average 4.2 days) revealed 31% with an occluded IRA. After revascularization (PTCA/CABG), 17% were still occluded at the time of randomization (ejection fraction 30% vs. 37%; p = 0.01). Significant predictors of composite end point (cardiovascular mortality and morbidity or decrease in ejection fraction by 9%) were occluded IRA (relative risk 1.73), number of diseased vessels (1.38), ejection fraction (relative risk 1.18), captopril (relative risk 0.77), and β-blocker use (0.67).

242. **Lenderink T**, et al. Benefit of thrombolytic therapy is sustained throughout 5 years and is related to TIMI perfusion grade 3 but not grade 2 flow at discharge. *Circulation* 1995;92:1110–1116.

This study showed the benefits of achieving TIMI grade 3 flow. Five-year follow-up data were analyzed on 923 hospital survivors enrolled in the European Cooperative Study Group (ECSG) studies. Patients with TIMI grade 3 flow had a 91% 5-year survival rate compared with 84% for the TIMI grade 0–1 and TIMI grade 2 groups (p^2 = 0.01).

243. **Anderson JL**, et al. Metaanalysis of 5 reported studies on the relation of early coronary patency grades with mortality and outcomes after acute MI. *Am J Cardiol* 1996;78:1–8.

This meta-analysis focused on five studies with 3,969 patients. The mortality rate was 8.8% for TIMI grade 0/1, 7% for grade 2, and only 3.7% for grade 2 patients (grade 3 vs. 2; p = 0.001). TIMI grade 3 flow also was associated with better ejection fractions and less time to CK peak.

244. **Brodie BR**, et al. Importance of infarct-related artery patency for recovery of left ventricular and late survival after primary PTCA for acute MI. *J Am Coll Cardiol* 1996;28:319–325.

This retrospective analysis focused on 576 patients; all had 6-month follow-up catheterization and assessment of ejection fraction. The patent group (TIMI grade 2/3) had higher ejection fractions (56% vs. 48%; p = 0.001). Better late survival was observed in patients with acute ejection fraction <45% (89% vs. 44%), although it was not an independent predictor (only the case in large anterior MIs).

245. **Reiner JS**, et al. Evolution of early TIMI 2 flow after thrombolysis for acute MI. *Circulation* 1996;94:2441–2446.

This analysis of the GUSTO Angiography Study showed the benefit of progressing from early TIMI grade 2 flow to grade 3 at follow-up. 278 of 914 patients with TIMI grade 2 flow underwent angiography at both 90 minutes and 5–7 days. In the group that improved to grade 3 flow by the second catheterization (67%), there was a higher mean ejection fraction (57.5% vs. 52.8%; p = 0.02), better infarct zone wall motion (p = 0.01) and less visible thrombus (26% vs. 38%; p = 0.04). However, TIMI grade 3 flow at 90 minutes remained the best, with less thrombus (42% vs. 58%; p <0.0001) and highest 5–7 day ejection fraction (61.7% vs. 57.5%; p = 0.002).

246. **Pilote L**, et al. Determinants of the use of angiography and revascularization after thrombolysis for acute MI. *N Engl J Med* 1996;335:1198–1205.

This post hoc analysis focused on 21,772 GUSTO I patients; 71% had predischarge angiography, of which 58% underwent revascularization (PTCA 73%). Overall, the best predictor of angiography use was age [if <73 years, 76% (vs. 53%)]. Among young patients, PTCA availability was the most important predictor [83% vs. 67% (no PTCA)]. The number two predictor was recurrent ischemia. Reassuringly, coronary anatomy was the top predictor of the use and type of revascularization. However, the study yielded several unexpected findings: (a) similar revascularization rate in those with three-vessel disease and left ventricular dysfunction as those with an ejection fraction >50% and one- or two-vessel disease and left anterior descending stenosis ≤50%; (b) many without symptoms had revascularization for one- or two-vessel disease; and (c) patients <80 years of age with CHF or cardiogenic shock had similar angiography rates as those without these findings.

247. **Selby JV**, et al. Variation among hospitals in coronary angiography practices and outcomes after MI in a large health maintenance organization. *N Engl J Med* 1996;335:1888–1896.

This retrospective cohort study was composed of 6,851 patients treated from 1990 to 1992 at 16 hospitals. By 3 months, 30% to 77% had undergone angiography. After multivariate analysis, angiography rates in all hospitals were found to be inversely related to the risk of death from heart disease and heart disease events ($p = 0.03; p < 0.001$). However, at higher angiography rate hospitals, angiography was associated with lower risks of death and any heart disease event (hazard ratios 0.67 and 0.72). In patients without indications for angiography, less benefit was seen at high volume centers (hazard ratios 0.85 and 0.90).

248. **Barbagelata NA**, et al. TIMI grade 3 flow and reocclusion after intravenous thrombolytic therapy: a pooled analysis. *Am Heart J* 1997;133:273–282.

Analysis of 15 TIMI flow studies with 5,475 angiograms and 27 reocclusion studies with 3,147 angiograms. TIMI grade 3 flow rates at 60 minutes and 90 minutes were as follows: with accelerated tPA, 57.1%/63.2%; standard tPA, 39.5%/50.2%; APSAC, 40.2%/50.1%; and streptokinase, 31.5% (90 minutes). Reocclusion rates were as follows: with accelerated TPA, 6.0%; standard tPA, 11.8%; APSAC, 3.0%; and streptokinase, 4.2%.

249. **Bates DW**, et al. Coronary angiography and angioplasty after acute MI. *Ann Intern Med* 1997;126:539–550.

This literature review covers the timing of angiography and angioplasty after thrombolysis, angiography in patients with MI-related complications, factors that affect the decision to perform angiography (e.g., age, severe left ventricular dysfunction, stress-induced ischemia, prior MI, non–Q-wave MI), and complications of angiography. It concludes with a brief discussion of the use and costs associated with these procedures.

250. **Brodie BR**, et al. Importance of time to reperfusion for 30-day and late survival and recovery of left ventricular function after primary angioplasty for acute MI. *J Am Coll Cardiol* 1998;32: 1312–1319.

This analysis focused on 1,352 consecutive patients treated with primary PTCA. Reperfusion was achieved at <2 hours in 12%; this group had the lowest 30-day mortality rate, 4.3% [vs. 9.2% (2 hours); $p = 0.04$]. Interestingly, this early reperfusion benefit was relatively independent of time to reperfusion after 2 hours (30-day mortality rates: 2–4 hours, 9.0%; 4–6 hours, 9.5%; >6 hours, 9.5%. The early reperfusion group also had a greater improvement in ejection fraction (+6.9% vs. +3.1%; $p = 0.007$). These results suggest that factors other than myocardial salvage contribute to survival benefit in patients undergoing primary PTCA at 2 hours after symptom onset.

251. **Puma JA**, et al. Support for the open-artery hypothesis in survivors of acute MI: analysis of 11,228 patients treated with thrombolytic therapy. *Am J Cardiol* 1999;83:482–487.

This analysis focused on 11,228 GUSTO-I patients with available IRA patency data. Both univariable and multivariable analyses showed that an open artery was associated with a significantly lower 30-day mortality rate ($p < 0.001$). This benefit appears to extend beyond that provided by myocardial salvage because the effect remained after adjustment for LVEF.

252. **Bauters C**, et al. Angiographically documented late reocclusion after successful coronary angioplasty of an infarct-related lesion is a powerful predictor of long-term mortality. *Circulation* 1999; 99:2243–2250.

Retrospective analysis of 528 patients who had a patent IRA after balloon angioplasty procedure 10 ± 6 days after MI. At 6-month follow-up angiography, IRA reocclusion occurred in 17% (TIMI flow grade 0 or 1). At long-term follow-up (median 6.4 years), the reocclusion group had a 2.5-fold higher mortality rate (20% vs. 8%; $p = 0.002$). The actuarial 8-year total mortality rates were 28% and 10% ($p = 0.0003$) and the cardiovascular mortality rates were 25% and 7% ($p < 0.0001$). Of note, the mortality differences between reoccluded and patent IRA patients were greater in patients with an anterior MI.

253. **Gibson CM**, et al. Relationship between TIMI frame count and clinical outcomes after thrombolytic administration. *Circulation* 1999;99:1945–1950.

Corrected TIMI frame count (CTFC) was measured in 1,248 patients in TIMI 4, 10A, and 10B trials. Patients who died in the hospital and by 30–42 days had higher CTFCs (69.6 vs. 49.5, $p = 0.0003$; 66.2 vs. 49.9, $p = 0.006$). In a multivariate model CTFC was an independent predictor of in-hospital mortality (odds ratio 1.21 per 10-frame rise). The risk of in-hospital mortality increased in a graded fashion from 0.0% in patients with the fastest flow (0 to 13 frames, hyperemia, TIMI grade 4 flow), to 2.7% in patients with CTFC of 14 to 40 (CTFC 40 is the cutoff for TIMI grade 3 flow), to 6.4% in patients with CTFC >40 ($p = 0.003$).

Pre- or Postinfarct Angina

254. **Ruocco NA Jr**, et al. Invasive vs. conservative strategy after thrombolytic therapy for acute MI in patients with antecedent angina. *J Am Coll Cardiol* 1992;20:1445–1451.

This retrospective analysis focused on 3,534 TIMI-2 patients. The antecedent angina group was characterized by more multivessel disease [37.9% vs. 26.4% (invasive group)] and a higher 1-year reinfarction rate (11.2% vs. 7.9%; $p = 0.001$). However, as in the rest of the trial, a similar rate of death and MI between conservative and invasive strategies was observed in those with or without antecedent angina.

255. **Anzai T**, et al. Preinfarction angina as a major predictor of left ventricular function and long-term prognosis after a first Q wave MI. *J Am Coll Cardiol* 1995;26:319–327.

This analysis of 291 patients showed that preinfarction angina was associated with lower peak CK, a decreased incidence of in-hospital ventricular tachycardia and ventricular fibrillation (anterior, 8% vs. 24%; inferior, 3% vs. 13%), and decreased cardiac mortality (anterior, 8% vs. 27%; inferior, 3% vs. 13%). Also, in multiple regression analysis, preinfarction angina was the most powerful predictor of cardiac mortality [relative risk 1.85 (vs. 1.83 for anterior location and 1.76 for absence of successful revascularization)].

256. **Andreotti F**, et al. Preinfarction angina as a predictor of more rapid coronary thrombolysis in patients with MI. *N Engl J Med* 1996;334:7–12 (editorial pp. 51–52).

This small study was composed of 14 (out of 23) MI patients with preceding unstable angina. Angiography was performed at 15 minutes, 35 minutes, 55 minutes, and 24 hours. The preinfarction angina group had higher TIMI grade 3 flow at 35 minutes (64% vs. 0%; $p = 0.006$) and lower peak CK-MB ($p < 0.01$). The time to reperfusion correlated with the indices of infarct size ($r = 0.53, p^2 = 0.02$). Of note, the preinfarction angina group had a faster time (by 27%) to initiation of thrombolytic therapy. These patients also had an increased incidence of prior coronary disease (43% vs. 22%) and thus were more likely to have a good collateral network. The accompanying editorial by Braunwald offers four possible explanations for this phenomenon: (a) coronary collaterals are closed in the absence of ischemia; (b) ischemic preconditioning (adenosine release) occurs; (c) patients on aspirin and heparin are more amenable to thrombolysis; and (d) more rapid reperfusion occurs (this study).

257. **Galli M**, et al. GISSI-3 Angina Precoce Post-Infarto (**APPI**). Early and 6 month outcome in patients with angina pectoris early after acute MI. *Am J Cardiol* 1996;78:1191–1197.

This prospective study was composed of 2,363 patients (at 31 of 200 GISSI-3 centers lacking revascularization capability); 74% were thrombolyzed. Multivariate predictors of post-infarction angina with ECG changes (14% incidence) were preinfarction angina, age 70 years, female gender, and history of MI. Early angina was associated with increased in-hospital and 6-month reinfarction [relative risks 3.1 (7% vs. 2%) and 2.9 (12% vs. 5%); both $p < 0.001$] and 6-month mortality [relative risk 2.3 (13% vs. 7%); $p < 0.001$]. Unfortunately, no factors predicted reinfarction after angina.

258. **Kobayashi Y**, et al. Previous angina reduces in-hospital death in patients with acute myocardial infarction. *Am J Cardiol* 1998; 81:117–122.

This retrospective analysis focused on 2,262 consecutive acute MI patients. In-hospital mortality was lower in those with previous angina than without (first MI, 6.9% vs. 11.4%, $p < 0.01$; prior MI, 17.7% vs. 25.3%, $p < 0.05$). In multivariate analysis, previous angina was an independent predictor of in-hospital death. In patients with a first MI, death due to cardiac rupture was less common in those with previous angina (1.4% vs. 5.0%; $p < 0.01$). Among those with a prior MI, there was a trend toward fewer deaths due to cardiogenic shock or CHF in patients with previous angina (12.8% vs. 19.0%; p = 0.05).

Thrombolysis-Specific Studies

259. **Hillis LD**, et al. Risk stratification before thrombolytic therapy in patients with acute MI. *J Am Coll Cardiol* 1990;16:313–315.

    This analysis focused on 3,339 TIMI II patients (78 excluded with shock or pulmonary edema). The low-risk group (26%; zero of eight risk factors) had a low 6-week mortality rate of 1.5%. The group with one risk factor (age 70 years, female gender, diabetes, prior MI, anterior MI, atrial fibrillation, SBP <100 mm Hg, or heart rate >100 beats/min) had a 6-week mortality rate of 5.3% (p < 0.001). If four risk factors, 17.2% mortality rate.

260. **Cragg DR**, et al. Outcome of patients with acute MI who are ineligible for thrombolytic theraphy. *Ann Internal Med* 1991;115: 173–177.

    This retrospective analysis focused on 1,471 patients; 16% were thrombolyzed on protocols (88% TIMI IIB) and 7% got non-protocol lysis, primary balloon angioplasty, or both. The non-thrombolyzed group was older, more likely to be female, and more frequently had hypertension and prior MIs. Ineligible patients had a fivefold higher mortality rate (19% vs. 4%; p < 0.001). Independent mortality predictors were age >76 years, stroke or other bleeding risk, ineligible ECG, or two exclusion criteria.

261. **Barbash GI**, et al. Significance of smoking in patients receiving thrombolytic therapy for acute MI: experience gleaned from the International tPA/Streptokinase Mortality Trial. *Circulation* 1993;87:53–58.

    This analysis of 8,259 International tPA/Streptokinase Trial patients found a protective effect of smoking in patients suffering acute MI (*see* also *Am J Cardiol* 1995;75:232). Both non-smokers (more diabetes, higher Killip class, and older) and exsmokers had more in-hospital reinfarctions (4.7% and 5% vs. 2.7%; p < 0.001) and decreased in-hospital and 6-month mortality rates (13%/18%, 8%/12%, 5%/8%).

262. **Grines CL**, et al. Effect of cigarette smoking on outcome after thrombolytic therapy for MI. *Circulation* 1995;91:298–303.

    This study showed that better outcomes in smokers suffering MI may be due to a low-risk profile. Analysis of 1,619 patients treated with tPA, urokinase, or both in six MI trials showed that smokers had similar 90-minute patency (but higher grade 3 flow: 41.1% vs. 34.6%; p = 0.03) but lower in-hospital mortality rates (4% vs. 8.9%; p = 0.0001). However, after adjustments [lower age (54 vs. 60 years), more inferior MIs (60% vs. 53%), less three-vessel disease (16% vs. 22%), and higher baseline ejection fraction (53% vs. 50%)], there was no independent prognostic significance associated with smoking.

263. **Lee KL**, et al. Predictors of 30-day mortality in the era of reperfusion for acute MI. Results from an international trial of 41,021 patients. *Circulation* 1995;91:1659–1668.

    Multivariate analysis showed the strong influence of age on mortality rate (only 1.1% if <45 years, 20.5% if >75 years). Other factors associated with mortality included lower systolic blood pressure, higher Killip class, elevated heart rate, and anterior infarct. These five factors contribute ~90% of prognostic information.

264. **Woodfield SL**, et al. Angiographic findings and outcome in diabetic patients treated with thrombolytic therapy for acute MI: the GUSTO-I experience. *J Am Coll Cardiol* 1996;28:1661–1669.

This analysis of 310 diabetics in the GUSTO Angiography Substudy showed diabetes to be an independent mortality predictor. This group had high-risk features (e.g., older, more CHF and hypertension, more prior bypass surgery and MIs), displayed a trend to more frequent reocclusion (9.2% vs. 5.3%; $p = 0.17$), and had a high raw 30-day mortality rate (11.3% vs. 5.9%). When adjustments were made for clinical and angiographic variables, diabetes remained an independent mortality predictor ($p = 0.02$).

265. **Woodfield SL**, et al. Gender and acute MI: is there a different response to thrombolysis? *J Am Coll Cardiol* 1997;29:35–42.

This GUSTO Angiography Substudy analysis showed female gender to be an independent risk factor for mortality. The women had some high-risk features (e.g., older, and more hypertension, diabetes, and heart failure) and some low-risk features (e.g., fewer prior MIs and bypass surgery, less smoking). The unadjusted 30-day mortality rate was nearly three times higher (13.1% vs. 4.8%; $p < 0.001$), and after multivariate analysis, female gender remained an independent mortality predictor.

Other

266. **Case RB**, et al. Living alone after MI. *JAMA* 1992;267:515–519.

This analysis of 1,234 MI patients with an average follow-up of 2.1 years showed that living alone was associated with 54% more end points (nonfatal MI plus cardiac death).

267. **Frasure-Smith N**, et al. Depression following MI. *JAMA* 1993; 270:1819–1825 (editorial pp. 1860–1861).

This small study was composed of 222 MI patients who survived to hospital discharge. Patients were interviewed at average 7 days (major depression, 2 weeks). Depression was associated with a 4.3-fold higher mortality rate ($p = 0.013$). Of note, the impact was at least equivalent to that of left ventricular dysfunction (Killip class) and a history of prior MI. The accompanying editorial points out that typically 15%–20% of post-MI patients have major depression.

268. **Jollis JG**, et al. Outcome of acute MI according to the specialty of the admitting physician. *N Engl J Med* 1996;335:1880–1887 (editorial pp. 1918–1919).

This retrospective analysis of 8,241 Medicare patients showed that cardiologists provide optimal care for MI patients. All-cause 1-year mortality hazard ratios (based on admitting physician) were: cardiologists, 0.88; family medicine, 0.98; general practitioner, 1.06; and other, 1.16. Of note, cardiologist-treated patients were younger and healthier and had less diabetes, more Killip Class I, lower predicted 30-day mortality rates (GUSTO I model; 18 vs. 20%), and longer hospital stay (9.3 vs. 7.3–8.6 days). Cardiologists used thrombolysis about twice as often; used angiography, revascularization, treadmill tests, nuclear imaging, Holter monitoring, and echocardiography more frequently; and put more patients on aspirin, β-blockers, and heparin. In an analysis of all

1992 Medicare claims (~220,000 patients), the same mortality pattern emerged: with cardiologists, 30%; internists, 37%; family medicine, 39%; and general practitioners, 40%. Of note, although 82% of the attending physicians were the same as the admitting physician, the role of consultants and transfers were not assessed.

269. **Chen J**, et al. Do America's best hospitals perform better for acute MI? *N Engl J Med* 1999;340:286–292.

This analysis focused on data from the Cooperative Cardiovascular Project on over 149,000 Medicare beneficiaries with acute MI in 1994 or 1995. Hospitals were classified as one of three types: (a) top-ranked, (b) similarly equipped (not in top rank but with on-site facilities for catheterization, PCI, and bypass surgery), and (c) nonsimilarly equipped. Patients admitted to a top-ranked hospital had a lower adjusted 30-day mortality rate [odds ratio 0.87 (vs. other two types), 95% CI 0.76–1.00; $p = 0.05$]. Top-ranked hospitals were more likely to prescribe aspirin and β-blockers to those without contraindications (96.2% vs. 88.6% and 83.4%; 75.0% vs. 61.8% and 58.7%). Not surprisingly, after adjusting for the increased appropriate use of these medications, the mortality benefit associated with admission to a top-ranked hospital was attenuated (odds ratio 0.94; $p = 0.38$).

270. **Thiemann DR**, et al. The association between hospital volume and survival after acute myocardial infarction in elderly patients. *N Engl J Med* 1999;340:1640.

This retrospective cohort analysis focused on 98,898 Medicare patients ≥65 years of age with a principal discharge diagnosis of acute MI. Patients admitted to hospitals in the lowest quartile of volume of invasive procedures had a 17% higher in-hospital mortality rate compared with patients at highest volume quartile hospitals (hazard ratio 1.17; 95% 1.09–1.26; $p < 0.001$).

Complications of MI

General Review Article

271. **Chatterjee K**. Complications of acute MI. *Curr Probl Cardiol* 1993;18:7–79.

Excellent review of the major complications occurring after acute MI. The largest section was dedicated to arrhythmias. Other major topics include pulmonary congestion with or without shock syndrome, right ventricular infarction, mechanical complications, postinfarct ischemia, and pericarditis.

Arrhythmias, Bundle Branch Block

272. **Antman EM**, Berlin JA. Declining incidence of ventricular fibrillation in MI: implications for prophylactic use of lidocaine. *Circulation* 1992;86:764–773 (editorial pp. 1033–1035).

This analysis focused on 18 randomized trials with 4,754 patients. Earlier year of publication (range 1969–1988) was a significant predictor of ventricular fibrillation ($p = 0.002$), even after adjusting for other variables. The incidence of ventricular fibrillation in controls fell from 4.5% in 1970 to only 0.35% in 1990. Based on the latter incidence and the trend toward excess mortality with lidocaine use, the authors recommend against routine prophylactic use of lidocaine.

273. **Solomon SD**, et al. Ventricular arrhythmias in trials of thrombolytic therapy for acute MI: a meta-analysis. *Circulation* 1993; 88:2575–2581.

This analysis focused on 15 randomized trials with 39,606 patients. Thrombolytic administration was associated with lower risk of ventricular fibrillation during entire hospitalization (odds ratio 0.83; 95% CI 0.76–0.90; $p < 0.0001$) but not in the first 6 or 24 hours after thrombolysis (odds ratios 0.98 and 1.00). Thrombolytic use also was associated with a higher incidence of ventricular tachycardia during hospitalization (odds ratio 1.34; 95% CI 1.15–1.55; $p < 0.0001$).

274. **Newby KH**, et al. Incidence and clinical relevance of the occurrence of bundle branch block in patients treated with thrombolytic therapy. *Circulation* 1996;94:2424–2428.

This study was composed of 681 TAMI-9 and GUSTO-I patients who underwent continuous 12-lead ECG monitoring for 36–72 hours. Bundle branch block occurred in 23.6% (right bundle branch block, 13%; left bundle branch block, 7%; alternating bundle branch block, 3.5%). Mortality was 2.5 times higher in bundle branch block patients compared with those without bundle branch block (8.7% vs. 3.5%; $p = 0.007$) The highest mortality rate was observed in those with persistent bundle branch block [19.4% vs. 5.6 (transient) and 3.5% (none); $p < 0.001$]. Bundle branch block patients also had decreased ejection fraction, increased peak CK, and more diseased vessels.

Cardiac Rupture

275. **Becker RC**, et al. Cardiac rupture associated with thrombolytic therapy: impact of time to treatment in the LATE (Late Assessment of Thrombolytic Efficacy) study. *J Am Coll Cardiol* 1995; 25:1063–1068.

This analysis of 5,711 LATE patients found that cardiac rupture was the listed cause of death in 53 of 547 patients (9.7%) who died in the first 35 days. There was no increased risk of rupture in the group receiving rt-PA at 6 to 24 hours compared with the placebo group. However, rupture events did occur earlier in the thrombolytic group (treatment by time to death interaction; $p = 0.03$).

276. **Becker RC**, et al. A composite view of cardiac rupture in the U.S. National Registry of MI. *J Am Coll Cardiol* 1996;27:1321–1326.

In this analysis of 350,755 patients, thrombolytic administration (~12,000 patients) was associated with 5.9% mortality (no thrombolytic therapy, 12.9%). Cardiac rupture was reported as the cause of death in 12% of thrombolyzed patients [vs. 6% (non-thrombolyzed)] and occurred more frequently within the first 24 hours.

277. **Anzai T**, et al. C-reactive protein as a predictor of infarct expansion and cardiac rupture after a first Q-wave acute MI. *Circulation* 1997;96:778–784.

Elevated C-reactive protein was shown to be a risk factor for cardiac rupture. C-reactive protein was measured every 24 hours in 220 patients. Among the rupture patients (n = 9), C-reactive protein levels were twice as high (23.7 vs. 12.2 mg/dL; $p = 0.001$). In a multivariate analysis, a C-reactive protein of ≥20 mg/dL was an independent risk factor for rupture (relative risk 4.72; $p = 0.004$), as well as left ventricular aneurysm (relative risk 2.11; $p = 0.03$), and 1-year cardiac death (relative risk 3.44; $p < 0.0001$).

278. **Becker RC**, et al. Fatal cardiac rupture among patients treated with thrombolytic agents and adjunctive thrombin antagonists. *J Am Coll Cardiol* 1999;33:479–487.

   This analysis of 3,759 patients enrolled in the TIMI 9A and 9B trials showed a 1.7% incidence of cardiac rupture. By multivariate analysis, independent predictors of rupture were age >70 years (odds ratio 3.77; 95% CI 2.06–6.91), female gender (odds ratio 2.87; 95% CI 1.44–5.73), and prior angina (odds ratio 1.82; 95% 1.05–3.16). There was no association between the intensity of anticoagulation or type of thrombin inhibition (e.g., heparin or hirudin) and cardiac rupture.

Cardiogenic Shock and CHF

279. **Goldberg RJ**, et al. Cardiogenic shock after acute MI: incidence and mortality from a community-wide perspective, 1975–88. *N Engl J Med* 1991;325:1117–1122.

   This retrospective analysis focused on 4,762 acute MI patients. Cardiogenic shock (incidence 7.5%) patients had a high rate of mortality: 77% vs. 13.5%. No significant changes were noted between 1975 and 1988.

280. **Califf RM**, Bengston JR. Current concepts: cardiogenic shock. *N Engl J Med* 1994;330:1724–30.

   This thorough review covers the definition, epidemiology, pathophysiology, clinical assessment, and management of cardiogenic shock. The management section focuses on the role of IABP, thrombolytic therapy, balloon angioplasty, and CABG surgery.

281. **Holmes DR Jr**, et al. Contemporary reperfusion therapy for cardiogenic shock: the GUSTO-I experience. *J Am Coll Cardiol* 1995;26:668–674.

   Cardiogenic shock occurred in 2,972 patients (7.2%), with 89% of cases developing after hospital admission. These shock patients had a higher reinfarction rate (11% vs. 3%) and much higher mortality rate [57% (shock upon presentation) and 55% (shock after admission) vs. 3%; *p* < 0.001]. Shock developed less frequently in patients treated by rt-PA (6.3% vs. 7.7% and 8.1% in streptokinase groups). Also, 30-day mortality was lower among the 19% who underwent angioplasty (31% vs. 61%).

282. **Holmes DR Jr**, et al. Difference in countries' use of resources and clinical outcome for patients with cardiogenic shock after MI: results from the GUSTO trial. *Lancet* 1997;349:75–78.

   Analysis of GUSTO data showed that the following features were evident among U.S. patients: younger (*p* < 0.001), more anterior MIs (49% vs. 53%), and treated earlier (3.1 vs. 3.3 hours; *p* < 0.01). They underwent procedures much more often: catheterization, 58% vs. 23%; PTCA, 26% vs. 8%; IABP, 35% vs. 7%; pulmonary artery use, 57% vs. 22%. Revascularization was associated with decreased mortality in all nations; however, the United States had a 24% lower 30-day mortality rate [50% vs. 66% (other nations); *p* < 0.001 (adjusted for revascularization rates)]. Authors suggest better U.S. outcomes due to earlier identification of patients as a result of closer monitoring.

283. **Berger PB**, et al. Impact of an aggressive invasive catheterization and revascularization strategy on mortality in patients with cardiogenic shock in the GUSTO-I trial. *Circulation* 1997;96: 122–127.

This analysis focused on 2,200 patients with SBP <90 mm Hg for 1 hour who survived 1 hour after onset of shock. The early angiography (≤24 hours) group had a lower 30-day mortality rate (38% vs.62%; p = 0.0001). After multiple logistic regression analysis, the early angiography group was found to be younger (63 vs. 68 years), to have had fewer prior MIs (19% vs. 27%), and to have been thrombolyzed earlier (2.9 vs. 3.2 hours). An aggressive strategy is still associated with a lower 30-day mortality rate (odds ratio 0.43; p = 0.0001). Of note, a subsequent GUSTO-I analysis showed that most patients (88%) with cardiogenic shock who were alive at 30 days survived at least 1 year, and that those who underwent revascularization within 30 days had better 1-year survival than patients not revascularized (*see Circulation* 1999;99:873–878).

284. **Goldberg RJ**, et al. Temporal trends in cardiogenic shock complicating acute MI. *N Engl J Med* 1999;340:1162–1168.

This observational study was composed of 9,076 patients admitted to all local hospitals at a metropolitan area (Worcester, MA) during 11 one-year periods between 1975 and 1997. The incidence of cardiogenic shock was relatively stable during this period (average 7.1%). Cardiogenic shock was associated with a 71.7% in-hospital mortality rate (vs. 12.0%; p < 0.001). There was a significant trend toward better in-hospital survival among patients treated in the mid-to-late 1990s compared with mid-to-late 1970s [odds ratios 0.49 (1993 and 1995) and 0.46 (1997)].

Stroke

285. **Maggioni AP**, et al. Risk of stroke in patients with acute MI after thrombolytic and antithrombotic therapy. *N Engl J Med* 1992; 327:1–6.

This analysis focused on GISSI-2 and International Study patients; complete data were available on 20,768 patients. The in-hospital stroke rate was 1.14% (hemorrhagic, 0.36%; ischemic, 0.48%; undefined cause, 0.30%). Patients treated with tPA had a small but significant excess of stroke vs. streptokinase-treated patients (1.33% vs. 0.94%, adjusted odds ratio 1.42; 95% CI 1.09–1.84). Factors associated with increased risk of stroke were older age, higher Killip class, and anterior infarction.

286. **Simoons ML**, et al. Individual risk assessment for intracranial hemorrhage during thrombolytic therapy. *Lancet* 1993;342:1523–1528.

This analysis focused on data from the Netherland registry, European Cooperative Study Group, GISSI-2 and International Study Group trials, TIMI II trials, TAMI trials, and ISAM study. By multivariate analysis, independent predictors of intracranial hemorrhage were age >65 years (odds ratio 2.2; 95% CI 1.4–3.5), body weight <70 kg (odds ratio 2.1; 1.3–3.2), hypertension on hospital admission (odds ratio 2. 0; 1.2–3.2), and administration of alteplase (odds ratio 1.6; 95% CI 1.0–2.5).

287. **Loh E**, et al. Ventricular dysfunction and the risk of stroke after MI. *N Engl J Med* 1997;336:251–257.

This analysis focused on 2,231 SAVE patients (all with ejection fraction ≤0.4), with a 5-year stroke rate of 8.1%. Independent stroke risk factors were lower ejection fraction (≤28% vs. >35%, relative risk 1.86), age (18% higher risk per 5 years), no aspirin or anticoagulation (with aspirin, relative risk 0.44; with anticoagulation, relative risk only 0.19). Limitations of the analysis were (a) aspirin and anticoagulation not randomly assigned, (b) no data on anticoagulation intensity, and (c) role of atrial dysfunction not assessable.

288. **Gurwitz JH**, et al. Risk for intracranial hemorrhage after tissue plasminogen activator for acute MI. *Ann Intern Med* 1998;129: 597–604.

This analysis focused on 71,073 patients from the National Registry of MI 2 treated with tPA between June 1994 and September 1996. The in-hospitalization intracranial hemorrhage rate was 0.95% [0.88% confirmed (CT or MRI)]. In multivariate models, the following were intracranial hemorrhage predictors: older age, female sex, black ethnicity, SBP >140 mm Hg, DBP >100 mm Hg, history of stroke, tPA dose >1.5 mg/kg, and lower body weight.

Reocclusion, Recurrent Ischemia, and Reinfarction

289. **Benhorin J**, et al. Prognostic significance of nonfatal myocardial reinfarction. *J Am Coll Cardiol* 1990;15:253–258.

This analysis focused on 1,234 placebo patients in the Multicenter Diltiazem Trial. At follow-up (1–4 years), nonfatal MI had occurred in 9.4%, with a higher frequency in women and those with prior cardiac symptoms. Nonfatal MI was associated with a threefold higher risk of subsequent cardiac mortality (5.4 times higher if the index event was a first MI).

290. **Ohman EM**, et al. Consequences of reocclusion after successful reperfusion therapy in acute MI. *Circulation* 1990;82:781–791.

This analysis focused on 810 TAMI patients with repeat angiography at average 7 days that showed a reoccluded IRA in 12.4% (58% with symptoms). At follow-up, occluded patients had a similar ejection fraction, but worse infarct-zone function and increased in-hospital mortality (11% vs. 4.5%; $p = 0.01$).

291. **Ellis SG**, et al. Treatment of recurrent ischemia after thrombolysis and unsuccessful reperfusion for acute MI: effect on in-hospital mortality and left ventricular function. *J Am Coll Cardiol* 1991;17:752–757.

Retrospective analysis of 405 TAMI patients treated within 6 hours followed by angiography (≤2 hours later). Successful reperfusion occurred in 75%, initial reperfusion followed by recurrent ischemia was seen in 18%, whereas 7% failed. In-hospital mortality rates for these three groups were 2%, 15%, and 32%. No significant difference in ejection fraction was observed between groups. Survival predictors if recurrent ischemia occurred were (a) initial treatment at <90 minutes (0% vs. 21% mortality) and (b) no cardiogenic shock at presentation.

292. **Kornowski R**, et al. Predictors and long-term prognostic significance of recurrent infarction in the year after a first MI. *Am J Cardiol* 1993;72:883–888.

This retrospective analysis focused on 3,695 SPRINT patients, with a 1-year reinfarction rate of 6% (associated in-hospital mortality 30%). Reinfarction predictors were peripheral vascular disease (adjusted relative risk 2.12), anterior MI (relative risk 1.62), angina prior to MI (relative risk 1.53), CHF on admission (relative risk 1.34), diabetes (relative risk 1.33), hypertension (relative risk 1.28), and age increment (relative risk 1.13). Reinfarction rates were as follows: zeri or one risk factor, 4.0%; five or six risk factors, 23.3%. Importantly, recurrent MI is the strongest long-term mortality predictor (adjusted relative risk 4.76).

293. **Mueller HS**, et al. Prognostic significance of nonfatal reinfarction during 3 year follow-up of the TIMI II Clinical Trial. *J Am Coll Cardiol* 1995;26:900–907.

The incidence of reinfarction was 10.1% (43 of 339 died). Relative risks of death were 1.9 if reinfarction occurred at <42 days, 6.2 at 43–365 days, and 2.9 at 1–3 years.

294. **Verheught FWA**, et al. Reocclusion: the flip of coronary thrombolysis. *J Am Coll Cardiol* 1996;27:766–773.

This analysis focused on 61 studies with 6,061 patients undergoing angiography twice. Reocclusion usually occurs within weeks. Overall, an 11% reocclusion rate was observed, but a 16% incidence was seen in true occlusion studies. Thus, initial occlusion is a risk factor. Aspirin and heparin were not associated with benefit in prevention (APRICOT, HART trials). Hirudin and hirulog appear beneficial (*see* TIMI-5 and *Circulation* 1994; 89:1567). Half of reocclusions are clinically silent. Revascularization is helpful, especially if symptoms are present (*see N Engl J Med* 1992;27:1825). The authors suggest a randomized trial of predischarge angiography versus no angiography.

Left Ventricular Thrombi

295. **Vecchio C**, et al. Left ventricular thrombus in anterior acute MI after thrombolysis. *Circulation* 1991;84:512–519.

This GISSI-2 ancillary echocardiography study was composed of 180 consecutive patients with first MI. Echocardiography was performed within 48 hours and prior to discharge. Left ventricular thrombi were found in 28% (no difference between the four treatment groups). Mural shape was more common, especially in heparinized patients. Only one in-hospital embolic event was documented.

296. **Vaitkus PT**, Barnathan ES. Embolic potential, prevention and management of mural thrombus complicating anterior MI: a meta-analysis. *J Am Coll Cardiol* 1993;22:1004–1009.

This analysis focused on 11 studies with 856 patients. Thrombus by echocardiography was associated with an odds ratio of embolization of 5.45 (11% vs. 2%). In anterior MI patients, the odds ratio was 8.0. Anticoagulation was associated with 86% less embolization. Primary anticoagulation led to 68% less embolization, whereas thrombolytic therapy was associated with 52% less embolization (16% vs. 32%).

297. **Greaves SC**, et al. Incidence and natural history of left ventricular thrombus following anterior wall acute MI. *Am J Cardiol* 1997;80:442–448.

This analysis focused on 309 Healing and Early Afterload Reducing Treatment (HEART) substudy patients, 78% with Q-wave anterior MIs. Echocardiography was performed on days 1, 14, and 90. Left ventricular thrombus rates were low: day 1, 0.6%; day 14, 3.7%; day 90, 2.5%. Only one thrombus was detected on two echocardiograms. Thrombus patients had a greater left ventricular size increase and wall motion abnormalities.

Valvular Damage and Septal Defects

298. **Radford MJ**, et al. Ventricular septal rupture: a review of clinical and physiologic features and an analysis of survival. *Circulation* 1981;64:545–553.

This retrospective analysis focused on 41 patients with ventricular septal rupture. Cardiogenic shock developed in 55%, usually secondary to right ventricular impairment. Perioperative survival was higher in patients not in shock (82% vs. 27%). The 4-year survival rate of perioperative survivors was 76%. Patients not undergoing surgery did poorly [11 of 13 (85%) dead within 3 months].

299. **Lehmann KG**, et al. Mitral regurgitation in early MI: incidence, clinical detection and prognostic implications. *Ann Intern Med* 1992;117:10–17.

This analysis focused on 206 TIMI I patients with contrast left ventriculography within 7 hours of symptom onset. Mitral regurgitation was present in 27 patients (13%) and associated with a markedly increased 1-year mortality rate (relative risks 12.2 and 7.5 by univariate and multivariate analyses, respectively).

300. **Tcheng JE**, et al. Outcome of patients sustaining acute ischemic mitral regurgitation during MI. *Ann Intern Med* 1992;117:18–24.

This inception cohort case study was composed of 1,480 consecutive patients who underwent catheterization within 6 hours of infarction. Acute ischemic moderately severe to severe (3+ to 4+) mitral regurgitation was associated with a mortality rate of 24% at 30 days and 52% at 1 year. Of note, physical examination did not identify 50% of these patients. Acute reperfusion by thrombolysis or angioplasty did not reliably reverse valvular incompetence.

301. **Lamas GA**, et al. Clinical significance of mitral regurgitation after acute MI. *Circulation* 1997;96:827–833.

This study was composed of 727 SAVE patients with catheterization and left ventriculography data (done within 16 days of MI). Mitral regurgitation patients (19.4%) were more likely to have a persistently occluded IRA (27.2% vs. 15.2%; $p = 0.001$). At follow-up (median 3.5 years), mitral regurgitation patients had a more than twofold higher cardiovascular mortality rate (29% vs. 12%; $p < 0.001$), more severe CHF (24% vs. 16%; $p = 0.015$), and a higher rate of cardiovascular mortality, severe CHF, and reinfarction (47% vs. 29%; $p < 0.001$). In multivariate analysis, mitral regurgitation was an independent cardiovascular mortality predictor [relative risk 2.0; 95% CI 1.28–3.04].

Congestive Heart Failure

EPIDEMIOLOGY

Although age-adjusted rates of congestive heart failure (CHF) for both men and women have decreased over the past decade (*see Am J Cardiol* 1998;82:76), the aging of the U.S. population has resulted in an increasing prevalence of CHF, which now affects nearly 5 million Americans. CHF is also responsible for more than 1 million hospital admissions each year at a cost of more than $20 billion. Overall, more women than men have CHF, primarily due to its higher prevalence in women over 80 years of age (15). There are conflicting data on the median survival of CHF patients; most studies show women surviving longer than men (9,10,12,15; *see* also *Arch Intern Med* 1999;159:1816), whereas the Studies of Left Ventricular Dysfunction (SOLVD) trial found the opposite (15). The likely explanation for this discrepancy is that the SOLVD trial enrolled a higher percentage of women with coronary artery disease, and CHF due to an ischemic etiology is associated with increased mortality.

Factors associated with an increased risk of CHF are advanced age, male gender, black race, diabetes, obesity, smoking, and hypertension (10–14). Among women, those with hypertension and diabetes are more likely than men to develop CHF (14). Echocardiographic findings associated with increased risk include low left and/or right ventricular ejection fraction (EF), left ventricular dilatation, and valvular disease (18).

Among those diagnosed with heart failure, progression of disease is predicted by functional class. The New York Heart Association (NYHA) classification is as follows:

Class I: no limitation

Class II: slight heart failure; comfortable at rest but ordinary activity causes fatigue, dyspnea, or angina

Class III: marked failure; less than ordinary activity causes symptoms

Class IV: severe failure; symptoms of CHF at rest

The mortality rate in NYHA class III patients with peak oxygen consumption of 10 to 15 mL/kg/min is 15% to 20% per year, and it rises to $\geq 50\%$/yr in class IV patients with oxygen consumption of less than 10 mL/kg/min.

HISTORY AND PHYSICAL EXAMINATION

Symptoms include dyspnea, fatigue, paroxysmal nocturnal dyspnea, orthopnea, and nocturia. Orthopnea appears to be the most sensitive symptom for predicting elevated pulmonary capillary wedge pressure (PCWP) (16). Impaired concentration may occur in individuals with decreased cardiac output at rest.

The physical examination may be notable for rales (often not present if chronic or gradual in onset), elevated jugular venous pressure, presence of third heart sound, peripheral edema, cool extremities, narrowed pulse pressure, and tachycardia. Hepatomegaly and ascites are often seen with right heart failure. Most of these signs have limited sensitivity at predicting elevated PCWP. In one study, jugular venous distention, at rest or inducible by an abdominojugular test, had a sensitivity of 80% for predicting elevated PCWP (17). In another study, low pulse pressure was an excellent predictor of poor cardiac output, with a pulse pressure of less than 25% having a 91% sensitivity and 83% specificity for a cardiac index of ≤2.2 L/min/m^2 (16). Of note, congestion with hypoperfusion is the most common presentation in patients hospitalized for CHF (Tables 5-1 and 5-2).

ETIOLOGY

Systolic dysfunction is due to pump failure, typically from ischemic cardiomyopathy, dilated cardiomyopathy, or valvular disease. High output causes of CHF are less common, and include anemia, hyperthyroidism, and pregnancy. Rare causes include Paget's disease, arteriovenous fistula, pheochromocytoma, and beriberi. Diastolic dysfunction is a component in approximately one third of CHF cases; it is typically associated with hypertension, hypertrophic cardiomyopathy, and infiltrative disease.

An important precipitating factor of CHF that must not be overlooked is noncompliance with a prescribed drug regimen and poor diet (e.g., high salt). In one study of patients hospitalized for heart failure, over 60% were found to be noncompliant with drugs and/or diet (1). Abrupt/acute precipitating causes of CHF include acute myocardial infarction (MI), acute pulmonary embolism, acute mitral regurgitation and aortic insufficiency, acute ventricular septal defect, and infection. (Tachycardia results in higher cardiac output.) More chronic precipitating causes of CHF include drugs [nonsteroidal antiinflammatory drugs; verapamil, diltiazem, and procainamide (negative inotropy), estrogens, androgens and minoxidil (water retention); and adriamycin and steroids (8) and worsening renal function (impaired sodium excretion).

TESTS

1. Laboratory tests. Low serum sodium is common (dilutional hyponatremia from expansion of extracellular fluid volume) and predictive of poor outcome (20); elevated creatinine and liver function tests are also predictors of poor outcome.

Table 5-1.

	Systolic Dysfunction	Diastolic Dysfunction
Third heart sound	Frequent	Rare
Fourth heart sound	Rare	Frequent
Rales	Occasional	Occasional
Peripheral edema	Frequent	Rare
Jugular venous distention	Frequent	Rare
Cardiomegaly	Usual	Rare

Modified from Braunwald E. *Heart Disease*. Philadelphia, W. B. Saunders, 1997.

Table 5-2.

	Acute Heart Failure	Decompensated Chronic Heart Failure	Chronic Heart Failure
Severity of symptoms	Severe	Severe	Mild to moderate
Pulmonary edema	Rare	Common	Rare
Peripheral edema	Rare	Common	Common
Weight gain	None to minimal	Moderate to severe	Mild to moderate

Modified from Braunwald E. *Heart Disease.* Philadelphia, W. B. Saunders, 1997.

2. Chest x-ray. Findings of increased pulmonary capillary pressure are seen in approximately 50% of patients; bilateral pleural effusions and cardiomegaly also may be present (14).
3. Electrocardiography (ECG). Q waves and left bundle branch block are good predictors of systolic dysfunction (18). A wide QRS (>220 msec) is predictive of increased mortality.
4. Echocardiogram (25,26). A simple and useful tool, echocardiography can help determine systolic versus diastolic dysfunction and left and/or right ventricular impairment.
5. Six-minute walk test. Short distance correlates with higher mortality and increased heart failure–related hospitalizations (24; *see* also *Chest* 1996;110:325 and *Am Heart J* 1998;136:449).
6. Metabolic stress testing. Used to measure oxygen consumption, a peak oxygen consumption of less than 12 to 14 mL/kg/min portends a poor prognosis (23).
7. Endomyocardial biopsy. Biopsy is useful in selected cases, such as suspected amyloidosis, sarcoidosis, and giant cell myocarditis.

TREATMENT
Acute
1. Nitrates. Nitrates are given sublingually or intravenously. In the case of severe heart failure, nitroprusside administration should be considered if both PCWP and systemic vascular resistance (SVR) are elevated.
2. Diuretics. Furosemide 20 to 240 mg is administered intravenously. (Initial dose should be based on prior diuretic history.) Addition of a thiazide (e.g., metolazone or chlorothiazide) may help potentiate diuresis. In cases of massive fluid overload that respond poorly to diuretics, ultrafiltration may be effective (*see J Am Coll Cardiol* 1993;21:424).
3. Inotropic agents. Choices include dobutamine (lowers systemic vascular resistance so need to be careful if blood pressure low), dopamine (especially if hypotensive), and milrinone.

Chronic
Diet
   Low sodium intake (≤2 g/day) and fluid restriction are particularly important in symptomatic and decompensated patients.

Angiotensin-Converting Enzyme Inhibitors

Clearly indicated if left ventricular dysfunction is present, angiotensin-converting enzyme (ACE) inhibitors should be initiated before aggressively diuresing the patients. The Cooperative North Scandinavian Enalapril Survival Study (CONSENSUS I) showed that enalapril reduced 1-year mortality by 31% in NYHA class IV patients (28), whereas the larger SOLVD trial enrolled NYHA class II and III patients and showed that enalapril reduced mortality by 16% (average follow-up 41 months) (29). Subsequent trials have shown similar benefits with other ACE inhibitors [e.g., Acute Infarction Ramipril Efficacy Study (AIRE) (31)]. Preliminary ATLAS results have shown that high doses are more efficacious: 8% lower mortality and 24% fewer hospitalizations (26). A meta-analysis of 32 studies found ACE inhibitor therapy to be associated with significant reductions in total mortality (odds ratio 0.77; 95% CI 0.67–0.88; $p < 0.001$) and mortality or hospitalization for CHF (odds ratio 0.65; 95% CI 0.57–0.74; $p < 0.001$) (Table 5-3) (27).

Angiotensin II Receptor Antagonists

If severe ACE-related cough develops, angiotensin II receptor antagonists should be considered. In the ELITE trial, losartan was associated with a lower mortality rate than was captopril among patients over 65 years of age. However, mortality was not the primary end point, and the trial was not large [only 722 patients (32)]. A larger trial with mortality as the primary end point in now underway [Evaluation of Losartan in the Elderly (ELITE II)]. Other agents are also being evaluated: candesartan has shown favorable results in a preliminary dose-ranging study [Symptoms Tolerability Response to Exercise Trial of Candesartan Cilexil in Patients with Heart Failure (STRETCH) (34)] and is now being evaluated in the CHARM trial, and the combination of valsartan and an ACE inhibitor is being studied in the ongoing VALIANT trial.

Diuretics

Diuretics are used to control and reduce fluid retention. In most cases, they should be used in conjunction with an ACE inhibitor with or without a β-blocker. A few small studies have found that a continuous intravenous infusion of furosemide in patients hospitalized with severe CHF may provide improved diuresis and natriuresis (35). The recently completed Randomized Aldactone Evaluation Study (RALES), which evaluated the potassium-sparing diuretic spironolactone in patients receiving optimal therapy (including a loop diuretic), showed a significantly lower mortality rate among spironolactone-treated patients compared with those treated with a loop diuretic (36).

Digoxin

Two digoxin withdrawal trials [the Randomized Assessment of Effect of Digoxin on Inhibitors of ACE (RADIANCE) and Prospective Randomized Study of Ventricular Failure and Efficacy of Digoxin (PROVED) (39,40)] showed that fewer hospitalizations for worsening CHF occurred in those who remained on digoxin.

Table 5-3. Total mortality for randomized trials of ACE inhibitors

Trials by Agent	Allocation, No. Events/ No. Randomized		O–E	Var of O–E	OR (95% CI)
	ACE Inhibitors	Controls			
Benazepril hydrochloride					
Colfer et al.	0/114	3/58	−1.99	0.66	0.05 (0–0.55)
McGarry*	2/29	1/32	0.57	0.72	2.21 (0.22–22.15)
Subtotal	2/143	4/90	−1.41	1.39	0.36 (0.07–1.90)
Captopril					
Magnani and Magelli	7/48	6/46	0.36	2.83	1.14 (0.35–3.64)
Bussman et al.	2/12	3/11	−0.61	1.02	0.55 (0.08–3.83)
Captopril Digoxin Multicenter Research Group	18/104	15/100	1.18	6.95	1.18 (0.56–2.49)
CMRG	2/53	11/52	−4.56	2.87	0.20 (0.06–0.65)
Barabino et al.‡	12/52	18/49	−3.45	5.32	0.52 (0.22–1.22)
Kleber et al.	22/83	22/87	0.52	8.20	1.07 (0.54–2.11)
Subtotal	63/352	75/345	−6.56	27.19	0.79 (0.54–1.14)
Cilazapril					
Drexler et al.	0/11	1/10	−0.52	0.25	0.12 (0–6.20)
Enalapril maleate					
Cleland et al.	0/10	0/10	—	—	—
Rucinska*	2/67	4/65	−1.05	1.44	0.48 (0.09–2.48)
CONSENSUS	50/127	68/126	−1.89	3.32	0.57 (0.19–1.66)
Enalapril CHF Investigators	5/126	9/130	−1.89	3.32	0.57 (0.19–1.66)

(continued)

Table 5-3. Continued

Trials by Agent	Allocation, No. Events/ No. Randomized		O–E	Var of O–E	OR (95% CI)
	ACE Inhibitors	Controls			
Dickstein et al.	0/20	1/21	−0.49	0.25	0.14 (0–7.16)
SOLVD	452/1285	510/1284	−29.19	150.50	0.82 (0.70–0.97)
Rucinska*	0/55	1/55	−0.50	0.25	0.14 (0–6.82)
Subtotal	509/1690	593/1691	−42.34	171.57	0.78 (0.67–0.91)
Lisinopril					
Zwehl et al.	5/183	3/92	−0.32	1.74	0.83 (0.19–3.67)
Giles	4/130	5/63	−2.06	1.90	0.34 (0.08–1.40)
Rucinska*	1/28	0/30	0.52	0.25	7.94 (0.16–400.92)
Gilbert et al.*	0/10	0/10	—	—	—
Subtotal	10/351	8/195	−1.87	3.88	0.62 (0.23–1.67)
Perindopril					
Lechat et al.*	0/61	1/64	−0.49	0.25	0.14 (0–7.16)
Quinapril hydrochloride					
Riegger	0/169	0/56	—	—	—
Northridge	0/21	0/11	—	—	—
Uprichard*	1/114	2/110	−0.53	0.74	0.49 (0.05–4.78)
Uprichard*	2/105	3/103	−0.52	1.23	0.65 (0.11–3.83)
Uprichard*	2/139	0/47	0.51	0.38	3.84 (0.16–94.01)
Subtotal	5/548	5/327	−0.55	2.34	0.79 (0.22–2.85)

Ramipril

Swedberg et al.	3/115	7/108	-2.16	2.40	0.41 (0.11–1.44)
Maass*	8/87	4/45	0.09	2.47	1.40 (0.30–3.61)
Gordon*	1/94	5/98	-1.94	1.46	0.27 (0.05–1.34)
Maass*,**	8/329	5/171	-0.55	2.86	0.82 (0.26–2.63)
Maass*	1/47	1/48	0.01	0.49	1.02 (0.06–16.58)
Lemarie*	1/42	0/43	0.51	0.25	7.57 (0.15–381.49)
Subtotal	22/714	22/513	-4.04	9.93	0.67 (0.36–1.24)
Total	611/3870	709/3235	-57.26	216.54	0.77 (0.67–0.88)

Test for heterogeneity for all trials across all agents, $p = 0.87$.

ACE, angiotensin-converting enzyme; O–E, summation of observed–expected overall trials; Var of O–E, sum of the individual variance over all trials; OR, odds ratio; CI, confidence interval; and CHF, congestive heart failure.

* Unpublished. Overall point estimate for the unpublished studies (OR, 0.79; 95% CI, 0.46–1.38) was similar to that for the published studies (OR, 0.77; 95% CI, 0.67–0.88).

[‡] Six months of the trial was double blind, whereas 42 months was an open trial with patients kept in their original randomized group.

** Although 535 patients were randomized in this trial, the data were provided for 500 patients because 35 patients were excluded because of missing source data.

(Adapted from Garg R, et al. [27], with permission.)

Although the large Digoxin Investigation Group (DIG) mortality trial (41) found that digoxin had no significant effect on total mortality (positive or negative), it also found that digoxin-treated patients had fewer hospitalizations than placebo patients.

Vasodilators

Hydralazine and Isosorbide Dinitrate

This combination was associated with a higher mortality rate than was enalapril in the Second VA Cooperative Heart Failure Trial (Ve-HeFT II; 25% vs. 18% at 2 years) (43), but yielded better results than placebo in Ve-HeFT I (42). Short-term use of high-dose transdermal nitrates appears to result in significant improvement in exercise tolerance and hemodynamics.

Calcium-Channel Blockers

Negative inotropic effects are not desirable in systolic dysfunction. However, in the Prospective Randomized Amlopidine Survival Evaluation (PRAISE) trial (44), amlodipine showed a trend toward lower mortality (-16%, $p = 0.07$), with a 46% lower mortality rate among patients with nonischemic cardiomyopathy. PRAISE 2 is focusing on the nonischemic group.

β-Blockers

Safe when given carefully in controlled fashion, recent Consensus Recommendations advocate the use of β-blockers in patients in NYHA functional classes II or III. However, they should not be used in those with congested, decompensated CHF. All β-blocker trials of more than 1 month duration have shown improved left ventricular function, and a meta-analysis of 17 randomized trials with approximately 3,000 patients showed an approximately 30% mortality reduction, mostly due to fewer sudden deaths (47). The Cardiac Insufficiency Bisoprolol Study (CIBIS II) enrolled over 2,600 NYHA class III or IV patients with an EF of less than 35% and found that bisoprolol-treated patients had a mortality rate approximately one third lower than that of placebo-treated patients (48), whereas the recently completed Metoprolol CR/XL Randomized Intervention Trial in HF (MERIT-HF) trial enrolled nearly 4,000 patients with an EF of less than 40% and found that metoprolol-XL reduced mortality by 35% compared with placebo (59). The BEST trial is still ongoing (bucindolol vs. placebo).

Carvedilol is a new nonselective β-blocker and α_1-agonist. The dose must be carefully titrated. Patients have dropped out of trials in the run-in phase due to intolerance. The largest published experience to date, which pooled data from different small studies (51–53), found an impressive 65% mortality reduction at 6 months in carvedilol-treated patients (54). The ongoing COMET trial is evaluating carvedilol versus metoprolol.

Amiodarone

One South American study, of the Grupo de Estudio de la Sobrevida en la Insuficiencia Cardiaca en Argentina (GESICA) (62), showed a mortality benefit, whereas the more recent and better designed Survival Trial of Antiarrhythmic Therapy in CHF (CHF-STAT) (63) found no mortality advantage in the amiodarone group. Of note, in the CHF-STAT, there was a trend toward a lower mortality rate with amiodarone in the subgroup of patients with nonischemic cardiomyopathy.

Other Agents

1. Oral milrinone. A higher mortality rate was found in the Prospective Randomized Milrinone Survival Evaluation (PROMISE) trial (65).
2. Vesnarinone. Despite one study that suggested a benefit with 60 mg/day (66), a recent larger study showed increased mortality with 60 mg/daily compared with placebo (70).
3. Flosequinan and pimobendan. These agents also have been shown to result in excess mortality. [Flosequinan was initially approved based on Flosequinan-ACE Inhibitor Trial (FACET) data (67) but was removed when postmarketing data showed increased mortality rates.]
4. Ambulatory dobutamine. Most small studies suggest increased mortality.

Surgical Options

Left Ventricular Assist Device

Useful as a bridging device to transplantation or long-term therapy, the left ventricular assist device (LVAD) significantly improves peak oxygen consumption (77). Failure of long-term therapy is predicted by several preoperative variables, including poor urine output, elevated central venous pressure, mechanical ventilation, prolonged prothrombin time, and reoperation (71).

Coronary Artery Bypass Graft Surgery

In CHF patients with coronary artery disease and moderate to severe left ventricular dysfunction (EF < 40%), CABG improves 3-year survival by 30% to 50% (6). It is not clear if this magnitude of benefit is obtained in patients with primarily heart failure symptoms and little or no angina.

Cardiac Transplantation

Heart transplantation should be considered if peak oxygen consumption is below 10 to 12 mL/kg/min on optimal therapy. Other eligibility criteria also must be met [e.g., age ≤65 years, no active infection, and no malignancy; *see* the American Heart Association/ American College of Cardiology (AHA/ACC) guidelines in *Circulation* 1995;92:3593].

Controversial or Experimental Treatment

1. Partial ventriculectomy (Batista procedure). A wedge of the left ventricular muscle is removed from apex to base, and the mitral valve apparatus is often repaired or replaced. Results at a few centers are promising, but 1-year mortality rates have ranged from 15% to 30%, and LVAD rescue is often necessary (73,74). Longer term follow-up and additional studies are needed.
2. Mitral valve repair. This option is used in patients with CHF due to dilated cardiomyopathy complicated by severe, refractory mitral regurgitation. In one study, mitral valve reconstruction resulted in significant NYHA class improvement and a 2-year survival rate of over 70% (75).

3. Cardiomyoplasty. A portion of the trapezius muscle is wrapped around the heart to assist pump function. Initial studies have been conducted in small, highly selected populations (72).

Miscellaneous

Tailored Therapy

Right heart catheterization is performed in patients with severe CHF, and intravenous and ultimately oral vasodilators are used to achieve optimal hemodynamics (*see Am J Cardiol* 1990;66:1348 and *J Heart Lung Transplant* 1991;10:468).

Exercise Training and Rehabilitation

Numerous studies have shown tolerability and benefits of exercise in most patients. Regular exercise typically results in increased peak oxygen uptake and increased peak workload. Patients with circulatory failure in addition to deconditioning may not respond to exercise training (79–83).

Multidisciplinary Approach

One study found that a comprehensive, nurse-directed management approach, consisting of patient and family education, prescribed diet, social service consult, medication review, and intensive follow-up, resulted in over 50% fewer CHF-related hospitalizations, improved quality of life, and significant cost savings (4).

New and Investigational Agents

1. Nesiritide. In preliminary results, use of this form of human b-type natriuretic peptide has resulted in rapid symptomatic and hemodynamic improvement in patients with acutely decompensated heart failure (48th ACC Scientific Session, New Orleans, LA, March 1999).
2. Eplerenone. This aldosterone antagonist has yielded a lower incidence of gynecomastia than spironolactone due to its minimal effect on serum testosterone levels.

COMPLICATIONS

Sudden Cardiac Death

Sudden cardiac death is responsible for 30% to 70% of deaths among those with CHF. The incidence is 2% to 3% per year in those with asymptomatic left ventricular dysfunction and up to 20%/yr in those with severe CHF. Patients with advanced CHF who experience a syncopal episode have a high incidence of subsequent sudden death [in one study, 45% at 1 year (86)]. The incidence of sudden cardiac death appears lower in patients receiving ACE inhibitors.

Atrial Fibrillation

The prevalence of atrial fibrillation is approximately 20% and it is associated with an increased risk of stroke (15%/yr if left ventricular dysfunction is present) and higher total mortality (85).

Embolism

Incidence is 1% to 2% per year in class II or III patients who are in normal sinus rhythm and 3% to 4% per year in patients awaiting transplantation. Oral anticoagulation should be considered if mural thrombus is present (embolic risk much higher).

REFERENCES

Review Articles, Miscellaneous

1. **Ghali JK**, et al. Precipitating factors leading to decompensation of heart failure: traits among urban blacks. *Arch Intern Med* 1988; 148:2013.

    This study of 101 patients admitted to an inner city hospital with a diagnosis of heart failure established precipitating factor(s) in 93%. The most common causes were noncompliance with diet and/or drugs (63%), uncontrolled hypertension (44%), arrhythmias (29%; mostly atrial fibrillation), environmental factors (19%), inadequate therapy (17%), pulmonary infection (12%), emotional stress (7%), and MI (6%).

2. **Gaasch WH**. Diagnosis and treatment of heart failure based on left ventricular systolic or diastolic dysfunction. *JAMA* 1994; 271:1276–1280.

    This review discusses the benefits of treating patients with a left ventricular ejection fraction (LVEF) of <40%, whether or not they have symptoms of heart failure. No large-scale therapeutic trials have been done in patients with diastolic dysfunction, but treatment options and its more favorable prognosis are reviewed.

3. Management of heart failure: pharmacologic therapy (part I); counseling, education and lifestyle modifications (part II); role of revascularization with moderate or severe left ventricular systolic dysfunction (part III); anticoagulation (part IV). *JAMA* 1994;272: 1361–1366, 1442–1446, 1528–1533, 1614–1618.

    The pharmacologic section emphasizes the proven benefits of ACE inhibitors. Topics discussed in the second part include sodium restriction and exercise training. Part three reviews the favorable data on bypass surgery in patients with both significant left ventricular dysfunction and limiting angina. The final section reports an incidence of arterial thromboembolism of ~2%/yr in large heart failure studies. The limited case series data on the effectiveness of anticoagulant therapy are reviewed.

4. **Rich MW**, et al. A multidisciplinary intervention to prevent the readmission of elderly patients with congestive heart failure. *N Engl J Med* 1995;333:1190–1195.

    This prospective, randomized trial was composed of 282 high-risk patients ≥70 years of age hospitalized with CHF. Patients were assigned to standard care (control group) or nurse-directed, multidisciplinary care, consisting of comprehensive education of the patient and family, a prescribed diet, social service consultation, medication review, and intensive follow-up. There was a trend toward improved survival without readmission (primary end point) in the multidisciplinary intervention group (64.1% vs. 53.6%; p = 0.09). The total number of hospital admissions was significantly lower in the multidisciplinary intervention group (53 vs. 94; p = 0.02), including 56% fewer CHF-related admissions (24 vs. 54; p = 0.04). The intervention group had an overall lower cost of care ($460 less per patient). Finally, in a subgroup of 126 patients, quality of life scores at 90 days improved significantly more in the intervention patients (p = 0.001).

5. **Cohn JN**. The management of chronic heart failure. *N Engl J Med* 1996;335:490–498.

This basic review includes sections on the mechanisms and diagnosis of left ventricular dysfunction, nonpharmacologic management, and drug therapy. The use of diuretics, vasodilators, and digoxin to alleviate symptoms is discussed. Among patients with left ventricular dysfunction, the data on ACE inhibitors improving mortality are reviewed. Other drugs with possible or no clear benefits are also mentioned, including antiarrhythmics, calcium antagonists, and anticoagulants. The limited data on β-blockers available at the time of publication are briefly discussed.

6. **Frazier OH,** Myers TJ. Surgical therapy for severe failure. *Curr Probl Cardiol* 1998;23:726–764.

This review covers heart transplantation, mechanical circulatory support measures, cardiomyoplasty, and myocardial revascularization (bypass surgery, transmyocardial laser).

7. **Cleland JGF**, et al. Successes and failures of current treatment of heart failure. *Lancet* 1998;352 (suppl):19–28.

This review focuses on pharmacologic therapy, including thorough sections on angiotensin II receptor antagonists (e.g., losartan), β-blockers (e.g., bisoprolol, carvedilol), and the newer calcium-channel blockers (e.g., felodipine, amlodipine).

8. **Feenstra J**, et al. Drug-induced heart failure. *J Am Coll Cardiol* 1999;33:1152–1162.

This review discusses the anthracyclines, cyclophosphamide, paclitaxel, mitoxantrone, other chemotherapeutic agents, nonsteroidal antiinflammatory drugs, immunomodulating agents (e.g., interferons, interleukin-2), and antidepressants. The contributory role of three major cardiac drug classes in causing heart failure are also reviewed: antiarrhythmics, β-blockers, and calcium-channel blockers.

Epidemiology

9. **Schocken DD**, et al. Prevalence and mortality rate of congestive heart failure in the United States. *J Am Coll Cardiol* 1992;20:301–306.

This analysis focused on prevalence data obtained from the National Health and Nutritional Examination Survey (NHANES I; 1971–1975) and mortality data from the NHANES-I Epidemiologic Follow-up Study (1982–1986). Prevalence based on clinical criteria was 2% for the noninstitutionalized U.S. population. Mortality increased with advancing age and was higher in men than in women (15-year rates in patients >55 years of age: men, 71.8%; women, 39.1%).

10. **Ho KKL**, et al. **Framingham Heart Study**. Survival after onset of CHF in Framingham Heart Study subjects. *Circulation* 1993;88: 107–115.

This study was conducted on an unselected population of 652 patients with a diagnosis of CHF made between 1948 and 1988. Shorter survival was seen in men (1.7 vs. 3.2 years). Higher mortality was seen with increasing age: 27% per decade in men, 61% per decade in women. Interestingly, no improved survival was observed over a four-decade study span.

11. **Levy D**, et al. The progression from hypertension to congestive heart failure. *JAMA* 1996;275:1557–1562.

This analysis focused on 5,143 Framingham Study subjects with a mean follow-up period of 14.1 years. Hypertension antedated 91% of new heart failure cases. After risk factor adjustment, hypertension was associated with relative risks of developing heart failure of ~2.0 (men) and 3.0 (women). Poor 5-year survival was observed among hypertensive CHF subjects: 24% in men and 31% in women.

12. **Adams KF Jr.**, et al. Relation between gender, etiology and survival in patients with symptomatic heart failure. *J Am Coll Cardiol* 1996;28:1781–1788.

This prospective, observational study was composed of 557 patients (177 women; nonischemic etiology in 68%). At a mean follow-up of 2.4 years, the all-cause mortality rate was 36%. Women with better survival ($p < 0.001$), primarily due to the lower mortality associated with a nonischemic etiology (men vs. women, relative risk 2.36; $p < 0.001$).

13. **Krumholz HM**, et al. Readmission after hospitalization for CHF among Medicare beneficiaries. *Arch Intern Med* 1997;157:99–104.

This analysis focused on 17,448 patients from all 33 Connecticut acute care hospitals treated from 1991 to 1994. The 6-month readmission rate was 44%, with CHF as the reason for readmission in 18% of cases. Readmission predictors included initial length of stay >7 days (odds ratio 1.32), one prior admission in prior 6 months (odds ratio 1.64), male gender (odds ratio 1.12), and high comorbidity score (odds ratio 1.56). Age was a significant predictor of readmission plus death.

14. **Petrie MC**. Failure of women's hearts. *Circulation* 1999;99:2334–2341.

This thorough review focused on the available epidemiologic data on CHF in women, including the higher risk of developing CHF among those with diabetes, hypertension, and obesity. The prevalence of heart failure in the U.S. population is higher in women because it is more common in elderly individuals. There are conflicting data on the median survival of CHF patients. Framingham Heart Study data showed that women had a longer survival than men, whereas the SOLVD trial found the opposite (latter enrolled more women with coronary artery disease). Women with CHF appear to have more associated morbidity, including greater functional impairment and higher risk of pulmonary embolism. Women are poorly represented in major treatment trials, but it appears that ACE inhibitors may be less effective in women with left ventricular dysfunction after acute MI.

15. **Adams KF**, et al. Gender differences in survival in advanced heart failure. *Circulation* 1999;99:1816–1821.

This analysis focused on 471 Flolan International Randomized Survival Trial (FIRST) patients, of whom 112 were women; 60% were NYHA class IV, and average EF was 18%. A Cox proportional-hazards model, which included adjustments for age, gender, and 6-minute walk results, showed a significant association between female gender and better survival. (Relative risk of death for men vs. women was 2.18; $p < 0.001$.)

Assessment and Prognosis

Physical Examination

16. **Stevenson LW**, Perloff JK. The limited reliability of physical signs for estimating hemodynamics in chronic heart failure. *JAMA* 1989;261:884–888.

This prospective study was composed of 50 patients with known chronic heart failure. Orthopnea within the preceding week was the most sensitive (91%) symptom for predicting elevated PCWP (≥22 mm Hg). Physical signs were not sensitive at predicting elevated PCWP because rales, edema, and elevated mean jugular venous pressure were absent in 18 of 43 patients (41.9%). A measured pulse pressure of <25% had a 91% sensitivity and 83% specificity for a cardiac index <2.2 L/min/m².

17. **Butman SM**, et al. Bedside cardiovascular exam with severe chronic heart failure: importance of rest or inducible jugular venous distention. *J Am Coll Cardiol* 1993;22:968–974.

This prospective study was composed of 52 patients with chronic CHF who underwent right heart catheterization. The presence of jugular venous distention had a 57% sensitivity and 93% specificity for a PCWP of 18 mm Hg. The combination of jugular venous distension at rest or inducible by an abdominojugular test had a sensitivity of 81%, specificity of 80%, and 81% predictive accuracy.

18. **Badgett RG**, et al. Can the clinical examination diagnose left-sided heart failure in adults? *JAMA* 1997;277:1712–1719.

This review of the literature asserts that the best findings for detecting increased filling pressure are jugular venous distention and radiographic redistribution. The best findings for detecting systolic dysfunction are abnormal apical impulse, cardiomegaly (by x-ray), and Q waves or left bundle branch block on ECG.

19. **Mcgee SR**. Physical examination of venous pressure: a critical review. *Am Heart J* 1998;136:10–18 (editorial pp. 6–9).

This review asserts that the failure to standardize the external reference point used to indicate a venous pressure of zero and the failure to recognize the importance of patient positioning in determining venous pressure are mainly responsible for the discrepancy between clinicians' estimates of jugular venous pressure and the central venous pressure measured at right heart catheterization. The authors emphasize that central venous pressure should be measured while the patient is in the supine position and recommend that it should be considered abnormally high (not quantified) if the top of the external or internal veins is >3 cm above the sternal angle of Lewis.

Other

20. **Lee WH**, et al. Prognostic importance of serum sodium concentration and its modification by converting enzyme inhibition in patients with severe chronic heart failure. *Circulation* 1986;73: 257–267.

This analysis focused on 30 clinical, hemodynamic, and biochemical variables in 203 consecutive severe heart failure patients. At follow-up (6–94 months), a regression analysis showed that pretreatment with a serum sodium concentration was the most powerful predictor of cardiovascular mortality [median survival 99 (serum Na ≤130 mEq/L) vs. 337 days; $p < 0.001$]. The poor outcomes in hyponatremic patients appeared to be related to high plasma renin levels because hyponatremic patients did better if treated with ACE inhibitors [median survival 108 (serum Na ≤137 mEq/L) vs. 232 days; $p = 0.003$].

21. **Cohn JN**, et al. Plasma norepinephrine as a guide to prognosis in patients with chronic congestive heart failure. *N Engl J Med* 1984;311:819–823.

A total of 106 patients with moderate to severe CHF had hemodynamics, plasma norepinephrine, and plasma renin activity measured at supine rest; follow-up lasted 1–62 months. Multivariate analysis found only plasma norepinephrine to be an independent predictor of mortality ($p = 0.002$).

22. **Gradman A**, et al. Predictors of total mortality and sudden death in mild to moderate heart failure. *J Am Coll Cardiol* 1989;14:546–570.

    This analysis focused on 295 patients with LVEF ≤40%, 81% in NYHA class II. The mean follow-up period was 16 months. In multiple regression analysis, LVEF was the strongest mortality predictor ($p = 0.006$): 27% with LVEF ≤20% died versus 7% with LVEF 30%. Ventricular tachycardia was also associated with increased mortality: 34% among those with >0.088 events/h vs. 12% in those with no events.

23. **Mancini DM**, et al. Value of peak exercise oxygen consumption for optimal timing of cardiac transplantation in ambulatory patients with heart failure. *Circulation* 1991;83:778–786.

    This study of 114 patients found a peak oxygen consumption of ≤14 mL/kg/min in 62 patients (35 were transplantation candidates and 27 had noncardiac issues) and >14 mL/kg/min in 52 patients. All three groups had similar NYHA functional class, LVEF, and cardiac index. Patients with an oxygen consumption >14 mL/kg/min had a lower PCWP and significantly better 1-year survival [94% vs. 70% (transplant candidates) and 47%]. A multivariate analysis found peak oxygen consumption to be the best survival predictor, whereas PCWP added further prognostic information.

24. **Bitner V**, et al. Prediction of mortality and morbidity with a 6-minute walk test in patients with left ventricular dysfunction. *JAMA* 1993;270:1702–1707.

    This analysis focused on 898 SOLVD patients with radiologic evidence of CHF and/or EF <45%; mean follow-up period was 8 months. There were no significant test-related complications. Highest versus lowest performance level (distance walked ≥450m vs. <300m): 71% lower mortality (3% vs. 10.2%), 51% fewer hospitalizations (19.9% vs. 40.9%), and 91% fewer heart failure hospitalizations (2% vs. 22.2%). Logistic regression analysis showed that EF and walk time were equally strong and independent predictors of mortality and hospitalization due to acute heart failure.

25. **Vasan RS**, et al. Left ventricular dilatation and the risk of congestive heart failure in people without MI. *N Engl J Med* 1997; 336:1350–1355 (editorial pp. 1381–1382).

    This analysis focused on 4,744 Framingham Study subjects, of whom 74 developed CHF during follow-up (mean 7.7 years). Adjusted hazard ratio of CHF for a 1 standard deviation increment in left ventricular end-diastolic dimension (by M-mode echocardiography) was 1.47 (range 1.25–1.73). Using left ventricular end-systolic dimension, the hazard ratio was 1.43. The authors assert that this method helps identify subclinical left ventricular dysfunction. The accompanying editorial points out that EF was not measured, the diagnosis of heart failure was based on clinical criteria with low sensitivity, and multivariate analysis did not include symptoms, physical examination findings, chest x-ray, ECG, or total cholesterol. Also, echocardiography for screening would be limited by low specificity.

26. **de Groote P**, et al. Right ventricular ejection fraction is an independent predictor of survival in patients with moderate heart failure. *J Am Coll Cardiol* 1998;32:948–954.

    This analysis focused on 205 consecutive NYHA class II or III patients who underwent exercise testing and radionuclide angiography. At follow-up (median 2 years), there were 44 cardiac-related deaths (21.5%). Multivariate analysis showed three variables to be independent predictors of both survival and event-free cardiac survival: NYHA classification, percentage of maximal predicted VO$_2$, and right ventricular EF.

Treatment

ACE Inhibitors and Angiotensin II Inhibitors

Meta-Analysis

27. **Garg R,** Yusuf S. Overview of randomized trials of angiotensin converting enzyme inhibitors on mortality and morbidity in patients with heart failure. *JAMA* 1995;273:1450–1456.

    This analysis focused on 32 studies with 7,105 patients. All studies were placebo-controlled, 8 weeks in duration and assessed all-cause mortality by intention to treat. ACE inhibitor therapy was associated with significant reductions in total mortality (odds ratio 0.77; 95% CI 0.67–0.88; $p < 0.001$) and mortality or hospitalization for CHF (odds ratio 0.65; 95% CI 0.57–0.74; $p < 0.001$). Patients with the lowest EF had the greatest benefit. The mortality reduction was mainly due to fewer deaths from progressive heart failure (odds ratio 0.69; 95% CI 0.58–0.83). There were nonsignificant reductions in the incidence of arrhythmic deaths (odds ratio 0.91; 95% CI 0.73–1.12) and fatal MI (odds ratio 0.82; 95% CI 0.60–1.12). There were no significant differences between several different agents (*see* Tables 5-1 and 5-2).

Studies

28. The Cooperative North Scandinavian Enalapril Survival Study **(CONSENSUS)** Group. Effects of enalapril on mortality in severe CHF. *N Engl J Med* 1987;316:1429–1435.
    Design: Prospective, randomized, double-blind, placebo-controlled, multicenter study. Average follow-up period was 6 months. Primary end point was all-cause mortality rate.
    Purpose: To evaluate the effect of enalapril, in addition to conventional therapy, on mortality in patients with severe CHF.
    Population: 253 NYHA class IV patients with heart size >600 mL/m^2 body surface area in men and >550 mL/m^2 in women.
    Exclusion Criteria: Acute pulmonary edema, MI in prior 2 months, unstable angina, planned cardiac surgery, and serum creatinine >300 μM.
    Treatment: Enalapril 2.5 mg/day orally up to 20 mg twice daily. All patients were on diuretics, 94% on digoxin, and 50% on vasodilators (mostly isosorbide dinitrate).
    Results: Trial was terminated early due to significant mortality benefit in the enalapril group: 40% relative risk reduction (RRR) in mortality at 6 months (26% vs. 44%; $p = 0.0002$), 31% RRR at 1 year (36% vs. 52%; $p = 0.001$), and 27% RRR at end of study (39% vs. 54%; $p = 0.003$). Of note, the entire mortality reduction was seen in patients with progressive heart failure (~50% lower mortality). No difference in sudden death rates was observed. A

significant mortality benefit was maintained at 2-year follow-up (*see Am J Cardiol* 1992;60:103).

29. The Studies of Left Ventricular Dysfunction **(SOLVD)** Investigators. Effect of enalapril on survival in patients with reduced ventricular ejection fraction and congestive heart failure. *N Engl J Med* 1991; 325:293–302 (editorial pp. 351–353).

Design: Prospective, randomized, double-blind, placebo-controlled, multicenter study. Average follow-up period was 41 months. Primary end point was all-cause mortality rate.

Purpose: To evaluate the effect of enalapril on mortality in patients with left ventricular dysfunction and heart failure symptoms.

Population: 2,569 NYHA class II and III patients 21–80 years of age with an EF ≤35%.

Exclusion Criteria: Active angina requiring surgery, unstable angina, or MI within preceding month; renal failure; pulmonary disease; and current ACE inhibitor therapy.

Treatment: Enalapril 2.5—5 mg twice daily initially then increased at 2 weeks to 5–10 mg twice daily; or placebo. Other drugs were not restricted (e.g., diuretics, digoxin, vasodilators).

Results: Enalapril group had 16% lower mortality (35.2% vs. 39.7%, 16% risk reduction; p = 0.0036). The majority of this effect was due to fewer deaths from progressive heart failure (16.3% vs. 19.5%; p = 0.0045). The enalapril group also had a lower rate of death and rehospitalization due to worsening heart failure (47.7% vs. 57.3%, 26% risk reduction; p < 0.0001). Sudden death rates were similar.

30. The SOLVD Investigators. Effect of enalapril on mortality and the development of heart failure in asymptomatic patients with reduced left ventricular ejection fractions. *N Engl J Med* 1992; 327:685–691.

Design: Prospective, randomized, double-blind, placebo-controlled, multicenter study. Follow-up period was 37 months. Primary end point was all-cause mortality rate.

Purpose: To evaluate effect of enalapril on mortality in patients with left ventricular dysfunction without overt heart failure.

Population: 4,228 patients 21–80 years of age with an EF ≤35% and on no medications for heart failure (diuretics allowed for hypertension and digoxin for atrial fibrillation).

Exclusion Criteria: See SOLVD trial (29).

Treatment: Enalapril 2.5–20 mg orally per day or placebo.

Results: Total mortality rates were 14.8% and 15.8% in the enalapril and placebo groups, respectively (p = 0.30). Most of this nonsignificant difference was due to 12% fewer cardiovascular deaths in the enalapril group (12.5% vs. 14.1%; p = 0.12). Fewer enalapril patients developed heart failure (20.7% vs. 30.2%; p < 0.001) and fewer required hospitalization due to heart failure (8.7% vs. 12.9%; p < 0.001).

31. The Acute Infarction Ramipril Efficacy Study **(AIRE)** Investigators. Effect of ramipril on mortality and morbidity of survivors of acute MI with clinical evidence of heart failure. *Lancet* 1993; 342:821–828.

Design: Prospective, randomized, double-blind, placebo-controlled, multicenter study. Mean follow-up period was 15 months. Primary end point was all-cause mortality.

Purpose: To compare the effects of ramipril with placebo on overall mortality in acute MI survivors with early evidence of CHF.

Population: 2,006 patients with an MI 2–9 days prior to study enrollment and clinical evidence of heart failure at any time since acute MI.

Exclusion Criteria: Severe CHF (usually NYHA class IV), unstable angina, and heart failure of primary valvular or congenital etiology.

Treatment: Ramipril 2.5 mg orally twice daily for 2 days, then 5 mg twice daily; or placebo.

Results: Ramipril group had a 27% risk reduction in mortality (17% vs. 23%; $p = 0.002$). Of note, this benefit was already apparent at 30 days. Sudden cardiac deaths were reduced by 30% ($p = 0.011$).

Comments: AIREX follow-up study analyzed 603 patients at a mean 59 months, and the ramipril group still had a significantly lower mortality rate (relative risk 0.64; 27.5% vs. 38.9; $p = 0.002$) (*see Lancet* 1997;349:1493).

32. **Pitt B**, et al. Evaluation of Losartan in the Elderly **(ELITE)**. Randomized trial of losartan vs. captopril in patients over 65 with heart failure. *Lancet* 1997;349:747–752.

Design: Prospective, randomized, double-blind, placebo-controlled, multicenter study. Primary end point was increase in creatinine clearance of 0.3 mg/dL.

Purpose: To compare the angiotensin II receptor inhibitor losartan with captopril on creatinine clearance and major cardiac events in elderly heart failure patients.

Population: 722 ACE inhibitor–naive patients in NYHA class II–IV and with EF ≤40%.

Exclusion Criteria: SBP <90 mm Hg, acute MI or coronary angioplasty in prior 72 hours, bypass surgery in prior 2 weeks, unstable angina in prior 3 months, and stroke or transient ischemic attack in prior 3 months.

Treatment: Losartan 12.5–50 mg daily or captopril 6.25–50 mg three times daily for 48 weeks

Results: Similar incidence of increased creatinine was observed in both groups (10.5%). Fewer losartan patients discontinued therapy: 12.2% vs. 20.8%; $p = 0.002$ (cough, 0 vs. 14 patients). The losartan group showed a trend toward lower rates of death and hospitalization (9.4% vs. 13.2%; $p = 0.075$) and a significant 45% lower overall mortality rate (4.8% vs. 8.7%, $p = 0.035$; sudden cardiac death: 5 vs. 14 patients). This mortality benefit was seen in all subgroups except women (240 patients, 7.6% vs. 6.6%).

Comments: Study was not designed to examine mortality. Of note, two placebo-controlled exercise studies with a total of 350 patients have also shown a mortality benefit for losartan (*see J Am Coll Cardiol* 1997;29 (suppl A):205A).

33. **ATLAS**. Preliminary results. Presented at the 47th ACC Scientific Session in Atlanta, GA, March 1998.

This prospective, randomized, multicenter trial was composed of 3,164 patients with moderate to severe heart failure. Patients received lisinopril 2.5–5 mg/day or 32.5–35 mg/day. The median follow-up period was 4 years. The high-dose group had 8% lower mortality (42.5% vs. 44.9%; $p = $ NS), 10% lower cardiovascular mortality (37.2% vs. 40.2%; $p = 0.073$), 24% fewer CHF hospitalizations, and a significant 12% reduction in death or all-cause hospitalization (79.8% vs. 83.9%; $p = 0.002$).

34. Symptoms Tolerability Response to Exercise Trial of Candesartan Cilexil in Patients with Heart Failure (**STRETCH**). Preliminary results presented at the 71st AHA Scientific Session in Dallas, TX, November 1998.

A total of 844 patients with NYHA class II or III heart failure and an EF of 30%–45% were randomized to one of three doses of candesartan (4, 8, or 16 mg/day) or placebo for 3 months. There was a prerandomization 4-week placebo run-in period to wash out the effects of ACE inhibitors that were discontinued. There appeared to be a dose-dependent effect of candesartan on exercise time (primary end point), although the difference versus placebo was significant only in the 16 mg/day group. There were no differences between groups in the incidence of adverse effects.

Diuretics

35. **Dormans TPJ**, et al. Diuretic efficacy of high dose furosemide in severe heart failure: bolus injection vs. continuous infusion. *J Am Coll Cardiol* 1996;28:376–382.

In this crossover study, 20 patients were randomized to an equal dosage by intravenous bolus or an 8-hour continuous infusion after a loading dose (20% total). Doses used ranged from 250 to 2,000 mg/24 h. The continuous infusion group had an increased urinary volume (2.9 vs. 2.3 L; $p < 0.001$) and better sodium excretion. Reversible hearing loss was seen in five intravenous bolus patients (maximal plasma concentration 95 vs. 24 µg/mL (*see also Chest* 1992;102:725: only nine patients, and the bolus plus 48-hour infusion yielded better results than intravenous boluses three times daily).

36. **Pitt B**, et al. Randomized Aldactone Evaluation Study (**RALES**) Investigators. The effect of spironolactone on morbidity and mortality in patients with severe heart failure. *N Engl J Med* 1999; 341:709–719 (editorial pp. 753–755).

Design: Prospective, randomized, double-blind, placebo-controlled, multicenter study. Mean follow-up was 24 months. Primary end point was all-cause mortality.

Purpose: To evaluate if spironolactone would significantly reduce mortality in patients with severe HF.

Population: 1,663 NYHA Class III (69%) or IV (31%) patients with an EF ≤35%. Ischemic etiology of HF in 54%.

Exclusion Criteria: Included valvular heart disease, unstable angina, hepatic failure, potassium ≥5 mm/L, creatine >2.5 mg/dL.

Treatment: Spironolactone 25 mg or placebo once daily. Dose could be increased to 50 mg if worsening HF with normal potassium. All patients were on loop diuretics, 95% were on ACE inhibitors, and 74% were receiving digoxin.

Results: Spironolactone group had a significant (30%) reduction in mortality compared to placebo (35% vs 46%, p <0.001). This benefit was attributable to a lower risk of sudden death from cardiac causes (29% relative risk reduction) and death from progressive HF (36% relative risk reduction). Spironolactone was associated with a higher incidence of gynecomostia (10% vs 1%, p <0.001); whereas, the incidence of serious hyperkalemia was similar (2% vs 1%).

Comments: Mortality benefit was evident at 3 months and gradually increased over a 2 year follow-up. Risk of gynecomostia may be reduced with the use of selective aldosterone-receptor antagonists (e.g. eplerenone).

Digoxin

Review Articles

37. **Rahimtoola SH,** Tak T. The use of digitalis in heart failure. *Curr Probl Cardiol* 1996;21:787–853.

    This review covers the following points: (a) numerous actions of digitalis (e.g., inotropic, electrophysiologic, neurohormonal); (b) results and implications of clinical studies in heart failure patients (including the RADIANCE, PROVED, and DIG trials); (c) digitalis use in acute MI; (d) pharmacokinetics, bioavailability, and dosing of digitalis; and (e) clinical manifestations and treatment of digitalis toxicity.

38. **Hauptman PJ,** Kelly RA. *Circulation* 1999;99:1265–1270.

    This review discusses the molecular and clinical pharmacology of cardiac glycosides, describes the clinical manifestations and treatment of digitalis toxicity, and examines recent trial data, with a focus on the DIG trial results.

Studies

39. **Packer M**, et al. Randomized Assessment of Effect of Digoxin on Inhibitors of ACE **(RADIANCE)** study. Withdrawal of digoxin from patients with chronic HF treated with ACE inhibitor. *N Engl J Med* 1993;329:1–7.

    Design: Prospective, randomized, double-blind, placebo-controlled, multicenter study. Primary end point was study withdrawal due to worsening heart failure, time to withdrawal, and changes in exercise tolerance.

    Purpose: To evaluate the effect of the withdrawal of digoxin from patients with chronic heart failure who were clinically stable while receiving digoxin, diuretics, and an ACE inhibitor.

    Population: 178 NYHA class II or III patients on digoxin, diuretics, and ACE inhibitors (captopril or enalapril).

    Exclusion Criteria: SBP ≥160 mm Hg or <90 mm Hg, DBP >95 mm Hg, history of supraventricular arrhythmias or sustained ventricular arrhythmias, MI in prior 3 months, and stroke in prior 12 months.

    Treatment: Patients were randomized to continue digoxin or to placebo for 12 weeks.

    Results: Cessation/placebo group had a markedly higher rate of worsening CHF requiring withdrawal from the study (24.7% vs. 4.7; relative risk 5.9; $p < 0.001$), lower EF ($p < 0.001$), decreased functional capacity (maximal exercise tolerance, $p = 0.033$; submaximal exercise endurance, $p = 0.01$; NYHA class, $p = 0.019$; and poorer quality of life scores ($p = 0.04$).

40. **Uretsky BF**, et al. Prospective Randomized Study of Ventricular Failure and Efficacy of Digoxin **(PROVED)**. Randomized study assessing effect of digoxin withdrawal in patients with mild-moderate chronic CHF. *J Am Coll Cardiol* 1993;22:955–962.

    Design: Prospective, randomized, double-blind, placebo-controlled, multicenter study. Primary end point was incidence of treatment failure, time to treatment failure, treadmill time, and 6-minute walk distance.

    Purpose: To evaluate the effects of digoxin withdrawal in patients with mild to moderate heart failure.

    Population: 88 NYHA class II or III patients in normal sinus rhythm and on digoxin and diuretics.

Exclusion Criteria: SBP <90 mm Hg, acute MI or coronary angioplasty in prior 72 hours, bypass surgery in prior 2 weeks, unstable angina in prior 3 months, and stroke or transient ischemic attack in prior 3 months.

Treatment: Patients were randomized to continue digoxin or to placebo for 12 weeks.

Results: Cessation/placebo group had lower exercise tolerance (–96 vs. –4.5 seconds; p = 0.003), twice as many treatment failures (39% vs. 19%; p = 0.039), decreased time to treatment failure (p = 0.037), lower EF (p = 0.016), and higher heart rate (p = 0.003).

41. Digoxin Investigation Group **(DIG)**. The effect of digoxin on mortality and morbidity in patients with heart failure. *N Engl J Med* 1997;336:525–533.

    Design: Prospective, randomized, double-blind, placebo-controlled, multicenter study. Follow-up period was 37 months. Primary end point was all-cause mortality rate.

    Purpose: To evaluate the effects of digoxin on mortality from any cause in heart failure patients.

    Population: 6,800 patients with an EF ≤45% and in normal sinus rhythm. Most patients were on ACE inhibitors (94%) and diuretics (82%).

    Treatment: Digoxin (average dose 0.25 mg/day) or placebo.

    Results: No significant difference in mortality rates (34.8% vs. 35.1%) was observed. The digoxin group did have fewer CHF hospitalizations (26.8% vs. 34.7%; risk ratio 0.72; p < 0. 001) and showed a trend toward fewer CHF deaths (risk ratio 0.88; p = 0.06), but this was offset by increased mortality due to other cardiac causes (not a prespecified outcome; 15% vs. 13%; p = 0.04). Subgroup analysis showed that greater reductions in death and hospitalization were due to worsening heart failure if EF <25% (–23% vs. –16%) or NYHA class III/IV (–22% vs. –18%). An overall decrease in hospital stays of only nine per 1,000 patient years was observed. An ancillary trial of 988 patients with EF >45% also showed no difference in mortality (both 23.4%).

Vasodilator Studies

42. **Cohn JN**, et al., VA Cooperative Heart Failure Trial **(V-HeFT I)**. Effect of vasodilator therapy on mortality in chronic congestive heart failure. *N Engl J Med* 1986;314:1547–1552.

    Design: Prospective, randomized, double-blind, placebo-controlled, multicenter study. Mean follow-up period was 2.3 years. Primary end point was all-cause mortality rate.

    Purpose: To determine whether two widely employed vasodilator regimens could alter life expectancy in men with stable chronic CHF.

    Population: 642 men 18–75 years of age with chronic heart failure (defined as cardiac dilatation by chest x-ray or echocardiography) or EF <45% in association with reduced exercise tolerance).

    Exclusion Criteria: Exercise tolerance limited by chest pain, MI in prior 3 months, and requirement for long-acting nitrates, calcium-channel antagonists, and/or β-blockers.

    Treatment: Prazosin 20 mg once daily, hydralazine 300 mg/day, and isosorbide dinitrate 160 mg/day; or placebo. Digoxin and diuretics were permitted.

    Results: Hydralazine-isosorbide dinitrate group had 38% lower mortality at 1 year (12.1% vs. 19.5% (placebo), 25% reduction at 2 years [25.6% vs. 34.3% y (placebo); $p < 0.028$], and 23% reduction at 3 years (36.2% vs. 46.9%). LVEF increased significantly at 8 weeks and at 1 year in the hydralazine-isosorbide dinitrate group (+2.9%, +4.2%; both $p < 0.001$). No significant benefits were seen with prazosin.

43. **Cohn JN**, et al. **V-HeFT II**. A comparison of enalapril with hydralazine-isosorbide dinitrate in the treatment of chronic CHF. *N Engl J Med* 1991;325:303–310.

Design: Prospective, randomized, double-blind, placebo-controlled, multicenter study. Average follow-up period was 2.5 years. Primary end point was 2-year all-cause mortality rate.

Purpose: To compare the efficacy of enalapril with hydralazine plus isosorbide dinitrate in heart failure patients.

Population: 804 men 18–75 years of age in mostly NYHA class II/III and on digoxin and diuretics.

Exclusion Criteria: MI or cardiac surgery in prior 3 months and angina limiting exercise or requiring long-term medical therapy.

Treatment: Enalapril 20 mg/day or hydralazine 300 mg/day plus isosorbide dinitrate 160 mg/day.

Results: Enalapril group had a 28% lower 2-year mortality rate (18% vs. 25%; $p = 0.016$) and a 14% lower overall mortality rate (32.8% vs. 38.2%; $p = 0.08$). This mortality difference was due to fewer sudden cardiac deaths (57 vs. 92 patients), mostly in NYHA class I or II patients. At 13 weeks, the enalapril group had a greater reduction in blood pressure, whereas the hydralazine-isosorbide dinitrate group had a greater increase in EF and exercise tolerance.

44. **Packer M**, et al. Prospective Randomized Amlopidine Survival Evaluation **(PRAISE)**. Effect of amlopidine on morbidity and mortality in severe chronic heart failure. *N Engl J Med* 1996;335:1107–1114.

Design: Prospective, randomized, double-blind, placebo-controlled, multicenter study. Average follow-up period was 14 months. Primary end point was mortality and cardiovascular morbidity (hospitalization for 24 hours for MI, pulmonary edema, severe hypoperfusion, ventricular tachycardia or ventricular fibrillation).

Purpose: To assess the safety and efficacy of the calcium-channel antagonist amlopidine in patients with severe chronic heart failure.

Population: 1,153 patients with an EF <30%. Heart failure was associated with ischemic disease in 732 patients (63.5%).

Exclusion Criteria: Unstable angina or MI in prior month, cardiac arrest or sustained ventricular tachycardia or ventricular fibrillation in prior year, stroke or cardiac revascularization in prior 3 months, SBP <85 mm Hg or ≥160 mm Hg, and primary valvular disease.

Treatment: Amlopidine 10 mg/day or placebo.

Results: Amlopidine group had a nonsignificant 16% mortality reduction (33% vs. 38%; $p = 0.07$) and 9% fewer major events (death or hospital due to cardiovascular events (39% vs. 42%; $p = 0.31$). Among nonischemic patients, amlopidine was associated with a 46% lower mortality rate ($p < 0.001$) and 31% fewer overall events ($p = 0.04$)

Comments: PRAISE-2 will focus on a nonischemic population. An interesting ancillary study of cytokines showed that high interleukin-6 levels correlated with increased CHF and death ($p = 0.048$) and were lowered by amlopidine ($p = 0.006$) but to values still more than five times normal (*see J Am Coll Cardiol* 1997; 30:35).

45. **Fonarow GC**, et al. **Hydralazine-Captopril study (Hy-C)**. Effect of direct vasodilation with hydralazine versus ACE inhibition with captopril on mortality in advanced heart failure. *J Am Coll Cardiol* 1992;19:842–850.

    This study was composed of 117 heart transplant evaluees with a mean EF of 20%. Patients were randomized to captopril (initial dose 6.25 mg, titrated to maximum 100 mg every 6 hours) or hydralazine (initial dose 25 mg, titrated up to 150 mg every 6 hours) with or without isosorbide dinitrate (discontinued if intolerable side effects occurred). Doses were titrated to achieve a PCWP of 15 mm Hg and systemic vascular resistance of 1,200 dynes sec/cm^5. The captopril group had a better 1-year survival rate (81% vs. 51%; $p = 0.05$). As seen in V-HeFT II, this benefit was due to fewer sudden deaths ($p = 0.01$).

46. **Elkayam U**, et al. Double-blind, placebo-controlled study to evaluate the effect of organic nitrates in patients with chronic heart failure treated with angiotensin-converting enzyme inhibition. *Circulation* 1999;99:2652–2657.

    This small study of 29 NHYA class II or III patients was of a prospective, randomized, double-blind, crossover design. Patients received high-dose transdermal nitroglycerin (50–100 mg) or placebo for 12 hours daily. Exercise tolerance (measured 4 hours after patch application) was significantly improved in the nitrate group at 1, 2, and 3 months (+38, +76, and +117 seconds). No significant changes were observed in the placebo group. The nitrate group also had decreased left ventricular end-diastolic and end-systolic dimensions and improved left ventricular fractional shortening. There were no significant differences in quality of life scores or CHF-related hospitalizations.

β-*Blockers*

Review Articles and Meta-Analyses

47. **Heidenreich PA**, et al. Effect of β-blockade on mortality in patients with heart failure: a meta-analysis of randomized clinical trials. *J Am Coll Cardiol* 1997;30:27–34.

    This analysis focused on 17 randomized trials enrolling a total of 3,039 patients with mortality data through at least 3 months. β-blocker use was associated with significantly lower mortality (odds ratio 0.69; 95% CI 0. 54–0.88), mostly due to fewer nonsudden cardiac deaths (odds ratio 0.58; 95% CI 0.4–0.83). For sudden cardiac death, the odds ratio was 0.84 (95% CI 0.59–1.2). Similar mortality reductions were observed for ischemic and nonischemic cardiomyopathy patients.

48. **Frishman WH**. Carvedilol. *N Engl J Med* 1998;339:1759–1765.

    This review describes the pharmacodynamic and pharmacokinetic properties of carvedilol, an agent that has both α- and β-adrenergic antagonism. The middle section discusses the clinical efficacy of carvedilol in CHF. The final two sections cover dose regimens and titration and side effects.

49. **Lechat P**, et al. Clinical effects of β-adrenergic blockade in chronic heart failure. *Circulation* 1998;98:1184–1191.

This meta-analysis focused on 18 double-blind, placebo-controlled, parallel-group studies with a total of 3,023 patients. β-blocker use was associated with a 29% increase in EF ($p < 0.0001$) and 37% reduction in the risk of death or hospitalization for heart failure ($p < 0.001$). All-cause mortality was decreased by 32% ($p = 0.003$). There was a greater reduction for nonselective β-blockers compared with β_1-selective agents (49% vs. 18%; $p = 0.049$). The effect of β-blocker use on NYHA functional class was of only borderline significance ($p = 0.04$).

Carvedilol Studies

50. Australian-New Zealand **(ANZ)** Heart Failure Research Collaborative Group. Effects of carvedilol, a vasodilator–β-blocker, in patients with congestive heart failure due to ischemic heart disease. *Circulation* 1995;92:212–218.
    Design: Prospective, randomized, double-blind, placebo-controlled, multicenter study. Primary end points were changes in LVEF and treadmill exercise duration from baseline to 6 months.
    Purpose: To evaluate the effects of carvedilol on symptoms, exercise performance, and left ventricular function in patients with CHF due to coronary artery disease.
    Population: 415 NYHA class II or III patients with an EF <45% and ischemic etiology of heart failure.
    Exclusion Criteria: SBP <90 mm Hg, heart rate <50 beats/min, heart block, coronary event or procedure within previous 4 weeks, primary myocardial or valvular disease, and verapamil and/or β-blocker therapy.
    Treatment: After a 2- to 3-week run-in period (3.125–6.25 mg twice daily; only 4% withdrawal rate), patients were randomized to carvedilol (target dose 25 mg twice daily), or placebo; 86% were on ACE inhibitors.
    Results: At 6 months, the carvedilol group had a 5.2% higher EF (by radionuclide ventriculography; $p < 0.0001$) and decreased left ventricular end-systolic and left ventricular end-diastolic dimensions [−2.6 mm ($p < 0.0001$) and −1.3 mm ($p = 0.048$)]. No changes were seen in exercise tolerance (6-minute walk test). NYHA class improvement was seen in 28% and 23% (placebo; $p = NS$), whereas worsening symptoms occurred in 5% vs. 12% ($p = 0.05$).

51. **Packer M**, et al. Prospective Randomized Evaluation of Carvedilol on Symptoms and Exercise **(PRECISE)**. Double-blind, placebo-controlled study of the effects of carvedilol in patients with moderate to severe heart failure. *Circulation* 1996;94:2793–2799.
    Design: Prospective, randomized, double-blind, placebo-controlled, multicenter study. Primary end point was exercise tolerance.
    Purpose: To evaluate the clinical effects of carvedilol in patients with moderate to severe CHF.
    Population: 278 patients with moderate to severe CHF (dyspnea or fatigue at rest or on exertion for 3 months), an EF ≤35% and receiving digoxin, diuretics, and an ACE inhibitor.
    Exclusion Criteria: MI, unstable angina, CABG surgery, or stroke in prior 3 months; uncorrected primary valvular disease; SBP <85 mm Hg or >160 mm Hg or DBP >100 mm Hg; heart rate <68 beats/min; and use of calcium-channel blockers or antiarrhythmic drugs.
    Treatment: During the open-label run-in period, carvedilol 6.25 mg twice daily for 2 weeks. If tolerated, the patient was randomized to

carvedilol 12.5 twice daily initially, with titration over 2–6 weeks to 25–50 mg twice daily for 6 months, or placebo.
Results: Carvedilol patients had more frequent improvement in symptoms, as evaluated by changes in NYHA functional class ($p = 0.014$) and global assessments by the patient ($p = 0.002$) and the physician ($p < 0.001$). Carvedilol patients also had a significant increase in EF (+8% vs. +3%; $p < 0.001$) and a significant decrease in morbidity and mortality (19.6% vs. 31.0%; $p = 0.029$). However, there was no significant effect on exercise tolerance or quality of life scores.

52. **Colucci WS**, et al. Carvedilol inhibits clinical progression in patients with mild symptoms of heart failure. *Circulation* 1996;94: 2800–2806.
Design: Prospective, randomized, double-blind, placebo-controlled, multicenter study. Primary end point was progression of heart failure (defined as death or hospitalization due to heart failure or need for sustained increase in heart failure medications).
Purpose: To determine if long-term treatment with carvedilol inhibits clinical progression in patients with mild symptoms of heart failure and receiving optimal therapy.
Population: 278 patients 18–85 years of age with an EF ≤35%.
Exclusion Criteria: MI, unstable angina, or CABG surgery in prior 3 months; SBP <85 mm Hg or >160 mm Hg or DBP >100 mm Hg; uncorrected primary valvular disease; and use of calcium-channel blockers or antiarrhythmic drugs.
Treatment: After the open-label run-in phase on carvedilol 6.25 mg twice daily, patients were randomized to carvedilol 12.5–50 mg twice daily or placebo for 6 months.
Results: Carvedilol group had a 48% reduction in clinical progression of heart failure (11% vs. 21%; $p = 0.008$). The carvedilol group also had a significant reduction in all-cause mortality (0.9% vs. 4.0%; risk ratio 0.23; $p = 0.048$) and improved EF (+10% vs. +3%; $p < 0.001$) and NYHA functional class ($p < 0.003$). However, there were no differences in exercise tolerance or quality of life, and no difference between idiopathic dilated cardiomyopathy and ischemic heart disease patients.

53. **Bristow MR**, et al. Multicenter Oral Carvedilol Heart Failure Assessment **(MOCHA)**. Carvedilol produces dose-related improvements in left ventricular function and survival in subjects with chronic heart failure. *Circulation* 1996;94:2807–2816.
Design: Prospective, randomized, double-blind, placebo-controlled, multicenter study. Follow-up period was 6 months. Primary end point was change in walk test distances (6-minute corridor test and 9-minute self-powered treadmill test).
Purpose: To evaluate the effects of carvedilol in addition to standard therapy on clinical events and quality of life in chronic heart failure patients.
Population: 345 patients 18–85 years of age with symptomatic, stable heart failure capable of walking 150–450 meters in 6 minutes.
Exclusion Criteria: MI or stroke in prior 3 months, uncorrected primary valvular disease, planned bypass surgery or balloon angioplasty, SBP <85 or >160 mm Hg, and use of calcium-channel blockers or antiarrhythmic drugs.
Treatment: Carvedilol 6.25–25 mg/day or placebo. Concomitant therapy included diuretics, digoxin, and ACE inhibitors.

Results: No differences were seen in submaximal exercise performance (as assessed by two walk tests) or heart failure symptoms. Carvedilol was associated with dose-dependent improvements in left ventricular function (+5%, +6%, and +8% in low-, medium-, and high-dose groups versus +2% with placebo; $p < 0.001$) and mortality (6.0%, 6.7%, and 1.1% vs. 15.5%; $p < 0.001$). When the three carvedilol groups were combined, the all-cause actuarial mortality risk was 73% lower ($p < 0.001$). Carvedilol patients also were hospitalized less frequently (by 58% to 64%; $p = 0.01$).

54. **Packer M**, et al. U.S. Carvedilol Heart Failure Study Group. The effect of carvedilol on morbidity and mortality in patients with chronic heart failure. *N Engl J Med* 1996;334:1349–1355 (editorial pp. 1396–1397).

    Design: Prospective, randomized, double-blind, placebo-controlled, multicenter study. Primary end point was mortality.

    Purpose: To evaluate the safety and efficacy of carvedilol in patients with chronic failure.

    Population: 1,094 chronic heart failure patients with an EF ≤35% and on digoxin, diuretics, and an ACE inhibitor.

    Exclusion Criteria: SBP <90 mm Hg, acute MI or coronary angioplasty in prior 72 hours, bypass surgery in prior 2 weeks, unstable angina in prior 3 months, and stroke or transient ischemic attack in prior 3 months.

    Treatment: After the 2-week open-label phase (5.6% failed to complete this period due to adverse events), patients were assigned to one of four treatment groups based on exercise capacity [6-minute walk: mild, 426–550 m; moderate, 150–425 m; severe, <150 m (fourth group dose-ranging protocol)] and randomized to carvedilol 6.25–50 mg twice daily (titrated over 2–10 weeks), or placebo.

    Results: At 6 months, carvedilol-treated patients had 65% lower mortality (3.2% vs. 7.8%; $p < 0.001$), 27% fewer cardiovascular-related hospitalizations (14.1% vs. 19.6%; $p = 0.036$), and a 38% reduction in death and hospitalization (15.8% vs. 24.6%; $p < 0.001$). Patients with an initial heart rate of >82 beats/min had the most benefit. More placebo patients had worsening heart failure.

    Comments: Analysis combined patients from three different studies [PRECISE, MOCHA, Colucci WS, et al. (52)]. This study had limited follow-up and only 53 total deaths; 7 carvedilol deaths occurred in the run-in period and 17 patients (1.4%) were excluded due to worsening heart failure [more problematic in severe heart failure patients (only 3% of this study population)].

55. Heart Failure Research Collaborative Group. **ANZ** (Australia/New Zealand). Randomized, placebo-controlled trial of carvedilol in patients with congestive heart failure due to ischaemic heart disease. *Lancet* 1997;349:375–380.

    Design: Prospective, randomized, double-blind, placebo-controlled, multicenter study. Average follow-up period was 19 months. Primary end point was changes in LVEF and treadmill exercise duration.

    Purpose: To evaluate the longer term effects on death and other serious clinical events of carvedilol in patients with chronic stable heart failure.

    Population: 415 NYHA class II or III patients with chronic stable heart failure.

    Exclusion Criteria: Current NYHA class IV; primary valvular disease; SBP <90 mm Hg or >160 mm Hg or DBP >100 mgHg; and

MI, unstable angina, bypass surgery, or coronary angioplasty in prior 4 weeks.

Treatment: 27 patients were withdrawn during the 2- to 3-week open label phase of carvedilol therapy (3.125 mg daily to 6.25 mg twice daily). Carvedilol was then given at 6.25–25 mg twice daily, or placebo.

Results: At 1 year, the carvedilol group had an increased EF (+5.3%; $p < 0.0001$) and decreased end-diastolic and end-systolic dimensions (−1.7 mm ($p = 0.06$) and −3.2 mm ($p = 0.001$)). However, there were no differences in exercise treadmill time, 6-minute walk distance, NYHA class, or specific activity score. At 19 months, there was no difference in the number of heart failure episodes, but the carvedilol group had a lower incidence of death and hospitalization (50% vs. 63%; relative risk 0.74; 95% CI 0.57–0.95).

Comments: ANZ echocardiographic substudy of 123 patients (echocardiograms at baseline and 6 and 12 months) showed that the carvedilol group had a left ventricular end-diastolic volume index 1 4mL/m^2 lower than placebo ($p = 0.0015$), left-ventricular end-systolic volume index 15.3 mL/m^2 lower than placebo ($p = 0.0001$), and EF 5.8% higher ($p = 0.0015$) (*see J Am Coll Cardiol* 1997;29:1060).

Other Studies

56. **Waagstein F**, et al. Metoprolol in Dilated Cardiomyopathy **(MDC)**. Beneficial effects of metoprolol in idiopathic dilated cardiomyopathy (DCM). *Lancet* 1993;342:1441–1446.

Design: Prospective, randomized, double-blind, placebo-controlled, parallel-group, multicenter study. Follow-up period was 12–18 months. Primary end point was death and need for cardiac transplantation.

Purpose: To evaluate the effects of metoprolol vs. placebo in patients with heart failure due to idiopathic dilated cardiomyopathy.

Population: 383 patients 16–75 years of age with left ventricular EF <0.40; 94% were in NYHA functional class II or III.

Exclusion Criteria: Use of β-blockers or calcium-channel blockers, coronary artery disease (>50% stenosis), SBP <90 mm Hg, heart rate <45 beats/min, obstructive lung disease requiring β-agonists, and insulin-dependent diabetes.

Treatment: If the test dose was tolerated (metoprolol 5 mg twice daily for 2–7 days), then patients were randomized to metoprolol [10 mg/day titrated up to 100–150 mg/day (mean 108 mg/day)], or placebo.

Results: Metoprolol group had 34% risk reduction in death or need for heart transplantation (22.5% vs. 36.5%; $p = 0.058$). At follow-up, the metoprolol group had a significantly better improvement in LVEF (+0.12 vs. +0.06 at 12 months; $p < 0.0001$), increased exercise duration (+76 vs. +15 seconds at 12 months; $p = 0.046$), and showed a trend toward lower PCWP (− 5 vs. −2 mm Hg; $p = 0.06$). The metoprolol group had better quality of life (based on patient assessment at 12 and 18 months; $p = 0.01$), and there was a significant correlation between the NYHA classification made by the physician and the quality of life assessment. A subsequent report showed that the metoprolol group had a significantly improved exercise oxygen consumption index ($p = 0.045$) (*see J Am Coll Cardiol* 1994;23:1397).

57. **Lechat P**, et al. Cardiac Insufficiency Bisoprolol Study **(CIBIS)**. A randomized trial of β-blockade in heart failure. *Circulation* 1994; 90:1765–1773.

    Design: Prospective, randomized, double-blind, placebo-controlled, multicenter study. Mean follow-up period was 1.9 years. Primary end point was total mortality rate.

    Purpose: To evaluate the effects of bisoprolol on all-cause mortality in heart failure patients.

    Population: 641 patients 18–75 years of age with an EF <40%; 95% were NYHA class III and 5% class IV.

    Exclusion Criteria: MI in prior 3 months, planned bypass surgery, heart failure secondary to mitral or aortic valve disease, insulin-dependent diabetes, SBP <100 or >160 mm Hg, and resting heart rate <65 beats/min.

    Treatment: Bisoprolol 1.25–5.0 mg/day or placebo. All patients were on diuretics and vasodilator therapy, and 90% were on ACE inhibitors.

    Results: Bisoprolol group had a nonsignificant 20% mortality reduction (16.6% vs. 20.8%; $p = 0.22$). Bisoprolol significantly improved the functional status of patients: fewer hospitalizations for cardiac decompensation (19% vs. 28%$p < 0.01$) and more with an improvement of one NYHA class (21% vs. 15%; $p = 0.04$).

    Comments: Study was underpowered and only half of patients were titrated to the target dose. In the subgroup of patients with no prior history of MI, there was a clear survival benefit ($p = 0.034$).

58. Cardiac Insufficiency Bisoprolol Study II **(CIBIS-II)** Investigators and Committees. *Lancet* 1999;353:9–12.

    Design: Prospective, randomized, double-blind, placebo-controlled, multicenter study. Mean follow-up period was 1.3 years. Primary end point was all-cause mortality rate.

    Purpose: To evaluate the efficacy of bisoprolol in decreasing all-cause mortality in patients with symptomatic chronic heart failure.

    Population: 2,647 NYHA class III or IV patients with LVEF <35%.

    Exclusion Criteria: Uncontrolled hypertension, MI, or unstable angina in prior 3 months, PTCA or CABG in prior 6 months, heart rate <60 beats/min, preexisting or planned therapy with β-blockers.

    Treatment: Bisoprolol 1.25–10.0 mg/day or placebo. All patients were on diuretics and ACE inhibitors.

    Results: Study was terminated because bisoprolol showed a significant mortality benefit: 11.8% vs. 17.3% (hazard ratio 0.66; $p < 0.0001$). The bisoprolol group also had a lower incidence of sudden death (3.6% vs. 6.3%, hazard ratio 0.56; $p = 0.0011$) and 20% fewer hospital admissions; treatment effects were independent of severity or cause of heart failure.

    Comments: No run-in period provided a better estimate of clinical effectiveness of bisoprolol. The low mortality rates suggest that not all patients were NYHA class III and IV patients. Further data are needed for many subgroups of patients: >80 years of age, post-MI, severe CHF, symptom-free with left ventricular dysfunction, and diastolic dysfunction.

59. **MERIT-HF** Study Group. Effect of metoprolol CR/XL in chronic heart failure: metoprolol CR/XL randomized intervention trial in congestive heart failure (MERIT-HF). *Lancet* 1999;353:2001–2007.

Design: Prospective, randomized, double-blind, placebo-controlled multicenter study. Mean follow-up period was 1 year. Primary end point was all-cause mortality.

Purpose: To evaluate whether metoprolol CR/XL, once daily, in addition to standard therapy, could lower mortality in symptomatic heart failure patients with impaired ejection fraction.

Population: 3,991 NYHA Class II–IV (II: 41%, III: 55%) patients with an ejection fraction ≤ 40%. Two thirds of patients that had an ischemic etiology of HF 89% were on an ACE inhibitor, 90% were on a diuretic, and 63% were receiving digoxin.

Treatment: Metoprolol CR/XL 12.5 mg (NYHA III or IV) or 25 mg (NYHA II) once daily; or placebo. Target dose was 200 mg/day with up-titration over 8 weeks. Of note: randomization was preceded by a 2 week single-blind placebo run-in period.

Results: All-cause mortality was significantly lower in the metoprolol group (7.2% vs 11.0%, relative risk 0.66, p < 0.001). The metoprolol group also had a 38% reduction in cardiovascular mortality (p < 0.001), a 41% reduction in sudden death (p < 0.001), and a 49% reduction in death due to progressive heart failure (p=0.002). The incidence of side effects was similar in both groups.

60. **Fisher ML**, et al. Beneficial effects of metoprolol in heart failure associated with coronary artery disease: a randomized trial. *J Am Coll Cardiol* 1994; 23:943–950.

   This small study was composed of 50 patients with known coronary artery disease and an EF ≤43%. The mean maximal dosage was 87 mg/day. At 6 months, the metoprolol group had increased EF (+4%), improved exercise tolerance (+193 seconds), and fewer hospital admissions (just 4% vs. 32%).

61. **Gilbert EM**, et al. Comparative, hemodynamic, left ventricular, functional and antiadrenergic effects of chronic treatment with metoprolol vs. carvedilol in the failing heart. *Circulation* 1996;94: 2817–2825.

   This analysis focused on 101 metoprolol patients from the MDC trial and 103 carvedilol patients from a phase II trial. Metoprolol 125–150 mg/day and carvedilol 50–100 mg/day were associated with similar reductions in exercise heart rates. Carvedilol patients had better NYHA and EF improvements, lower coronary sinus norepinephrine levels [vs. no change (metoprolol)], and no change in cardiac β-receptor density (vs. increased for metoprolol).

Amiodarone

62. **Doval HC**, et al. Grupo de Estudio de la Sobrevida en la Insuficiencia Cardiaca en Argentina **(GESICA)**. Randomized trial of low-dose amiodarone in severe CHF. *Lancet* 1994;344:493–498.

   Design: Prospective, randomized, open, parallel group, multicenter study. Follow-up period was 2 years. Primary end point was total mortality.

   Purpose: To evaluate the effect of low-dose amiodarone on mortality in patients with severe heart failure without symptomatic ventricular arrhythmias.

   Population: 516 NYHA class II–IV patients with stable functional capacity and not requiring antiarrhythmic therapy.

   Exclusion Criteria: Amiodarone treatment during prior 3 months; MI, heart failure onset, or syncope in prior 3 months; and history of sustained ventricular tachycardia or ventricular fibrillation.

Treatment: Amiodarone 500 mg/day for 14 days then 300 mg once daily for 2 years; or standard therapy (diuretics, digoxin, ACE inhibitors).

Results: Amiodarone group had 28% risk reduction in mortality at 2 years (33.5% vs. 41.4%; *p* = 0.024) and 31% risk reduction in hospitalization due to worsening heart failure (45.8% vs. 58.2%; *p* = 0.0024). There were reductions in both sudden death (27% risk reduction; *p* = 0.16) and death due to progressive heart failure (23% risk reduction; *p* = 0.16). These benefits were present in all examined subgroups and were independent of the presence of nonsustained ventricular tachycardia. Side effects were reported in 17 amiodarone patients (6.1%), of whom 12 discontinued therapy.

Comments: The study was blinded only to coordination center personnel, had a unique population (10% with Chagas' disease), and was terminated at the two-thirds point.

63. **Singh SN**, et al. Survival Trial of Antiarrhythmic Therapy in CHF **(CHF-STAT)**. Amiodarone in patients with congestive heart failure and asymptomatic ventricular arrhythmia. *N Engl J Med* 1995;333:77–82 (editorial pp. 121–122).

Design: Prospective, randomized, double-blind, placebo-controlled, multicenter study. Follow-up period was 45 months. Primary end point was overall mortality and sudden death from cardiac causes.

Purpose: To evaluate the effect of antiarrhythmic therapy on mortality in patients with CHF and asymptomatic ventricular arrhythmia.

Population: 674 patients with symptoms of CHF, cardiac enlargement, ≤10 premature ventricular contractions, and EF ≥40%.

Exclusion Criteria: MI in prior 3 months, history of cardiac arrest or sustained ventricular tachycardia, need for antiarrhythmic therapy, and SBP <90 mm Hg.

Treatment: Amiodarone 800 mg/day for 14 days, 400 mg/day for 50 weeks, then 300 mg/day; or placebo. Other therapy consisted of vasodilators (all patients), with or without digoxin or diuretics.

Results: There were no significant differences in mortality or sudden death [30.6% (amiodarone) vs. 29.2%; 15% vs. 19%; *p* = 0.43]. However, amiodarone was associated with a trend toward lower mortality in the subgroup of patients with nonischemic cardiomyopathy (*p* = 0.07). The amiodarone group also had better suppression of ventricular arrhythmias and a greater increase in EF at 2 years (+10.5% vs. +4.1%).

Comments: This VA-based trial had notable differences compared with GESICA: older patients (+6 yrs), more men (GESICA, 48% lower mortality in females vs. 26% in men), and healthier patients with higher EFs. However, subgroup analysis showed that the greatest benefits in CHF-STAT occurred in NYHA class II patients.

Inotropic and Other Agents

64. **Dibianco**, et al. A comparison of oral milrinone, digoxin and their combination in the treatment of patients with chronic heart failure. *N Engl J Med* 1989;320:677–683.

This prospective, randomized trial was composed of 230 patients comparing 12 weeks of digoxin, milrinone, and their combination. Both agents alone improved exercise tolerance (+64 vs. +82 seconds) and lowered frequency of decompensation [15% and 34% vs. 47% (placebo)]. Overall, there was no significant difference between the effects of the two drugs. Milrinone and digoxin were no better than digoxin alone.

65. **Packer M**, et al. Prospective Randomized Milrinone Survival Evaluation **(PROMISE)**. Effect of oral milrinone on mortality in severe chronic heart failure. *N Engl J Med* 1991;325:1468–1475. *Design:* Prospective, randomized, double-blind, placebo-controlled, multicenter study. Mean follow-up period was 6.1 months. Primary end point was all-cause mortality.
Purpose: To evaluate the effect of oral administration of the phosphodiesterase milrinone on mortality in patients with severe CHF.
Population: 1,088 NYHA class III or IV patients and EF <35%.
Exclusion Criteria: Obstructive valvular disease; history of serious ventricular arrhythmia; MI in prior 3 months; SBP <85 mm Hg; and requirement for β-blockers calcium-channel blockers, and antiarrhythmic drugs.
Treatment: Milrinone 40 mg/day orally or placebo. All patients were on digoxin, diuretics, and ACE inhibitors.
Results: Study was terminated early. Milrinone was associated with significantly higher all-cause mortality (30% vs. 24%; *p* = 0.038) and cardiovascular mortality rates (29.4% vs. 22.6%; *p* = 0.016). The milrinone group had a 69% increased risk of sudden cardiac deaths (*p* = 0.005), whereas there was no increased risk of death due to progressive heart failure. Adverse effects were worst among class IV patients (53% higher mortality; *p* = 0.006).

66. **Feldman AM**, et al. Effects of vesnarinone on morbidity and mortality in patients with heart failure. *N Engl J Med* 1993;329: 149–155.
This prospective study randomized 477 patients to vesnarinone 60 mg/day or placebo. Vesnarinone is a class III antiarrhythmic and anticytokine and an inotrope at high doses. The vesnarinone group had 48% lower mortality at 6 months. However, the drug has a narrow therapeutic range, with a higher mortality rate associated with 120 mg/day. Neutropenia was seen in 2.5% of patients on vesnarinone.

67. **Massie BM**, et al. Flosequinan-ACE Inhibitor Trial **(FACET)**. Can further benefit be achieved by adding flosequinan to patients with CHF who remain symptomatic on diuretic, digoxin and an ACE inhibitor? *Circulation* 1993;88:492–501.
This prospective, randomized trial was composed of 322 mostly NYHA class II or III patients with an EF ≤35% and on an ACE inhibitor, diuretic, and digoxin. Patients received flosequinan 100 mg once daily or 75 mg twice daily or placebo. Flosequinan is an arterial and venous vasodilator and has dose-dependent inotropic properties (undefined mechanism). At 16 weeks, only the 100-mg group had better exercise tolerance (+64 seconds), whereas the 75-mg group had a high incidence of palpations (17%) and headache (42%).

68. **Hampton JR**, et al. Prospective Randomised Study of Ibopamine on Mortality and Efficacy **(PRIME II)**. Randomised study of effect of ibopamine on survival in patients with advanced severe HF. *Lancet* 1997;349:971–977 (editorial pp. 966–967).
This prospective, randomized, multicenter trial was composed of 1,906 NYHA II–IV patients. The average follow-up period was

1 year. The trial was terminated early because the ibopamine group had increased mortality (25% vs. 20%; $p = 0.017$). In multivariate analysis, antiarrhythmic use was associated with increased mortality in ibopamine patients.

69. **Califf RM**, et al. Flolan International Randomized Survival Trial (**FIRST**). A randomized controlled trial of epoprostenol therapy. *Am Heart J* 1997;134:44–54.

    This prospective, randomized trial was composed of 471 patients with an EF <25% (<30% if on inotropes); NYHA class IIIB or IV symptoms for 1 month on digoxin, diuretic, and ACE inhibitor; and cardiac index ≤2.2 mL/kg/m² and PCWP 15 mm Hg. Patients were randomized to epoprostenol (initial dose 2 ng/kg/min, median 4.0) or standard care. A central line was placed for home infusion. The epoprostenol group had an increased cardiac index (1.81–2.61) and decreased PCWP (24.5–20.0 mm Hg), but showed a trend toward increased mortality ($p = 0.055$), prompting early termination of the trial.

70. **Cohn JN**, et al. for the Vesnarinone Trial Investigators. A dose-dependent increase in mortality with vesnarinone among patients with severe heart failure. *N Engl J Med* 1998;339:1801–1806 (editorial pp. 1848–1850).

    Design: Prospective, randomized, double-blind, placebo-controlled, multicenter study. Mean follow-up period was 286 days. Primary end point was all-cause mortality rate.

    Purpose: To determine the effects of vesnarinone on mortality and morbidity among patients with depressed left ventricular function and symptoms of severe heart failure.

    Population: 3,833 patients with NYHA class III or IV heart failure and an LVEF ≤30% despite optimal treatment (any regimen of diuretics, vasodilators, ACE inhibitor, and digitalis).

    Exclusion Criteria: MI or cardiac surgery in prior 2 months, significant valvular disease, and treatment with β-blockers.

    Treatment: Vesnarinone (30 or 60 mg) or placebo once daily.

    Results: Placebo group had significantly fewer deaths than the 60 mg vesnarinone group (18.9% vs. 22.9%; $p = 0.02$). Increased mortality with vesnarinone was mostly due to increased sudden death rate (12.3% vs. 9.1%). Quality of life (assessed by Minnesota Living with Heart Failure Questionnaire) improved significantly more in the 60 mg vesnarinone group than in the placebo group at 8 weeks ($p < 0.001$) and 16 weeks ($p = 0.003$), but by 26 weeks the differences were no longer significant. Agranulocytosis occurred in 1.2% and 0.2% of those given vesnarinone 60 mg/day and 30 mg/day, respectively.

    Comments: Inotropic agents should be avoided in patients in whom it is possible to modify disease progression and lower mortality. The accompanying editorial suggests that in the small portion of patients (~100,000 out of >4 million) in whom all therapies fail there may yet be a place for selected agents that cause sufficient relief of symptoms to justify a small increase in the risk of death.

Surgical Options

71. **Oz MC**, et al. Screening scale predicts patients successfully receiving long-term implantable left ventricular assist devices. *Circulation* 1995;92 (suppl II):II-169–II-173.

    A risk factor selection scale (range 0–10) was developed based on an analysis of easily obtainable preoperative risk factors in 56 patients undergoing LVAD insertion. Points were assigned as follows: urine output <30 mL/h (weight, 3), central venous pressure >16 mm Hg (weight, 2), mechanical ventilation (weight, 2), prothrombin time >16 seconds (weight, 2), and reoperation (weight, 1). The mortality rate among those with a score of 5 was 67%. The average score of nonsurvivors was 5.43 vs. 2.45 among survivors ($p < 0.0001$).

72. **Furnary AP**, et al. Multicenter trial of dynamic cardiomyoplasty for chronic heart failure. *J Am Coll Cardiol* 1996;28:1175–1180 (editorial pp. 1181–1182).

This analysis focused on 68 patients from eight North American and six South American centers, 47 with idiopathic etiology and 29 with ischemic cause of CHF. The in-hospital mortality rate was 12% and the 1-year mortality rate was 32%. At 6 months, better EF (25% vs. 23%; $p = 0.05$), stroke volume (56 vs. 50 mL/beat; $p = 0.02$), and NYHA functional class (3.0 vs. 1.8; $p = 0.0001$) were observed. No significant changes in peak oxygen consumption, cardiac index, PCWP, or heart rate were observed. The accompanying editorial points out that the study lacked a control group, that the results were worse than those typically seen with drugs, and that the technique is not applicable to NYHA class IV ("those who need it don't survive it, those who survive it don't need it").

73. **Batista RJV**, et al. Partial left ventriculectomy to treat end-stage heart disease. *Ann Thorac Surg* 1997;64:634–638.

A total of 120 patients with end-stage dilated cardiomyopathy of varying causes underwent surgical removal of a wedge of the left ventricular muscle, and the mitral valve apparatus was either preserved, repaired, or replaced with tissue prosthesis, depending on the distance between the two papillary muscles. Mortality at 30 days was 22%. At 2 years, mortality was 55%, with most of the survivors in NYHA class I (57%) or II (33%).

74. **McCarthy JF**, et al. Partial left ventriculectomy and mitral valve repair for end-stage congestive heart failure. *Eur J Cardiothorac Surg* 1998;13:337–343.

In this study of 57 NYHA class III or IV patients, 54 were listed for transplantation. All had a left ventricular end-diastolic diameter >7 cm. At the time of ventriculectomy, concomitant mitral valve repair was performed in 55 patients, tricuspid valve repair in 31, and CABG in 5. LVAD rescue was required in 17%, and 1-year actuarial survival was 82%. At 3 months, LVEF among survivors had improved to 23. 2% from 14.4%, and left ventricular end-diastolic diameter had decreased from 8.4 to 6.3 cm. There was also significant improvement in NYHA class at 3 months (2.2 vs. 3.6).

75. **Bolling SF**, et al. Intermediate-term outcome of mitral construction in cardiomyopathy. *J Thorac Cardiovasc Surg* 1998;115:381–386.

A total of 48 NYHA class III or IV patients with severe dilated cardiomyopathy and 4+ mitral regurgitation underwent surgery; all had annuloplasty rings inserted, 7 had CABGs for incidental disease, and 11 had tricuspid valve repair. Postoperative transesophageal echocardiography showed no mitral regurgitation in 41 patients and mild mitral regurgitation in 7 patients. One-and 2-year actuarial survival rates were 82% and 71%. At a median follow-up of 22 months, NYHA class had improved significantly from 3.9 to 2.0.

76. **Hunt SA**, et al. Mechanical circulatory support and cardiac transplantation. *Circulation* 1998;97:2079–2090.

    This review article discusses several specific mechanical circulatory support devices and the complications associated with their use. The transplantation section discusses recipient selection and survival rates and provides a brief overview of immunosuppression and rejection surveillance. The review concludes with a section on alternatives to transplantation, including long-term mechanical circulatory support, cardiomyoplasty, partial left ventricular reduction, and xenotransplantation.

77. **Mancini D**, et al. Comparison of exercise performance in patients with chronic severe heart failure versus left ventricular assist devices. *Circulation* 1998;98:1178–1183.

    Metabolic exercise testing was performed in 65 CHF and 20 LVAD patients. Peak oxygen consumption was significantly higher in the LVAD group (15.9 vs. 12.0 mL/kg/min; $p < 0.001$). At peak exercise, the LVAD group also had a significantly higher heart rate, blood pressure, and cardiac output, whereas PCWP was lower (14 vs. 31 mm Hg; $p < 0.001$). LVAD patients also had better hemodynamic measurements at rest, including higher cardiac output and lower PCWP.

78. **Mancini DM**, et al. Low incidence of myocardial recovery after left ventricular assist device implantation in patients with chronic heart failure. *Circulation* 1998;98:2383–2389.

    A retrospective chart review of 111 LVAD recipients identified only five successfully explanted patients. A prospective attempt to identify explantable patients using exercise testing was then undertaken on 39 consecutive patients, of whom 15 were able to exercise with maximal device support. Peak average oxygen consumption was 14.5 mL/kg/min and Fick cardiac output 11.4 L/min. Seven patients remained normotensive while exercising at 20 cycles/min and their peak oxygen consumption decreased from 17.3 to 13.0 mL/kg/min. In one of these patients, the LVAD was successfully explanted.

Exercise/Training

79. **Hambrecht R**, et al. Physical training in patients with stable chronic heart failure: effects of cardiorespiratory fitness and ultrastructural abnormalities of leg muscles. *J Am Coll Cardiol* 1995; 25:1239–1249.

    This small study showed the benefits of exercise and described accompanying physiologic changes. Twenty-two patients were randomized to training or inactivity. Average EF was 26%. At 6 months, trained patients had a 31% increase in oxygen uptake, a 19% increase in volume density of mitochondria, and a 41% increase in volume density of cytochrome-c oxidase–positive mitochondria (i.e., training delays anaerobic metabolism).

80. **Belardinelli R**, et al. Low intensity exercise training in patients with chronic HF. *J Am Coll Cardiol* 1995;26:975–982.

    This small study (27 patients) showed the tolerability and benefits of exercise in heart failure patients. Patients were randomized to low-intensity exercise (40% peak oxygen uptake), exercise three times per week for 8 weeks, or no exercise. The trained group had a 17% higher peak oxygen uptake and 21% increased peak workload. No differences are observed in cardiac output or stroke volume. A high correlation ($r = 0.77$) was observed between peak oxygen consumption and the volume density of mitochondria of the vastus lateralis (large thigh muscle).

81. **Keteyiajn SJ**, et al. Exercise training in patients with heart failure. *Ann Intern Med* 1996;124:1051–1057.

    This small randomized controlled trial was composed of 40 men with an EF ≤35%. The treatment regimen was composed of three sets of three exercises, each performed for 11 minutes (target heart rate 60% maximum) for 2 weeks, then up to 80% as tolerated. At 24 weeks, the exercise group had increased exercise duration (+2.8 minutes), 16% higher peak oxygen consumption, and increased power output (+20 watts). Of note, impact on activities of daily living was not assessed. Long-term benefits also need to be studied.

82. **Wilson JR**, et al. Circulatory status and response to cardiac rehabilitation in patients with heart failure. *Circulation* 1996;94:1567–1572.

    This study showed that only some patients respond well to exercise and offered insights into the pathophysiology of non-responders. Thirty-two patients underwent maximal exercise treadmill testing then rehabilitation for 3 months. Twenty-one had a normal cardiac output response to exercise, of whom 43% responded to the rehabilitation regimen (>10% increase in peak oxygen consumption and anaerobic threshold). Of the other 11 patients, 3 stopped rehabilitation (due to exhaustion) and 1 responded (9%; $p < 0.04$). The former group was likely limited by deconditioning, whereas the latter group was impaired by circulatory failures.

83. **Hambrecht R**, et al. Regular physical exercise corrects endothelial dysfunction and improves exercise capacity in patients with chronic heart failure. *Circulation* 1998;98:2709–2715 (editorial pp. 2652–2655).

    This small prospective randomized study of 20 patients showed that exercise training resulted in increased peak oxygen uptake (+26% at 6 weeks; $p < 0.01$). This increase correlated with endothelium-dependent changes in peripheral blood flow ($r = 0.64$; $p < 0.005$), suggesting that improved endothelial function contributes modestly to increased exercise capacity.

Complications

84. **Middlekauff HR**, et al. Prognostic significance of atrial fibrillation in advanced heart failure: a study of 390 patients. *Circulation* 1991;84:40–48.

    This retrospective analysis focused on 390 consecutive NYHA class III or IV patients with a mean EF of 19%. Actuarial survival and sudden death-free survival was significantly worse in the atrial fibrillation patients compared with those in normal sinus rhythm (52% vs. 71%; 69% vs. 82%, both $p = 0.0013$).

85. **Middlekauff HR**, et al. Syncope in advanced heart failure: high sudden death regardless of etiology. *J Am Coll Cardiol* 1993;21:110.

    This retrospective analysis focused on 491 NYHA class III or IV heart failure patients with no history of cardiac arrest and a mean EF of 20%. Sixty patients (12%) had a history of syncope. At follow-up (mean 1 year), sudden death had occurred in 14% and 13% had died of progressive heart failure. The 1-year actuarial incidence of sudden death was more than threefold higher in patients with a history of syncope than in those without syncope (45% vs. 12%; $p < 0.00001$). The incidence of sudden death was similar in patients with either cardiac syncope or syncope from other causes (49% vs. 39%; p = NS).

86. **Natterson PD**, et al. Risk of arterial embolization in 224 patients awaiting cardiac transplantation. *Am Heart J* 1995;129:564–570.

This analysis focused on 224 consecutive outpatients awaiting cardiac transplantation. Mean EF was 20%, and mean left ventricular end-diastolic diameter was 7.6 cm. During follow-up (301 ± 371 days), arterial embolization only occurred in six patients (2.7%). The risk of embolization was not significantly different between patients on warfarin, those with left ventricular thrombus on transthoracic echocardiography, or those with a history of embolization.

6

Ventricular Arrhythmias and Atrial Fibrillation

VENTRICULAR ARRHYTHMIAS (see pages 328, 329)

The field of management of ventricular arrhythmias and resuscitated sudden cardiac death has had many advances with the publication of several major clinical trials. This brief section is included to highlight a few of the major trials that illustrate three major points:

1. In patients with ventricular ectopic activity after MI, the Cardiac Arrhythmia Suppression Trials (CAST I and II), and survival with oral d-sotalol (SWORD) showed a significantly increased mortality with the class IC antiarrhythmics encainide and flecainide (1), moricizine (2), and d-sotalol (3).
2. In MI patients with ventricular ectopy and/or low ejection fraction (i.e., at increased risk of ventricular tachycardia), the class III agent amiodarone does not appear to increase mortality, and may reduce arrhythmic deaths (EMIAT and CAMIAT trails [4, 5]).
3. Implantable defibrillators are associated with significantly and dramatically improved survival compared with antiarrhythmic therapy, thus far demonstrated in patients with inducible VT (6–8). Many ongoing trials will help to further refine this area of therapy in the years to come.

ATRIAL FIBRILLATION

Epidemiology (see pages 330–332)

Atrial fibrillation (AF) is the most common sustained arrhythmia in the U.S. population. The prevalence of AF increases with age; the lifetime risk is approximately 7%. Prevalence is highest in those with clinical cardiovascular disease. Average age of onset is 70 to 74 years of age (age 65 for lone AF). AF also leads to more hospitalizations than any other arrhythmia. Patients with AF are at an increased risk of thromboembolic complications, especially stroke. Stroke rates are several-fold higher than normal, resulting in all-cause mortality being more than twice the normal rate (14). Patients at highest risk of stroke include those with a history of prior stroke, recent heart failure, hypertension, left atrial enlargement, and left ventricular dysfunction (19). In patients with atrial flutter, stroke risk appears to be modestly higher compared with individuals in normal sinus rhythm (21,23).

Natural History

Spontaneous conversion rates are variable (<15% to as high as 78%). Higher rates are associated with short duration (<12 hours), young age (≤years), and/or lone AF (no associated heart disease). Normal sinus rhythm can usually be successfully restored, but 50% revert to AF within 1 year.

Etiologies and Risk Factors (see page 331)

Many new cases of AF do not have a single clear etiology. In fact, 3% to 11% of AF patients have structurally normal hearts (*see JAMA* 1985;254:3449 and *N Engl J Med* 1987;317:669). Rather, several entities are associated with a significant, increased incidence of AF and thus are best described as being risk factors for the arrhythmia. In some instances, acute events such as cardiac ischemia are the clear cause of the arrhythmia. Below is a list of causes of AF classified by prevalence:

Major Causes:
    Ischemic heart disease
    Hypertension
    Postcardiac surgery
Common Causes
    Alcohol intoxication
    Pulmonary disease
    Rheumatic heart disease
    Valvular heart disease
    Cardiomyopathy
    Medications/drugs
    Thyrotoxicosis
    Low magnesium
Uncommon to Rare Causes
    Pericarditis
    Infiltrative disease
    Atrial myxoma
    Autonomic dysfunction
    Ventricular/atrial septal defect
    Pulmonary embolism

Patients with hypertension are four to five times more likely to have AF, whereas heart failure patients have an 8- to 20-fold increased risk. Patients with coronary disease frequently have AF, and patients with acute ischemia, particularly MI, are at significantly increased risk of developing new-onset AF. In one study of 517 MI patients, over 10% had new-onset AF (*see Clin Cardiol* 1996; 19:180).

AF also occurs commonly after cardiac surgery, especially coronary artery bypass grafting (CABG). In one study of 587 coronary bypass surgery patients, one third had new, postoperative-onset AF (20). Predictors of post-CABG AF were advanced age, male gender, intraaortic balloon pump, postoperative pneumonia, mechanical ventilation for >24 hours, and return to the intensive care unit. In another study of patients undergoing isolated valvular surgery, postoperative AF occurred in more than one third of patients; independent predictors were advanced age, mitral stenosis, and left atrial enlargement.Two recently randomized studies have evaluated the prophylactic use of oral d, 1 sotalol and low dose intravenous amiodarone (1 gm/day for 2 days) to *prevent* post-CABG and post-open heart surgery AF, respectively (*see JACC* 1999;34: 334–343). Both agents reduced the incidence of in-hospital AF; however, these reductions did not translate into significantly shorter hospital stays.

Alcohol intoxication is clearly associated with an increased risk of AF and contributes to the greatest percentage of cases among those under 65 years of age (*see Arch Intern Med* 1983;143:1882). Although the prevalence of rheumatic heart disease (RHD) has decreased recently in developed countries, when it is present it carries a significant increased risk of AF. In the Framingham Study, RHD was associated with a 17-fold increased risk of AF; patients with mitral stenosis are at the greatest risk. Non-rheumatic valve disease, especially mitral regurgitation, also carries a higher risk of AF. Thyrotoxicosis also causes some cases of new-onset AF. A recent large-scale AF registry found that many patients without clinical thyroid disease had a low thyroid-stimulating hormone level. However, the positive predictive value of the test was only approximately 10% (*see Arch Intern Med* 1996;156:2221). Patients with cardiomyopathy also have an increased risk of developing AF. Several medications and substances have been associated with AF, including morphine, caffeine, and herbal tea; little or no hard data are available to support or refute these associations. The association of pulmonary embolism (PE) with AF is controversial. The most common electrocardiographic (ECG) changes associated with PE are nonspecific T-wave and ST changes; S1Q3T3, right bundle branch block, and/or right axis deviation are also seen, particularly in massive pulmonary embolism. However, new-onset AF in the setting of PE is uncommon. In one study of 90 patients from the Urokinase-PE Trial National Cooperative Study, no patients had AF. However, other smaller studies and case reports assert an increased risk of acute fibrillation in the setting of PE.

Stroke Risk Factors (see page 335)
    The Stroke Prevention in Atrial Fibrillation (SPAF I) trial found the following risk factors to be significant for stroke among patients with atrial fibrillation (33): (a) prior cerebrovascular accident, (b) congestive heart failure within the preceding 100 days, (c) hypertension, and, among the echocardiographically assessed features, (d) left atrium >5 cm, and (e) left ventricular dysfunction. If one clinical factor was present, the risk of stroke was 7%/yr; if three factors were present, the risk was 18%/yr. No risk factors (clinical or echocardiographic) were demonstrated in 26%; this group had a stroke rate of only 1%/yr.

Presentation
    The most common presenting symptoms include palpitations, chest pain, dyspnea, and syncope. Typical physical findings include an irregular pulse, absence of a wave in the jugular venous pulse, and variability of the first heart sound. Several factors determine whether a patient becomes symptomatic from the arrhythmia, including the rapidity of the ventricular response and underlying cardiac status.

Workup
    Twelve-lead ECG and electrolytes are the usual tools of assessment. Other useful parameters are cardiac isoenzymes (if MI suspected), arterial blood gas (if hypoxemia suspected), echocardiogram (to assess for organic heart disease), thyroid function tests (if thyrotoxicosis suspected), and/or a ventilation perfusion scan (if pulmonary embolism is suspected).

Treatment

Pharmacologic Agents that Can Lead to the Restoration of Normal Sinus Rhythm (see pages 338–340)

1. Amiodarone (400 mg orally every 8 hours for 10–14 days, then 200–400 mg orally once daily or 5 mg/kg intravenously over 10–40 minutes). The Canadian Trial of Atrial Fibrillation (CTAF) showed a 57% reduction in recurrence compared with propafenone and sotalol (46).
2. Procainamide [loading of 1 g intravenously (or 15 mg/kg) at 20 mg/min, then 2–6 mg/min intravenously or 500–750 mg orally every 6 hours]. This treatment is more effective if AF is of short duration [90% (≤1 day) vs. 9% (>1 day) in one study]. Hypotension occurs in 10% to 15% of patients so treated.
3. Propafenone (150 mg orally every 4 hours or 600 mg orally once daily). Hypotension and QRS widening are uncommon.
4. Ibutilide (1–2 mg intravenously over 10 minutes; can repeat one time). Initial studies showed high conversion rates, but a 5% to 10% risk of torsades de pointes was observed (highest incidence in women) (41,42; *see* also *Am Heart J* 1998;136:642).
5. Quinidine (324 mg orally every 2 hours for two to three doses, then 324 mg every 8 hours).
6. Flecainide (≤400 mg given within 3 hours): Side effects are hypotension (8%) and QRS widening (4%).

Intravenous magnesium repletion should also be undertaken if serum levels are low.

Pharmacologic Agents that Can Achieve Ventricular Rate Control

1. Calcium-channel blockers: diltiazem (half-life 1–2 hours) 15 to 20 mg intravenously over 2 minutes, then 5 to 15 mg/h; verapamil (half-life <30 minutes) 2.5 to 10 mg intravenously over 2 minutes or 40 to 120 mg orally.
2. β-blockers: metoprolol 5 to 15 mg intravenously; esmolol 500 µg/kg over 1 minute, then 50 mg/min. β-blockers should not be used in patients with asthma, chronic obstructive pulmonary disease, or left ventricular dysfunction.
3. Digoxin (0.5 mg intravenously, then 0.25 mg intravenously every 4 hours for two to six doses, then 0.125–0.375 mg orally once daily). Digoxin is most affective for chronic AF, not paroxysmal AF. It takes hours to achieve effect and works poorly if high sympathetic tone is present. It should not be used in patients with left ventricular diastolic dysfunction.

The ongoing National Heart, Lung, and Blood Institute (NHLBI)-sponsored AF Follow-up Investigation of Rhythm Management (AFFIRM) study is randomizing patients with recent-onset AF to rate control or rhythm maintenance.

Cardioversion (see page 332)

If duration of AF is uncertain or >2 days, one series of patients suggests that if transesophageal echocardiography is performed and no thrombi are visible, the risk of subsequent thromboembolism is low (25). Most experts still recommend the more conservative approach of anticoagulation for 3 to 4 weeks before attempting cardioversion. A recent study in atrial flutter patients found an initial energy of 100 J was more efficient than 50 J for restoration of normal sinus rhythm.

Indications for cardioversion are low blood pressure, angina, and congestive heart failure in an unstable patient setting. For stable patients, cardioversion is used when the patient is refractory to drugs, as well for rate control, to avoid embolization, for hemodynamic improvement, and for improved functional capacity [in one study, a 14% increase in anaerobic threshold was observed (*see Br Heart J* 1988;59:572)].

Predictors of failure include long duration of AF and the presence of advanced pulmonary disease or valve disease.

Relative contraindications for cardioversion include (a) left atrial size >6 cm, (b) AF duration >1 year, (c) severe mitral valve disease, (d) slow ventricular response (heart rate ≤60 beats/min), (e) intolerance to antiarrhythmic drugs, and (f) failure to maintain normal sinus rhythm.

Postcardioversion drug therapy usually consists of anticoagulation for 3 weeks. (Atria take time to recover normal mechanical function.)

Long-term Anticoagulation (see pages 328, 332–334)

In a meta-analysis (2), anticoagulation reduced stroke risk by more than 50% compared with approximately 25% with aspirin. There was no difference in stroke rate between paroxysmal AF and chronic AF. When anticoagulation is employed, a target international normalized ratio (INR) of 2.0–2.5 should be targeted (23–30), as the SPAF III trial (31) showed an increased rate of ischemic stroke and embolic complications with lower INR (Table 6–1).

Recommendations for long-term anticoagulation are listed as follows:

1. If the patient has lone AF [i.e., no risk factors (history of prior stroke, transient ischemic attack, diabetes, hypertension)] and is less than 60 years of age, aspirin alone is considered by most experts to be adequate. (Without therapy, risk is ~0.5%/yr if <60 years of age and ~2%/yr if 60–75 years of age.)
2. If the patient is over 75 years of age or under 75 years of age with risk factors, anticoagulation with warfarin is recommended [target international normalized ratio (INR) of 2.0–2.5].

Other Treatment Measures

1. Ablation (*see J Am Coll Cardiol* 1995;25:39, *J Am Coll Cardiol* 1995;25:1365, *J Am Coll Cardiol* 1997;27:113, and *J Am Coll Cardiol* 1999;33:1217).
2. Surgical maze procedure. Atrial incisions are made to stem reentrant circuits that cause AF (*see J Am Coll Cardiol* 1996; 28:985).
3. Implantable atrial defibrillator (*see Circulation* 1998;98:1651).
4. Atrioventricular junction ablation with permanent pacemaker (*see Am Heart J* 1996;131:499 and *Am J Cardiol* 1999; 83:1437).
5. Atrial pacemakers. In one study, this experimental device showed no reduction in the time to first recurrence of paroxysmal AF (*see Circulation* 1999;99:2553).

REFERENCES

Ventricular Arrhythmias

1. The Cardiac Arrhythmia Suppression Trial (**CAST**) Investigators. Preliminary report: effect of encainide and flecainide on mortality in a randomized trial of arrhythmia suppression after myocardial infarction. *N Engl J Med* 1989;321:406–412 (*see also* Chapter 4, ref. 169).

   In 1,727 post-MI patients, encainide and flecainide led to a significantly higher mortality rate through 10 months follow-up (7.7% vs. 3.0% for placebo; relative risk 2.5; 95% CI 1.6–4.5).

2. The Cardiac Arrhythmia Suppression Trial II (**CAST II**) Investigators. Effect of the antiarrhythmic agent moricizine on survival after myocardial infarction. *N Engl J Med* 1992;327:227–233 (*see* Chapter 4, ref. 170).

   CAST-II was terminated early because of increased 14-day mortality associated with moricizine use (relative risk 5.6; adjusted $p < 0.02$). Incidence of long-term deaths was similar (15% vs 12%.). The authors concluded that the use of moricizine post-MI was not only ineffective but also harmful.

3. **Waldo AL**, et al. Survival with oral d-sotalol (**SWORD**) investigators. Effect of d-sotalol on mortality in patients with left ventricular dysfunction after recent and remote myocardial infarction. *Lancet* 1996;348:7–12 (*see* Chapter 4, ref. 171).

   In 3,121 post-MI patients with an EF ≤40%, there was an increased mortality rate associated with d-sotalol (5%) versus placebo (3.1%; $p = 0.006$).

4. **Julian DG**, et al. Randomised trial of effect of amiodarone on mortality in patients with left ventricular dysfunction after recent myocardial infarction: **EMIAT**. *Lancet* 1997;349:667–674.

   In 1,486 post-MI patients with an EF ≤4%, all-cause mortality was similar for amiodarone versus placebo, but there was a 35% risk reduction ($p = 0.05$) in arrhythmic deaths. The authors concluded that the systematic prophylactic use of amiodarone post-MI (with low ejection fraction) was not indicated, but the lack of proarrhythmia supports the use of amiodarone in patients for whom antiarrhythmic therapy is indicated.

5. **Cairns JA**, et al. Randomised trial of outcome after myocardial infarction in patients with frequent or repetitive ventricular premature depolarisations: **CAMIAT**. *Lancet* 1997;349:675–682 (*see* Chapter 4, ref. 173).

   Results were nearly identical to those observed in EMIAT (amiodarone group with nearly 50% fewer arrhythmic deaths plus resuscitated VF).

6. **Moss AJ**, et al. Improved survival with an implanted defibrillator in patients with coronary disease at high risk for ventricular arrhythmia. *N Engl J Med* 1996;335:1933–1940.

   A total of 196 patients with prior MI, ejection fraction ≤35%, a documented episode of asymptomatic unsustained VT, and inducible, nonsuppressible ventricular tachyarrhythmia on electrophysiologic study were randomized to implanted defibrillator (n = 95) or conventional medical therapy (n = 101). During 2-year follow-up, the mortality rate was 17% in the defibrillator group vs. 39% in the conventional therapy group, a 54% reduction ($p = 0.009$).

7. The Antiarrhythmics versus Implantable Defibrillators (**AVID**) Investigators. A comparison of antiarrhythmic-drug therapy with

implantable defibrillators in patients resuscitated from near-fatal ventricular arrhythmias. *N Engl J Med* 1997;337:1576–1583.

Among the 1,016 patients, survival was greater with the implantable defibrillator, 75% versus 64% in the antiarrhythmic-drug therapy group (using primarily amiodarone) at 3 years ($p = 0.02$).

8. Multicenter Unsustained Tachycardia Trial **(MUSTT)**. Preliminary results presented at the American College of Cardiology Scientific Sessions, New Orleans, LA, March 1999.

Patients with nonsustained VT on Holter monitoring were randomized to electrophysiology (EP) testing–guided drug or implantable cardioverter-defibrillator (AICD) therapy versus conventional treatment. Overall, the EP group showed a lower rate of cardiac or arrhythmic death ($p = 0.043$) and lower mortality (hazard ratio 0.80; $p = 0.06$). However, all the benefit was achieved among patients who had received an AICD, whereas patients treated with EP-guided antiarrhythmic therapy had a slightly higher mortality rate compared with placebo.

Atrial Fibrillation
Review Articles and Miscellaneous

9. Stroke Prevention in Atrial Fibrillation (**SPAF**) group. Predictors of thromboembolism in atrial fibrillation: echocardiographic features of patients at risk. *Ann Intern Med* 1992;116:6–12.

In this cohort study, 568 SPAF patients were assigned to placebo and underwent baseline echocardiography; the median follow-up period was 1.3 years. Left ventricular dysfunction as shown on two-dimensional echocardiograms ($p = 0.003$) and left atrial size shown on M-mode echocardiograms ($p = 0.02$) were the strongest independent predictors of subsequent thromboembolism. The relative risk of thromboembolism associated with moderate to severe global or regional left ventricular dysfunction was 3.2 [95% confidence interval (CI) 1.6–6.3], whereas the relative risk with a left atrial size of 5.7 cm was 2.7 (95% CI 1.1–6.2). Compared with risk stratification using only clinical variables (e.g., history of hypertension, recent congestive heart failure, prior thromboembolism), echocardiographic findings changed risk stratification in 38% of those without any of the three clinical risk factors (history of hypertension, recent heart failure, prior thromboembolism). Overall, if a patient had three of the five clinical and echocardiographic risk factors, the thromboembolic risk was 18.6%/yr versus 1.0%/yr if no risk factors present and 6.0%/yr if one or two risk factors present.

10. **Albers GW**. Atrial fibrillation and stroke: 3 new studies, 3 new questions. *Arch Intern Med* 1994;154:1443–1448.

Analysis of the trials showed that anticoagulation therapy was associated with a reduction in stroke rates of ~50% compared with placebo, whereas aspirin reduced the risk by ~25%. There was no significant difference in stroke rates between those with paroxysmal and chronic AF. Based on these data, the following recommendations were proposed: (a) in individuals <60 years of age with no risk factors (history of previous stroke, transient ischemic attack, diabetes, hypertension), no therapy is required (stroke risk is <0.5%/yr); (b) in patients 60–75 years of age with lone AF, aspirin only is adequate (risk is 2%/yr without therapy); and (c) in patients >75 years of age or <75 years of age with risk factors, anticoagulation should be performed.

11. **Lauapacis A**, et al. Risk factors for stroke and efficacy of antithrombotic therapy in atrial fibrillation: an analysis of pooled data from 5 randomized controlled trials (AFASAK, SPAF, BAATAF, SPINAF, CAFA). *Arch Intern Med* 1994;154:1449–1457.

    Pooled data from these five trials showed that warfarin use was associated with a 68% reduction in stroke risk (to 1.4%/yr) and 33% lower all-cause mortality. This significant benefit of warfarin was also present in patients with paroxysmal/intermittent AF [1.7%/yr (warfarin) vs. 5.7%/yr (placebo)]. Risk factors for thromboembolism were history of hypertension, prior stroke or transient ischemic attack, diabetes, and age >65 years. There was a nonsignificant increase in the frequency of major bleeding. Of note, only two of these five trials randomized patients to an aspirin group.

12. **Prystowsky EN**, et al. Management of patients with atrial fibrillation: a statement for healthcare professionals from the Subcommittee on Electrocardiography and Electrophysiology, American Heart Association. *Circulation* 1996;93:1262–1277.

    A number of recommendations were made: (a) selection of antiarrhythmic therapy should be individualized (minimal randomized trial data); (b) for acute rate control, intravenous verapamil, diltiazem, or β-blockers should be used [procainamide if conduction is over an accessory pathway (e.g., in Wolff-Parkinson-White syndrome)]; (c) for antithrombotic therapy, aspirin alone is adequate in low-risk patients, whereas warfarin should be used in higher risk patients (with frequent INR monitoring in patients >75 years of age); and (d) for cardioversion, in patients with AF of unknown duration or >48 hours, anticoagulation should be performed for 3 weeks before and at least 4 weeks after cardioversion. (Alternatively, if transesophageal echocardiography shows no atrial thrombi, cardioversion may be undertaken without 3 weeks of preceding anticoagulation.)

13. **Golzari H**, et al. Atrial fibrillation: restoration and maintenance of sinus rhythm and indications for anticoagulation therapy. *Ann Intern Med* 1996;125:311–323.

    This thorough review discusses the efficacy and safety of electrical and pharmacologic conversion of AF, strategies for maintenance of normal sinus rhythm, and antithrombotic therapy. The authors concluded that cardioversion is the preferred method of reestablishing normal sinus rhythm, that antiarrhythmic therapy should be used only if recurrences or initial clinical instability occur, and that antithrombotic therapy is indicated in all patients >60 years of age.

14. **Viskin S**, et al. The treatment of atrial fibrillation: pharmacologic and nonpharmacologic strategies. *Curr Probl Cardiol* 1997;22: 44–108.

    This extensive review begins with a discussion of antiarrhythmic agents (procainamide, quinidine, flecainide, propafenone, β-blockers, amiodarone, sotalol, ibutilide, verapamil, diltiazem, digoxin) and cardioversion for treatment of new-onset AF. There is a section on AF in specific patient subgroups, including those with long-standing AF, postcardiac surgery, Wolff-Parkinson-White syndrome, acute MI, and thyrotoxicosis. Other sections include prevention of AF recurrence after cardioversion, prevention of thromboembolic events in patients with chronic AF, and newer, experimental treatment modalities (e.g., catheter ablation, surgical maze procedure, atrial pacing, implantable atrial defibrillators).

15. **Ezekowitz MD**, et al. Preventing stroke in patients with atrial fibrillation. *JAMA* 1999;281:1830–1835.

     This analysis of 10 studies found that AF in patients <65 years of age, with no risk factors, and not receiving antithrombotic therapy, is associated a 1%/yr risk of stroke. The stroke risks in individuals 65–75 years of age with no risk factors and on aspirin and warfarin are 1.4%/yr and 1.1%/yr, respectively. Stroke risk in older patients and/or those with risk factors (e.g., hypertension, diabetes, prior stroke or transient ischemic attack, poor ventricular function) ranges from 4.3%/yr to >12%/yr (untreated) to 1.2% to 4.0%/yr with the use of warfarin.

Epidemiology

16. Framingham Study. Kannel WB, et al. Epidemiologic features of chronic atrial fibrillation. *N Engl J Med* 1982;306:1018–1022.

     This extensive 22-year follow-up study was composed of 5,191 Framingham Heart Study participants who were initially free of AF. AF developed in only 0.24% of those initially 25–34 years of age, whereas the rates were 3.79% (men) and 2.99% (women) in those initially 55–64 years of age. The most powerful predictors of AF were rheumatic heart disease [risk ratios 8.3 (men) and 15.3] and cardiac failure (risk ratios 17.5 and 5.7).

17. **Kopecky SL**, et al. The natural history of lone atrial fibrillation. *N Engl J Med* 1987;317:669–674.

     In this population-based study of Olmstead County, Minnesota, residents, between 1950 and 1980, 3,623 persons were found to have AF, of whom 97 (2.7%) were <60 years of age (mean age 44 years at diagnosis) and had no overt cardiovascular disease or precipitating illness. Among these lone AF patients, 21% had an isolated episode, 58% had recurrent AF, and 22% had chronic AF. At 15-year follow-up, only 1.3% of patients had had a stroke on a cumulative actuarial basis, and there was no difference in survival or stroke-free survival among patients with the three types of lone AF. Based on these findings, the authors suggest that routine anticoagulation may not be indicated in individuals with lone AF.

18. **Benjamin EJ**, et al. Left atrial size and the risk of stroke and death: the Framingham Heart Study. *Circulation* 1995;92:835–841.

     This analysis focused on 3,099 patients ≥ 50 years of age. For each 1-cm increase in left atrial size, the relative risk of stroke was 2.4 in men and 1.4 in women and for death 1.3 and 1.4 in men and women, respectively.

19. **Krahn AD**, et al. The natural history of atrial fibrillation: incidence, risk factors, and prognosis in the Manitoba Follow-up Study. *Am J Med* 1995;98:476–484.

     In this observational study of 3,983 male air crew recruits, the average follow-up was 38.7 years. The incidence of AF rose from <0.5 per 1,000 person-years before age 50 to 9.7 per 1,000 person-years after age 70. Risk factors for AF included MI (relative risk 3.6), angina (relative risk 2.8), ST- or T-wave abnormalities in the absence of ischemic heart disease (relative risk 2.2), and hypertension (relative risk 1.4). AF was associated with higher all-cause mortality (relative risk 1.3) and cardiovascular mortality (relative risk 1.4), as well as an increased risk of stroke (relative risk 2.1) and congestive heart failure (relative risk 3.0).

20. **Aranki SF**, et al. Predictors of atrial fibrillation after coronary artery surgery: current trends and impact on hospital resources. *Circulation* 1996;94:390–397.

This analysis focused on 587 patients, of whom 33% developed postoperative AF. Independent predictors of AF were increased age (70–80 years, odds ratio 2.0; >80 years, odds ratio 3.0), male gender (odds ratio 1.7), hypertension (odds ratio 1.6), intraoperative intraaortic balloon pump (odds ratio 3.5), postoperative pneumonia (odds ratio 3.9), mechanical ventilation >24 hours (odds ratio 2.0), and return to the intensive care unit (odds ratio 3.2). The AF group had a longer hospital stay (15.3 vs. 9.3 days) and had $10,000 higher hospital charges.

21. **Wood KA**, et al. Risk of thromboembolism in chronic atrial flutter. *Am J Cardiol* 1997;79:1043–1047.

    Retrospective analysis of 86 patients referred for radiofrequency ablation. The annual risk of embolic events was 3% (1.6% after exclusion of patients with transient ischemic attack and pulmonary embolism). In a logistic regression model, there were no significant independent predictors of increased thromboembolic risk.

22. **Benjamin EJ**, et al. Impact of atrial fibrillation on the risk of death. *Circulation* 1998;98:946–952 (editorial pp. 943–945).

    Of 5,209 Framingham Study participants, 296 men and 325 women developed AF during 40 years of follow-up. AF patients were more likely (at baseline) to smoke and have hypertension, left ventricular hypertrophy on ECG, history of MI, congestive heart failure, valvular disease, and stroke or transient ischemic attack. AF was associated with an adjusted odds ratio for death of 1.5 (95% CI 1.2–1.8) in men and 1.9 (95% CI 1.5–2.2) in women. The presence of AF increased the risk of dying at all ages. Of note, most of the excess mortality was seen in the first 30 days after AF developed.

23. **Seidl K**, et al. Risk of thromboembolic events in patients with atrial flutter. *Am J Cardiol* 1998;82:580–583.

    This retrospective analysis focused on 191 consecutive patients with atrial flutter. At an average follow-up of 26 months, embolic events had occurred in 11 patients (7%). Acute (<48 hours) embolism occurred in 4 patients (3 after DC cardioversion, 1 after catheter ablation). In multivariate analysis, the only independent predictor of embolic events was hypertension (odds ratio 6.5; 95% CI 1.5–45).

Cardioversion

Review Article

24. **Silverman DI,** Manning WJ. Role of echocardiography in patients undergoing elective cardioversion of atrial fibrillation. *Circulation* 1998;98:479–486.

    This review article focuses on the transesophageal echocardiography–guided approach to early cardioversion. Available data suggest that the safety of this approach is similar to that of conventional therapy (1 month of precardioversion anticoagulation). Advantages of the transesophageal echocardiography–guided approach include better cost effectiveness if transthoracic echocardiography is omitted, and earlier restoration of normal sinus rhythm allows for more rapid recovery of atrial mechanical function

Anticoagulation Studies and Miscellaneous

25. **Manning WJ**, et al. Cardioversion from atrial fibrillation without prolonged anticoagulation with the use of transesophageal

echocardiography to exclude the presence of atrial thrombi. *N Engl J Med* 1993;328:750–755.

This study was composed of 94 patients with AF of >2 days duration (average 4.5 weeks). Eighty patients received heparin before cardioversion; 14 thrombi were seen by transesophageal echocardiography versus only 2 of 14 seen on transthoracic echocardiography (two of these patients died suddenly, whereas the other 10 were cardioverted after prolonged oral anticoagulation). No embolic events occurred in the other patients [78 of 82 successfully cardioverted (47 by drugs)].

26. **Manning WJ**, et al. Transesophageal echocardiography facilitated early cardioversion form atrial fibrillation using short-term anticoagulation: final results of a prospective 4.5-year study. *J Am Coll Cardiol* 1995;25:1354–1361.

In this study of 230 patients (inclusion criteria was AF of >2 days duration or of unknown duration), transesophageal echocardiography identified 40 atrial thrombi in 34 patients, of whom 18 had successful cardioversion after prolonged anticoagulation. Among patients without thrombi, 95% had successful cardioversion without a thromboembolic event. Among patients without prolonged anticoagulation (i.e., warfarin for 1 month), none experienced thromboembolic events.

27. **Klein AL**, et al. Assessment of Cardioversion Using Transesophageal Echocardiography **(ACUTE)**. Cardioversion guided by transesophageal echocardiography: the ACUTE Pilot Study. *Ann Intern Med* 1997;126:200–209.

This randomized, multicenter trial was composed of 126 patients with AF of >2 days duration. Patients received conventional therapy (warfarin for 3 weeks) or transesophageal echocardiography–guided cardioversion. (Warfarin treatment for 4 weeks was initiated only if left atrial or left atrial appendage thrombus was present.) The transesophageal echocardiography group had a 13% incidence of atrial thrombi. Among patients undergoing immediate cardioversion (success rate 84%), there were no embolization events. In the conventional group, 58% had cardioversion (success rate 76%), and one peripheral embolic event and more hemodynamic instability and bleeding complications occurred.

Drug Therapy after Cardioversion

28. **Coplen SE**, et al. Efficacy and safety of quinidine therapy for maintenance of sinus rhythm after cardioversion: a meta-analysis of randomized controlled trials. *Circulation* 1990; 82:1106–1116.

This analysis focused on six trials with 808 patients. Quinidine use was associated with less AF recurrence. At 3, 6, and 12 months, 69%, 58%, and 50% of quinidine-treated patients were in normal sinus rhythm versus 45%, 33%, and 25% of controls. Despite the lower recurrence rates, the quinidine group had a higher all-cause mortality rate (2.9% vs. 0.8%; $p < 0.05$).

29. **Gosselink TM**, et al. Low-dose amiodarone for maintenance of sinus rhythm after cardioversion of atrial fibrillation or flutter. *JAMA* 1992;267:3289–3293.

This study was composed of 89 AF patients who had failed previous therapy. A loading dose of amiodarone (600 mg over 4 weeks) was followed by an average daily dose of 204 mg/day. Fifteen patients (16%) converted to normal sinus rhythm during loading;

90% were in sinus rhythm after cardioversion and 53% remained in normal sinus rhythm at 3-year follow-up. No proarrhythmias were documented.

30. **Catherwood E**, et al. Cost-effectiveness of cardioversion and antiarrhythmic therapy in nonvalvular atrial fibrillation. *Ann Intern Med* 1999;130:625–636.

This Markov decision-analytic model of a hypothetical cohort of 70-year-old patients was based on data from the published literature and hospital accounting information. For patients with a high risk of ischemic stroke (5.3%/yr), cardioversion alone followed by repeated cardioversion and amiodarone upon relapse was most cost effective ($9,300 per quality-adjusted life year). In the moderate-risk cohort (stroke risk 3.6%/yr), this same strategy was also optimal, but it was more expensive ($18,900 per quality-adjusted life year). Cardioversion alone plus aspirin was the best strategy in the low-risk cohort (stroke risk 1.6%/yr).

Pharmacologic Studies

Anticoagulation

31. **Peterson**, et al., Atrial Fibrillation, Aspirin, Anticoagulation **(AFASAK)** study. Placebo-controlled, randomized trial of warfarin and aspirin for prevention of thromboembolic complications in chronic atrial fibrillation. *Lancet* 1989;333:175–178.
Design: Prospective, randomized, partially open (warfarin), partially blinded (aspirin vs. placebo) study. Follow-up period was 2 years. Primary end point was thromboembolic complications (transient ischemic attack, minor stroke, nondisabing stroke, fatal stroke, or embolism to viscera or extremities).
Purpose: To assess the efficacy of low-dose warfarin in preventing strokes in patients with nonrheumatic AF.
Population: 1,007 patients 18 years of age with chronic AF.
Exclusion Criteria: Prior anticoagulation for 6 months, cerebrovascular events in prior 1 month, blood pressure (BP) >180/100 mm Hg.
Treatment: Low-dose warfarin [target prothrombin time (PT) 1.2–1.5 times control (approximate INR 2.8–4.2)], aspirin 75 mg/day, or placebo.
Results: Warfarin group had significantly fewer thromboembolic complications [1.5% vs. 6.0% (aspirin) and 6.3% (placebo)]. Vascular death occurred in 0.9%, 3.6%, and 4.5% of the warfarin, aspirin, and placebo groups ($p < 0.02$). Warfarin patients had more frequent nonfatal bleeding (6.3% vs. 0.6% and 0% of aspirin and placebo patients).

32. Boston Area Anticoagulation Trial for Atrial Fibrillation **(BAATAF)**. The effect of low-dose warfarin on the risk of stroke in patients with nonrheumatic atrial fibrillation. *N Engl J Med* 1990; 323:1505–1511.
Design: Prospective, randomized, open, controlled, multicenter study. Mean follow-up period was 2.2 years. Primary end point was ischemic stroke.
Purpose: To assess the efficacy of low-dose warfarin in preventing strokes in patients with nonrheumatic AF.
Population: 420 patients (mean age of 63 years) with chronic or intermittent AF.
Exclusion Criteria: Prosthetic valves, severe heart failure, stroke in prior 6 months, and contraindications to or requirement for aspirin or warfarin therapy.

Treatment: Warfarin (target PT 1.2–1.5 times normal or nothing); aspirin was allowed in the control group,

Results: Target adjusted thromboplastin time was achieved in 83%. The warfarin group had 86% fewer strokes [0.41%/yr vs. 2.98%/yr (control group); $p = 0.002$] and a 62% lower death rate (2.25%/yr vs. 5.97%/yr, $p = 0.005$). The warfarin group had more minor hemorrhages (38 vs. 21 patients).

Comments: The trial was terminated early because of strong evidence in favor of warfarin.

33. **SPAF** Investigators. Stroke Prevention in Atrial Fibrillation Study: final results. *Circulation* 1991;84:527–539.

Design: Prospective, randomized, partially open (warfarin), partially blind (aspirin vs. placebo), multicenter study. Mean followup period was 1.3 years. Primary events were ischemic stroke and systemic embolism.

Purpose: To determine the efficacy and safety of warfarin and aspirin compared with placebo for the prevention of ischemic stroke and systemic embolism in patients with nonrheumatic AF.

Population: 1,330 patients with chronic or intermittent AF.

Exclusion Criteria: Prosthetic valves, mitral stenosis, MI in prior 3 months, and stroke or transient ischemic attack in prior 2 years.

Treatment: Group 1 [627 patients (most ≤75 years of age)]: warfarin (target PT 1.3–1.8 times normal (approximate INR 2.0–4.5)], aspirin 325 mg/day, or placebo. Group 2 (703 non-anticoagulation candidates): aspirin or placebo.

Results: Aspirin-treated patients had 67% fewer primary events than placebo patients (3.6%/yr vs. 6.3%/yr; $p = 0.02$). In the warfarin-eligible patients, warfarin reduced the risk of primary events by 67% compared with placebo (2.3%/yr vs. 7.4%/yr; $p = 0.01$).

Primary events or death were reduced 58% by warfarin ($p = 0.01$) and 32% by aspirin ($p = 0.02$). Disabling stroke or vascular death was reduced 54% by warfarin and a nonsignificant 22% by aspirin ($p = 0.33$). Significant bleeding rates were similar in all three groups (1.4%–1.6%/yr). Significant risk factors for stroke were (a) prior cerebrovascular accident, (b) CHF within preceding 100 days, (c) hypertension, and among the echocardiographically assessed features, (d) left atrium >5 cm, and (e) left ventricular dysfunction. If one clinical factor was present, the risk of stroke was 7%/yr; if two or all three factors were present, the risk was 18%/yr. The group without any risk factors (26%) had an event rate of only 1%/yr.

Comments: Placebo arm of group 1 was discontinued in late 1989 due to strong evidence of superiority of both warfarin and aspirin over placebo.

34. **Connolly SJ**, et al. Canadian Atrial Fibrillation Anticoagulation study **(CAFA)**. *J Am Coll Cardiol* 1991;18:349–355 (editorial pp. 301–302).

Design: Prospective, randomized, double-blind, placebo-controlled, multicenter study. Primary end point was nonlacunar ischemic stroke, other systemic embolism, and intracranial or fatal hemorrhage.

Purpose: To evaluate the effectiveness and safety of warfarin in AF patients.

Population: 378 patients with recurrent paroxysmal or chronic AF.

Exclusion Criteria: Clear indications or contraindications to anticoagulation, stroke, or transient ischemic attack in prior year,

MI in prior month, use of antiplatelet drug(s), and uncontrolled hypertension.

Treatment: Warfarin (target INR 2–3) or placebo.

Results: Target INR was achieved with only 44% frequency (subtherapeutic values in 39.6%). The warfarin group had a nonsignificant 37% risk reduction in primary outcome events (3.5%/yr vs. 5.2%/yr; $p = 0.26$). Major/fatal and minor bleeding events were common with warfarin use (2.5%/yr vs. 0.5%/yr and 16%/yr vs. 9.4%/yr).

Comments: Trial was terminated early due to the AFASAK and SPAF results.

35. **Ezekowitz MD**, et al., VA Stroke Prevention in Nonrheumatic Atrial Fibrillation (**SPINAF**). Warfarin in the prevention of stroke associated with nonrheumatic atrial fibrillation. *N Engl J Med* 1992;327:1406–1412.

Design: Prospective, randomized, double-blind, placebo-controlled, multicenter study. Average follow-up period was 1.8 years. Primary end point was cerebral infarction.

Purpose: To evaluate whether low-intensity anticoagulation will decrease the risk of stroke in patients with nonrheumatic AF.

Population: 571 men, 46 with prior stroke, without echocardiographic evidence of rheumatic heart disease and AF on two ECG tracings 4 weeks apart.

Exclusion Criteria: Contraindications to or requirement for anticoagulation, BP >180/105 mm Hg, and use of nonsteroidal antiinflammatory drugs.

Treatment: Warfarin (target INR 1.4–2.8) or placebo.

Results: A 79% risk reduction was observed among patients without a history of stroke (0.9%/yr vs. 4.3%/yr; $p = 0.001$). Significant benefit also was seen in patients >70 years of age (0.9% vs. 4.8%/yr; $p = 0.02$) and with a history of prior stroke (6.1%/yr vs. 9.3%/yr). Major hemorrhage rates were similar [1.3%/yr (warfarin) vs. 0.9%/yr]. Cerebral infarction occurred more frequently among patients with a history of cerebral infarction [9.3%/yr (placebo group) and 6.1%/yr (warfarin group)].

Comments: An analysis of 516 evaluable admission computed tomography (CT) scans showed that 14.7% had one silent infarct. Strokes during the study were not predicted by infarct on admission CT scan, but rather by active angina [placebo group, 15% (angina) vs. 5%] (*see Circulation* 1995;92:2178).

36. European Atrial Fibrillation Trial (**EAFT**). Secondary prevention in non-rheumatic fibrillation after transient ischemic attack or minor stroke. *Lancet* 1993;342:1255–1262.

Design: Prospective, randomized, partially open (anticoagulant therapy), double-blind aspirin treatment, placebo-controlled, multicenter study. Mean follow-up period was 2.3 years. Primary end points were death from vascular disease, any stroke, MI, and systemic embolism.

Purpose: To evaluate and compare the effectiveness of oral anticoagulation and aspirin in AF patients with recent minor cerebrovascular events.

Population: 1,007 patients with nonrheumatic AF and minor stroke or transient ischemic attack in previous 3 months.

Exclusion Criteria: Use of non-steroidal antiinflammatory or other antiplatelet drugs, MI in prior 3 months, and scheduled coronary surgery or carotid endarterectomy within next 3 months.

Treatment: Group 1 (669 patients): warfarin (target INR 2.5–4.0) or aspirin 300 mg daily, or placebo. Group 2: Contraindications to anticoagulation; 338 patients.

Results: Anticoagulation was more effective than aspirin and placebo: 8% vs. 15% and 17% annual rates of primary outcome events; risk of stroke was especially lower in warfarin-treated patients [4%/yr vs. 12%/yr (placebo)]. Overall, warfarin use was associated with 90 fewer vascular events per 1,000 patient years (vs. 40 with aspirin). Bleeding events were common in warfarin-treated patients [2.8%/yr vs. 0.9%/yr (aspirin patients). Analysis of group 2 patients showed that the optimal INR range was 2.0–3.9, with most bleeding complications occurring when the INR was >5.0, and no significant treatment effect was seen if INR was <2.0 (*see N Engl J Med* 1995;333:5).

37. **SPAF II**. Warfarin versus aspirin for prevention of thromboembolism in atrial fibrillation. *Lancet* 1994;43:687–691.

    Design: Prospective, randomized, open, parallel-group, multicenter study. Mean follow-up period was 2.3 years. Primary events were stroke and systemic embolism.

    Purpose: To define the long-term benefits and risks associated with warfarin compared with aspirin, according to age and risk of thromboembolism.

    Population: 1,100 patients, 715 patients ≤75 years of age and 385 > 75 years of age, with AF in prior 12 months.

    Exclusion Criteria: Lone AF if <60 years of age, stroke or transient ischemic attack in prior 2 years.

    Treatment: Warfarin (target INR 2.0–4.5) or aspirin 325 mg daily.

    Results: No significant difference was observed between groups. However, 12 of 28 events in the warfarin group occurred while patients were not on warfarin. Thus, a 50% difference in favor of warfarin is evident if these events are excluded. Event rates per year for patients ≤75 years of age were 1.3% vs. 1.9% ($p = 0.24$); >75 years of age, 3.6% vs. 4.8% ($p = 0.39$). Low-risk younger patients (no hypertension, recent heart failure, or prior thromboembolism) had a low 0.5%/yr primary event rate. Among older patients, stroke rates were similar in the two treatment groups (aspirin, 4.3%/yr; warfarin, 4.6%/yr). Among warfarin-treated patients, the intracranial hemorrhage was significantly higher in older vs. younger patients (1.6% vs. 4.2%; $p = 0.04$).

    Comments: Randomization was performed separately for the two age groups.

38. **Hylek EM**, et al. An analysis of the lowest effective intensity of prophylactic anticoagulation for patients with nonrheumatic atrial fibrillation. *N Engl J Med* 1996;335:540–546.

    This retrospective, case-control analysis focused on 74 consecutive patients with ischemic strokes on warfarin (INR measured at admission) and 222 controls (INR measured closest to admission day of case patient). The risk of stroke rose significantly at INRs <2.0; the adjusted odds ratio for stroke was 2.0 if INR 1.7–2.0, 3.3 if INR 1.5–2.0, and 6.0 if INR 1.3–2.0. Other independent risk factors were prior stroke (odds ratio 10.4), diabetes (odds ratio 2.9), hypertension (odds ratio 2.5), and smoking (odds ratio 5.7).

39. **SPAF III**. Adjusted-dose warfarin vs. low-intensity, fixed-dose warfarin and aspirin for high-risk patients with atrial fibrillation: SPAF III randomised clinical trial. *Lancet* 1996;348:633–638.

Design: Prospective, randomized, partially open, multicenter study. Mean follow-up period was 1.1 years. Primary events were ischemic stroke and systemic embolism.

Purpose: To compare the safety and effectiveness of a combination of low-intensity, fixed-dose warfarin plus aspirin with adjusted-dose warfarin in AF patients at high risk of stroke.

Population: 1,044 AF patients with one of the following: congestive heart failure or ejection fraction ≤25%, prior thromboembolism, systolic blood pressure (SBP) >160 mm Hg, or female >75 years of age.

Exclusion Criteria: Conditions requiring standard anticoagulation therapy and contraindications to aspirin or warfarin.

Treatment: Fixed-dose warfarin [initial INR 1.2–1.5 (mean 1.3)] and aspirin (325 mg/day) or adjusted-dose warfarin [INR 2–3 (mean 2.4)].

Results: Trial was terminated early. The low INR group had four times more ischemic strokes and systemic emboli (7.9%/yr vs. 1/9%/yr; $p < 0.0001$). Rates of disabling stroke (5.6%/yr vs. 1.7%/yr; $p = 0.0007$) and of primary or vascular death (11.8%/yr vs. 6.4%/yr; $p = 0.002$) were also higher with combination therapy. Bleeding rates were similar. The greatest benefits of standard adjusted-dose warfarin were seen in patients with prior thromboembolism.

40. **Gullov Al**, et al., **AFASAK II**. Fixed minidose warfarin, aspirin alone and in combination versus adjusted-dose warfarin for stroke prevention in atrial fibrillation. *Arch Intern Med* 1998;158: 1513–1521 (editorial pp. 1487–1491).

    Design: Prospective, randomized, controlled, single-center study. Primary end point was stroke and systemic thromboembolic events.

    Purpose: To investigate the effects of mini-dose warfarin alone and in combination with aspirin in chronic AF patients.

    Population: 677 patients (median age 74 years) with chronic AF documented by ECG tracings at least 1 month apart.

    Exclusion Criteria: Lone AF in patients ≤60 years of age, SBP >180 mm Hg, diastolic blood pressure >100 mm Hg, and stroke or transient ischemic attack in prior 6 months.

    Treatment: Warfarin 1.25 mg/day, warfarin 1.25 mg/day and aspirin 300 mg/day, aspirin alone, or warfarin alone (target INR 2–3).

    Results: Trial was terminated early due to SPAF III results. One-year cumulative primary event rates were as follows: mini-dose warfarin, 5.8%; warfarin plus aspirin, 7.2%; aspirin alone, 3.6%; and adjusted-dose warfarin, 2.8% ($p = 0.67$). No significant differences were seen at 3 years. Major bleeding events were rare.

Other Drug Studies

41. **Galve E**, et al. Intravenous amiodarone in the treatment of recent-onset atrial fibrillation: results of a randomized, controlled trial. *J Am Coll Cardiol* 1996;27:1079–1082.

    One hundred patients with AF <1 week in duration and not taking any antiarrhythmics were randomized to amiodarone 5 mg/kg over 30 minutes then 1, 200 mg over 24 hours, or placebo. Both groups were given intravenous digoxin. At 24 hours, there were no differences in the incidence of normal sinus rhythm (68% vs. 60%; $p = 0.53$). Among nonconverters, the amiodarone group had a decreased average ventricular rate (82 vs. 91 beats/min).

There were also no differences in the 15-day recurrence rate (12% vs. 10%).

42. **Stambler BS**, et al. Efficacy and safety for repeated intravenous doses of ibutilide for rapid conversion of atrial flutter of fibrillation. *Circulation* 1996;94:1613–1621 (editorial pp. 1499–1502).

    This randomized trial was composed of 266 patients with sustained (3 hours to 45 days) AF or flutter. Patients received one or two 10-minute infusions [1.0 mg plus 0.5 mg (separated by 10 minutes) or 1 mg plus 1 mg]; or placebo. Ibutilide converted 47% (vs. 2%), with the best success in the flutter patients (63% vs. 31%). The average time to termination was 27 minutes. No significant differences were seen between regimens. Polymorphic VT occurred in 8.3%.

43. **Falk RH**, et al. Intravenous dofetilide, a class III antiarrhythmic agent, for the termination of sustained atrial fibrillation or flutter. *J Am Coll Cardiol* 1997;29:385–390 (editorial pp. 391–393).

    Randomized trial of 107 patients with AF (n = 75) or atrial flutter (n = 16) for 2 weeks to 6 months. Patients received dofetilide 4 or 8 µg/kg (over 15 minutes) or placebo. Conversion rates were 31%, 12.5% (vs. 31%: $p = 0.05$), and 0%. Atrial flutter patients had the best response to dofetilide (54% vs. 14.5%; $p < 0.001$). The accompanying editorial questions whether there will be lower efficacy in patients with AF of <6 months duration and if dofetilide is cost effective given that DC cardioversion is typically successful in 75% to 95% of patients.

44. **Bianconi L**, et al. for the Propafenone in Atrial Fibrillation Italian Trial **(PAFIT-3)** Investigators. Comparison between propafenone and digoxin administered intravenously to patients with acute atrial fibrillation. *Am J Cardiol* 1998;82:584–588.

    In this study, 123 patients with AF of <72 hours duration were randomized to 10-minute infusion of propafenone (2 mg/kg), digoxin (0.007 mg/kg), or placebo. After 1 hour, if AF persisted, drug patients were switched to another drug and placebo patients to propafenone or digoxin. At 1 hour, the conversion rates were 49% in the propafenone group, 32% in the digoxin group ($p = 0.12$), and 14% in the placebo group [$p < 0.001$ (propafenone vs. placebo); $p = 0.08$ (propafenone vs. digoxin)]. After crossover, digoxin converted only 5% of the propafenone patients, whereas propafenone converted 48% of the digoxin patients. In 36 nonconverted placebo patients, propafenone was effective in 53% (vs. only 5% with digoxin; $p < 0.05$). In nonconverters, propafenone use was associated with faster and more prominent ventricular rate reduction (15 vs. 45 minutes; –24% vs. –14%). Overall, in 116 patients treated with drug first, propafenone was twice as successful (50% vs. 25%; $p < 0.01$).

45. Azimilide Supraventricular Arrhythmia Program **(ASAP)**. Preliminary results presented at the 71st AHA Scientific Session in Dallas, TX, November 1998.

    This prospective, randomized, placebo-controlled trial enrolled 367 patients in sinus rhythm but with a documented history of AF. Patients received azimilide (three dose groups: 50, 100, or 125 mg twice daily for 3 days, then once daily for 6 months), or placebo. There was a dose-dependent increase in the primary end point of time to AF recurrence (outside the initial 3-day loading period): 17 days in the placebo group, 22 days in the azimilide 50 mg group,

41 days in the 100 mg group, and 130 days in the 125 mg group. Over 90% of patients began therapy in an outpatient setting, and only one patient had an episode of torsades de pointes.

46. Canadian Trial of Atrial Fibrillation **(CTAF)** Preliminary results presented at the 48th ACC Scientific Session in New Orleans, LA, March 1999.

    This prospective, randomized, multicenter trial of 403 patients with symptomatic AF showed the significant benefits associated with amiodarone therapy. Patients were randomized to amiodarone or sotalol or propafenone. The average daily doses at 1 year were amiodarone 194 mg, propafenone 554 mg, and sotalol 231 mg. At a mean follow-up of 15 months, only 35% of the amiodarone patients experienced 1 electrophysiogically documented recurrence(s) of AF versus 63% on the other antiarrhythmics. The mean time to recurrence was 340 days in the amiodarone group and 207 days with sotalol or propafenone. Amiodarone was stopped in 33% (vs. 45%). Discontinuation was due to adverse effects in 16% and 10%, respectively.

47. **Platia EV**, et al. Esmolol versus verapamil in the acute treatment of atrial fibrillation or flutter. *Am J Cardiol* 1989;63:925–929.

    This randomized, parallel-group, open-label study was composed of 45 patients. Esmolol-treated patients had similar rate control compared with verapamil patients (139 beats/min to 100 beats/min vs. 142 beats/min to 97 beats/min), but with a higher conversion rate in new-onset patients [50% (occurred at a mean of 29 minutes and with infusion rates of 8–16 mg/min) vs. 12% (verapamil 5–10 mg for one or two doses); $p < 0.03$].

48. **Chun SH**, et al. Long-term efficacy of amiodarone for the maintenance of normal sinus rhythm in patients with refractory atrial fibrillation or flutter. *Am J Cardiol* 1995;76:47–50.

    This retrospective study was composed of 110 patients with AF or atrial flutter (53 chronic, 57 paroxysmal) who were refractory to class I agents and received amiodarone 268 ± 100 mg/day. Maintenance of normal sinus rhythm was achieved in 87%, 70%, and 55% at 1, 3, and 5 years, respectively. Higher recurrence rates were observed among paroxysmal AF patients (40% vs. 9%). Drug discontinuation rates were 8%, 22%, and 30%. Reasons for discontinuation included skin discoloration, pulmonary fibrosis, and thyroid toxicity.

49. **Halinen MO**, et al. Comparison of sotalol with digoxin-quinidine for conversion of acute atrial fibrillation to sinus rhythm (the Sotalol-Digoxin-Quinidine trial). *Am J Cardiol* 1995;76:495–498.

    This randomized trial was composed of 61 patients with paroxysmal AF randomized at <48 hours to sotalol 80–320 mg (80-mg doses repeated if AF persisted, heart rate ≥80 beats/min, BP ≥ 120 mm Hg) or quinidine 200–600 mg [digoxin given first (0.25–0.75 mg) if heart rate >100 beats/min]. The quinidine group had an increased conversion rate (86% vs. 52%). Sotalol was discontinued in 16 of 33 patients secondary to asymptomatic bradycardia or hypotension. Asymptomatic wide complex tachycardia occurred in 13% (sotalol 27%).

50. **Zarembski DG**, et al. Treatment of resistant atrial fibrillation: a meta-analysis comparing amiodarone and flecainide. *Arch Intern Med* 1995;155:1885–1891.

This meta-analysis focused on six amiodarone trials and two flecainide trials. Results were compared with those from the quinidine meta-analysis. At 3 and 12 months, the amiodarone-treated
patients were in normal sinus rhythm significantly more often than
the quinidine patients (72.6% and 59.8% vs. 70% and 50%). In contrast, the flecainide patients were in normal sinus rhythm significantly less often than the quinidine patients (48.5% and 34%).

51. **Maisel WH**, et al. Risk of initiating antiarrhythmic drug therapy
    for atrial fibrillation in patients admitted to a university hospital.
    Ann Intern Med 1997;127:281–284.

    Retrospective chart analysis of 417 consecutive patients with 550
    hospital stays and 597 drug trials (procainamide, n = 189; quini-
    dine, n = 179; disopyramide, n = 20; propafenone, n = 110; fle-
    cainide, n = 2; sotalol, n = 72; amiodarone, n = 25). Adverse events
    occurred in 13.4%, bradyarrhythmia in 7.9%, QT prolongation war-
    ranting drug discontinuation in 1.5%, and ventricular arrhythmia
    in 1.3%. Highest risk was seen in the first 24 hours. Multivariate
    analysis showed that prior MI (odds ratio 1.9) and age (odds ratio
    1.29/decade) were independent predictors of adverse events. Based
    on these data, the authors recommend that patients be observed in
    the hospital for 24–48 hours.

52. **Kochiadakis GE**, et al. Amiodarone versus propafenone for con-
    version of chronic atrial fibrillation: results of a randomized, con-
    trolled study. *J Am Coll Cardiol* 1999;33:966–971.

    Prospective, randomized, placebo-controlled study of 101 pa-
    tients with AF of >3 weeks duration. Patients received amio-
    darone (300 mg intravenously over 12 hours and then 20 mg/kg
    over the next hour, followed by 200 mg orally three times daily for
    1 week, then 400 mg/day for 3 weeks), propafenone (2 mg/kg intra-
    venously over 15 minutes, followed by 10 mg/kg over 24 hours, then
    450 mg/day orally for 1 month), or placebo. Amiodarone and pro-
    pafenone were equally effective in terminating AF. Conversion to
    sinus rhythm occurred in 47% of amiodarone patients and 40.6%
    of propafenone patients versus 0% of control patients ($p < 0.001$).

Table 6–1. Major Randomized Trials of Warfarin for Prevention of Thromboembolism in Nonvalvular Atrial Fibrillation

Study	Primary Endpoint(s)	Annual Event Rate (%)			
		Target INR	Warfarin	Control	p
AFASAK (28)	stroke, TIA, embolic complications to viscera and extremities	2.8-4.2	2.0	5.5*	<0.05
BAATAF (29)	ischemic stroke	1.5-2.7	0.4	3.0**	0.002
SPAF I (30)	ischemic stroke, systemic emboli	2.0-3.5	2.3	7.4*	0.01
CAFA (31)	nonlacunar stroke, non-CNS embolic event, ICH, other fatal hemorrhage	2.0-3.0	3.5	5.2*	NS
SPINAF (32)	cerebral infarction	1.4-2.8	0.9	4.3	0.001
EAFT (33)	vascular death, any stroke, MI, recent stroke/TIA, systemic embolism	2.5-4.0	8.0	15.0*	0.001
SPAF II (34)	ischemic stroke, systemic emboli	2.0-4.5	1.9	2.7†	0.15
SPAF III (36)	ischemic stroke, systemic emboli	2.0-3.0	1.9	7.9#	<0.0001
AFASAK II (37)	stroke, systemic emboli	2.0-3.0	2.8	3.6‡	NS

*: placebo group; **: no treatment but aspirin allowed; †: aspirin; #: aspirin and fixed low dose warfarin (mean INR 1.3); ‡: low-dose warfarin.
CAF = chronic atrial fibrillation, PAF = paroxysmal atrial fibrillation, INR = international normalized ratio, ICH = intracranial hemorrhage, MI = myocardial infarction, TIA = transient ischemic attack, CNS = central nervous system, NS = not significant.

Subject Index

Page numbers followed by f indicate figures; page numbers followed by t indicate tables.
Discontinuous topics are indicated by italicized reference numbers following the page number(s).